Proceedings of the
XIXth International Congress on Electrocardiology

ELECTROCARDIOLOGY '92

Lisbon, Portugal
24 – 27 June 1992

Proceedings of the
XIXth International Congress on Electrocardiology

ELECTROCARDIOLOGY '92

Lisbon, Portugal
24 – 27 June 1992

Editors

Peter W Macfarlane
University of Glasgow, Scotland

Fernando de Padua
University of Lisbon, Portugal

World Scientific
Singapore • New Jersey • London • Hong Kong

Published by

World Scientific Publishing Co Pte Ltd
5 Toh Tuck Link, Singapore 596224
USA office: 27 Warren Street, Suite 401-402, Hackensack, NJ 07601
UK office: 57 Shelton Street, Covent Garden, London WC2H 9HE

British Library Cataloguing-in-Publication Data
A catalogue record for this book is available from the British Library.

ELECTROCARDIOLOGY '92

ISBN-13 9789810213879
ISBN-10 9810213875

The XIXth International Congress was organised under the auspices of the

INTERNATIONAL COUNCIL ON ELECTROCARDIOLOGY (INTERNATIONAL SOCIETY)

LOCAL ORGANISING COMMITTEE

Presidents:	Fernando de Padua A. Bayes de Luna
Vice-President:	Mario G. Lopes
Treasurer:	Manuel Carrageta
Secretary:	Armando Pereirinha
Assistant Secretary:	Manuela Fiuza

Organising Committee:

A. Vaz Carneiro
Antonio Brandao
Carlos Franca
Cassiano Abreu Lima
Isabel Dionisio
Jose Correia
Madalena Carvalho
Mario Jose Correia
Paula Fong
Vitor Camilo
Vitor Gil
Zelia C. Zilva

Scientific Committee:

Alvaro Pimenta
Bastos Machado
Carlos Ribeiro
Cerqueira Gomes
Chorao de Aguia
Falcao de Freitas
Fernanda Sampayo
Jose A. Rato
Salomao S. Amram

PREFACE

The 19th International Congress on Electrocardiology was held in Lisbon from 24th to 27th June, 1992. Twelve years previously, the 7th International Congress on Electrocardiology was also held in Lisbon in June. The present Proceedings, therefore, afford an opportunity to compare progress over the past twelve years with the work published in *New Frontiers of Electrocardiology* (Research Studies Press, Wiley, Chichester). *Electrocardiology '92* contains almost ninety papers which reflect the wide variety of topics presented in Lisbon.

As in 1980, the Congress attracted many physicians and scientists from around the World. Delegates from Japan and Russia were able to exchange ideas with colleagues from North America and Europe. The Proceedings, therefore, reflect a variety of approaches to research in electrocardiology in different schools.

On this occasion, it was felt that the Proceedings should be produced by the photo-offset process in order to avoid six months of retyping the contributions as happened in 1980. This does lead to some differences in presentation but the time saved is thought to represent a significant advantage. It does also mean that the papers are not able to be refereed in the usual way and there may be some shortcomings in presentation as viewed by the purist. However, this should not detract from the advantages of allowing a free flow and rapid distribution of information among researchers in the same discipline.

The Organisers of the 19th International Congress on Electrocardiology would wish to thank all those who assisted with the organisation of the Congress. This is never an easy task and involves many months of hard work. In particular, the local Organising Committee, whose names are to be found elsewhere, deserve the sincere thanks of all the participants in the Congress.

Finally, the Editors would like to thank World Scientific Publishing for producing the Proceedings so expeditiously.

P.W. Macfarlane, Glasgow
F. de Padua, Lisbon

CONTENTS

PART I

Theoretical Electrocardiology

BOUNDARY PROBLEMS OF DIPOLAR ELECTROCARDIOTOPOGRAPHY

IVAN RUTTKAY-NEDECKÝ, RÓBERT OSVALD
Institute of Normal and Pathologic Physiology,
Slovak Academy of Sciences, Sienkiewiczova 1, 813 71 Bratislava,
Czech and Slovak Federative Republic.
and
IGOR RIEČANSKÝ, EVA VANŽUROVÁ
Institute for Cardio-Vascular Diseases, Partizánska 2,
813 26 Bratislava, Czech and Slovak Federative Republic.

ABSTRACT

Dipolar electrocardiotopographic presentation of physically corrected orthogonal lead signals was studied in 77 patients with angina pectoris, pre and postoperativelly in 55 patients with right ventricular enlargement due to secundum type atrial septum defect, and in 36 healthy subjects. Application of fuzzy mathematics for evaluation of the image of ventricular activation allowed to recognize and quantify in addition to normal and abnormal activation 2 respective intermediary classes i.e. marginally normal, and marginally abnormal. This approach makes it possible to represent and evaluate conditions when the activation front is situated partly outside and partly inside normal limits. It may be applied also to other kinds of topographic representation of myocardial activation. In both groups of patients the incidence of marginally normal activation showed a symmetrical distribution throughout ventricular activation with a peak at 30 - 40ms after QRS onset, while the distributions of marginally abnormal and abnormal activations were two - peaked with the minimum corresponding to the maximum of the former.

1. Introduction

The front of myocardial activation is an irregular, bounded surface, represented in vectorcardiography by a point in space: the end-point of the instantaneous vector. As a consequence, in cases where the front is situated partly within and partly outside normal limits, it cannot be adequately evaluated since the vector end-point is situated either within or outside the limits of the reference distribution. This problem may be overcome by dipolar electrocardiotopographic representation of vectorcardiographic lead signals: here the activation front is represented by a bounded set of points (elements) on a discretized spherical image surface encopassing the heart [1] and so the set of activated points may be situated around the boundary of a reference distribution. Treatment of the set of activated points as a fuzzy subset of all activable points on the image surface allows to quantify the degree of normality of the activation front under study. Results obtained by this method were studied in 2 groups of patients, one with angina pectoris and another with right ventricular enlargement, as well as in a sample of healthy subjects.

2. Methods and Material

In dipolar electrocardiotopography, the projection of the instantaneous spatial vector onto a discretized spherical surface encompassing the heart, called image surface (IS), becomes the center of a spherical segment, the radius of which is proportional to the spatial magnitude of the vector. This circular surface is considered to be activated and consequently, the set of elements (points) within its boundary is also activated. Relative frequencies of activation of points on the discretized IS were computed in healthy subjects and in this manner probabilistic ISs were constructed for 10ms intervals of QRS, taking 5% relative frequency as the limit of norm [2].

In the individual case, the set of activated points is considered as a fuzzy subset of all activable points. The characteristic membership functions of its elements are made equal to values of relative frequencies at respective points on the probabilistic IS. Their sum is called the probability function (PF), its normalized value characterizes the degree of normality of the set of activated points. Zero membership function indentifies an abnormally activated point (AP) [3].

Values of x,y,z components of instantaneous vectors at 10ms time intervals from onset to the end of QRS were processed by a IBM PC/AT microcomputer in order to obtain maps of activated points on the IS, to indentify abnormally activated points and to compute the sum of membership functions of points lying within normal limits.

Each set of activated points was included into one of the following categories: (i) normal: no AP, PF greater or equal to $\bar{X}$ - 2SD of its normal reference distribution, (ii) marginally normal: no AP, PF less than $\bar{X}$ - 2SD, (iii) marginally abnormal: AP present, PF greater or equal to $\bar{X}$ - 2SD, (iv) abnormal: AP present, PF less than $\bar{X}$ - 2SD.

The group of patients with angina pectoris consisted of 77 subjects (66 men, 11 women) aged 25 to 59 years. In the group of patients with right ventricular enlargement were 55 subjects with ostium secundum - type atrial septum defect, aged 5 to 25 years (mean 14 years, SD 5). The sample of healthy subjects was formed by 30 men and 6 women, aged 10 to 67 years (median 46 years).

The data were obtained in both groups of patients by manual measurement of optically magnified McFee axial lead system VCG loops, recorded by a Hewlett-Packard 1520A vectorcardiograph. In the sample of healthy subjects, they were computed directly from Frank lead x,y,z signals by the electrocardiologic diagnostic system Cardiag (ZPA, Čakovice).

3. Results

All 77 patients with angina pectoris underwent selective coronary arteriography, the criterion of significant stenosis was more than 50% luminal narrowing. 26 of patients were without significant stenosis, 10 had one vessel, and 31 more than one vessel disease. The frequency of marginally normal activation versus abnormal activation (marginally abnormal and abnormal) is illustrated for the 3 subgroups in Fig. 1.

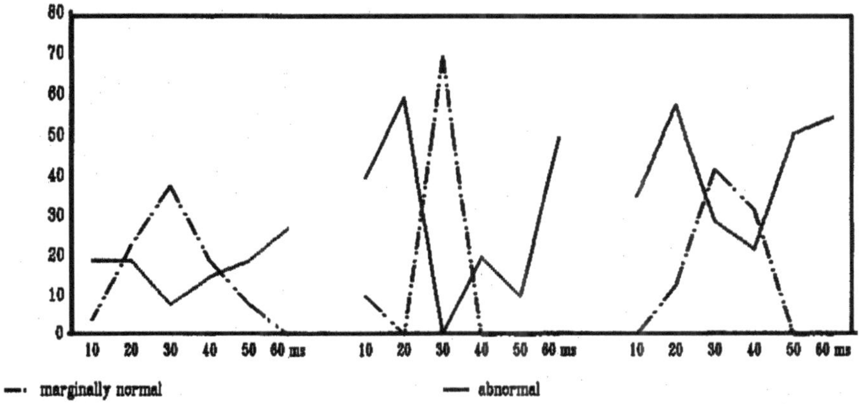

Fig.1 Frequency (%) of marginally normal activation and of abnormal activation in the course of ventricular activation in 3 subgroups of patients with angina pectoris. Left panel: without significant stenosis, middle panel: one vessel disease, right panel: more than one vessel disease Abscissa: ms QRS.

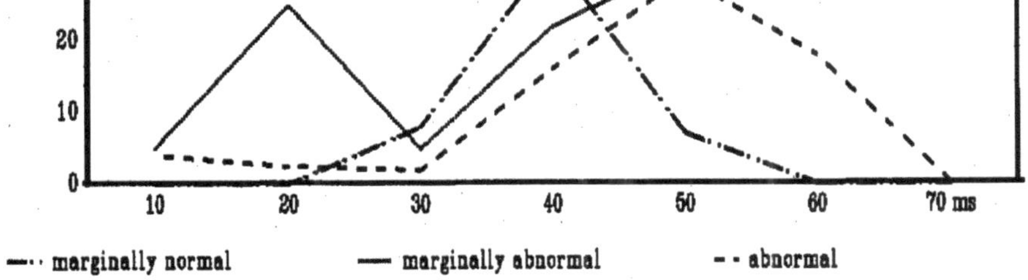

Fig.2 Frequency (%) of marginally normal activation , of marginally abnormal activation and of abnormal activation in the course ofventricular activation in patients with right ventricular enlargement. Abscissa: ms QRS.

The peak incidence of marginally normal activation occurring at 30ms QRS was accompanied by a minimum of abnormal activation, it attained 38% even in the subgroup without significant stenosis, increased significantly ($p < 0,05$) to 70% in patients with one vessel disease and decreased due to an overall increase of abnormal activation in patients with more than one vessel disease.

All patients with right ventricular enlargement were subjected to surgical repair of the atrial septum defect. The classification of activation throughout QRS, prior to intervention,is shown on Fig.2.The frequency of marginally normal acivation had a symmetrical course with a peak at 40ms QRS (33%), abnormal activation had a maximum (29%) at 50ms, and marginally abnormal activation was two - peaked, 25% at 20ms and 55% at 60ms Significant decreases ($p < 0,05$) of the incidence of the various categories of activation occurred after a postoperative period of 1 to 9 years.

In healthy subjects, classificational changes of QRS were studied due to held deep inspiration. The statistics of PF obtained in the expiratory chest position served as the reference. The change of the heart - to - body surface geometry did not change normal activation to marginally normal one, but led in some cases to occurrence of abnormally activated points toward the end of QRS, probably due to the rotation of the heart around its long axis.

4. Discussion

Application of fuzzy sets for evaluation of sequential images of ventricular activation is not restricted to dipolar electrocardiotopography. It allows to delineate two categories of activation which cannot be identified by vectorcardiography: marginally normal and marginally abnormal activation. It seems that the marginally normal activation carries independent diagnostic information. Since its frequency throughout the QRS period has a generally inverse course as compared to abnormal activation, as demonstreted in our subgroup of patients with angina pectoris without significant coronary stenosis, it may be a sensitive indicator of myocardial alteration in cases with no signs of focal lesion. Marginally abnormal activation, on the other hand, may indicate that in spite of abnormal activation of some part of myocardium the front is situated to a sufficient extent within normal limits. This may occur e.g. in cases of ventricular enlargement. In our patients in this category, it was influenced in a favorable way by surgical correction of the hemodynamic status.

5. References

1. L.I. Titomir and I. Ruttkay-Nedecký, *Int.J.Bio-Medical Computing* **20** (1987) 275.
2. I.Ruttkay-Nedecký, L.I. Titomir, O.V. Baum and L.Bachárová, in *Electrocardiology 87*, ed. E. Schubert (Akademie-Verlag, Berlin, 1988).
3. I. Ruttkay-Nedecký, in *Computers in Cardiology 1991* (IEEE Computer Society Press, Los Alamitos, 1992).

A Direct Inverse Solution with Specific Anatomy

D.M. Budgett[*], D.M. Monro[†], and M.J.K. Grimnes[†]

[*]*Department of Electrical Engineering, Imperial College, London SW7 2AY, England*

[†] *School of Electrical Engineering, University of Bath, Bath BA2 7AY, England*

ABSTRACT

We report the achievement of a direct inverse solution recovering an epicardial distribution from body surface measurements, based on the specific anatomy of the subject.

A patient specific model was formulated using a whole thoracic MRI scan from a normal subject. The thorax was classified into appropriate tissue categories in 5mm cubes. A forward solution from epicardial sources was implemented on a SIMD parallel computer using this anatomy. A finite difference model computes a full forward solution using a volume grid of constant size voxels. This allows classified MRI data to be easily incorporated into the model. The inverse model was assembled from these results. Using a Tikhonov regularization technique, inverse calculations to recover epicardial potentials were made from body surface measurements of the same subject at rest.

The comparison of the potential distribution obtained with chimpanzee epicardial distributions measured by others suggests that the results are physiologically reasonable. The major features were evident in both measured epicardial distributions and recovered epicardial distributions at all stages of the cardiac cycle.

1. Introduction

To recover the heart's electrical generators from non-invasive body surface measurements is known as the inverse problem of electrocardiography. We choose to represent the heart generators in terms of epicardial potentials because there is evidence that they closely mirror underlying cardiac electrical events[1,2], the solution is unique (without introducing simplifying assumptions), and epicardial distributions can be verified experimentally by direct epicardial mapping.

In previous work, knowledge of the epicardial potential distribution on the human heart has been use to determine the locations of accessory pathways of patients with the Wolff-Parkinson-White syndrome[3]. Experimental investigations have studied localisation of myocardial infarction[4], conduction abnormalities and mechanisms of arrhythmias[3].

The inverse solution is calculated by first solving the forward problem (calculating the body surface potential distributions from specified epicardial sources) to obtain a transfer matrix. This matrix, which relates epicardial activity to body surface activity, must be inverted to find the inverse solution. The ill-posed nature of the inverse problem means that a small amount of body surface noise (instrumentation noise, electrode miss-placement) will be amplified to cause large variations in recovered epicardial distributions. To overcome this requires some form of constrained inverse solution[5].

2. Methods

2.1. Forward Model

We implement a Finite Difference Model (FDM) which enables the macroscopic properties of the thorax (heart, lungs, trunk, liver, spine, fat, and ribs) to be represented as a regularly spaced array of cubic elements or voxels. This formulation of the forward model from accurate geometrical data contained in the MRI is relatively easy compared with the finite element or boundary element methods. The effect of thoracic anisotropy is receiving much current attention[6], and is easily incorporated into FDMs[7]. The traditional limitation of FDMs was their computational burden. By using a variation of the coloured SOR iteration, our FDM can be arranged to be data parallel to take full advantage of the performance of massively parallel computers[7].

2.2 Anatomical Model

The anatomical model contains thoracic conductivity information which is passed to the FDM. It is formulated from MRI data of the subject being studied. The thorax is subdivided into 457232 voxels which are 5mm cubes. MRI scans with a 5mm separation, ranging from the suprasternal notch to the umbilicus, are processed by an Automatic Tissue Classification (ATC) system to classify the voxels. The ATC system is at a prototype stage using information from the preceding classified slice, simple thresholding, and an interactive editor. The classification remains labour intensive, requiring about 20 hours at the console.

The FDM calculates potentials at nodes located at the corners of each voxel. The conductivity between nodes is obtained from the classified MRI data and the conductivities in Table 1.

Tissue	$\sigma, (\Omega\text{-}cm)^{-1}$	Tissue	$\sigma, (\Omega\text{-}cm)^{-1}$
Lung	4.76×10^{-4}	Liver	1.43×10^{-3}
Heart	N/A	Trunk	2.16×10^{-3}
Bone	4.76×10^{-4}	Blood	6.17×10^{-3}

Table 1. Tissue types and conductivity

2.3 Inverse Model

The inverse solution requires the forward transfer matrix A, to be formulated. To construct this matrix, the heart surface is sub-divided into 26 patches of unequal size. Sequentially each patch is set to a unit potential while all other patches are clamped to zero potential. The body surface potential distribution is calculated using the forward model for each patch activation, this contributes a column to A. After the transfer matrix has been inverted (using a regularization technique), epicardial potentials at the 26 epicardial patches, can be calculated from a body surface potential map.

To reduce the condition number of A, the body surface measurements are interpolated (using cubic splines) to the body location where the greatest potential was calculated for each patch, thus increasing the signal to noise ratio. The matrix A is still ill-conditioned, so that direct inversion will produce results very sensitive to noise. The Tikhonov regularization method is used and has been investigated for inverse solutions previously[3]. The epicardial potentials e, are produced from body surface potentials s, using Eq. 1:

$$e = (AA^T + kI)^{-1}A^T . s \tag{1}$$

where I is the identity matrix, and k controls the amount of regularization - chosen to produce stable maps for the amount of body surface noise present.

Results

Measured BSPMs and their corresponding calculated epicardial maps from a normal subject are shown in Figure 1, with measured chimpanzee epicardial maps by Spach et al[1] for comparison. Major features are consistent throughout the cardiac cycle. The left ventricular activation on the chimpanzee map must be shifted to the right to align with the human epicardial map, similarly for the right ventricle.

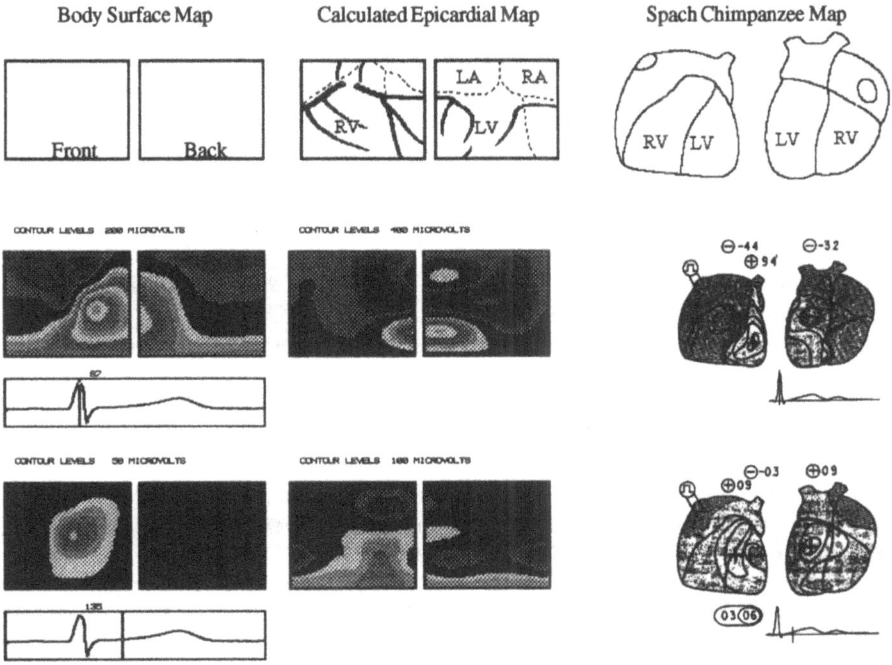

Figure 1. Potential distributions for peak R wave and ST segment, darker contours negative.

Summary

Epicardial potential maps have been calculated using a patient specific anatomical model based on MRI scans.

The finite difference model is able to model macroscopic properties of the thorax accurately, including anisotropy. Patient specific finite difference models are now feasible due to the relative ease of incorporating MRI data and the parallel implementation of the forward solution.

The major features shown on the non-invasive epicardial maps from the normal human subject agree with those measured directly from a chimpanzee[1] at all stages of the cardiac cycle.

Work is in progress to evaluate the model's accuracy by comparison of calculated epicardial potentials with directly measured epicardial potentials from the same subject, using the individual's own MRI data to formulate the model.

Acknowledgements

We are grateful to Dr Keith Straughan for the acquisition of the MRI data, Stuart Edwards for his assistance with the mapping work, and David Wilson for computational support. This work is supported by the Wellcome Trust in the form of a Wellcome Prize Studentship for D M Budgett, and also by a donation from Ciba-Geigy UK limited.

References

[1] MS Spach, RC Barr, CF Lanning and PC Tucek *Origin of Body Surface QRS and T Wave Potentials from Epicardial Potential Distributions in the Intact Chimpanzee* Circ **55**, 1977, p 268

[2] D Durrer, RT van Dam, GE Freud, MJ Janse, FL Meijler and RC Arzbaecher *Total excitation of the isolated human heart* Circ **41**, 1980, p 899

[3] HS Oster and Y Rudy *The Use of Temporal Information in the Regularization of the Inverse Problem of Electrocardiography* IEEE BME **39**, 1992, p 65

[4] DM Monro and DM Budgett *Computed Epicardial Potentials in cases of Myocardial Infarction* Proceedings of the XIXth International Congress on Electrocardiology, 1992

[5] RO Martin and TC Pilkington *Unconstrained Inverse Electrocardiography: Epicardial Potentials* IEEE BME **19**, 1972, p 276

[6] H Zhou and A van Oosterom *Computation of the Potential Distribution in a Four-Layer Anisotropic Concentric Spherical Volume Conductor* IEEE BME **39**, 1992, p 154

[7] DM Monro and DM Budgett *Parallel Computation of ECG Fields* ISCE, 1992

MODELLING OF THE INFLUENCE OF CARDIAL AND EXTRACARDIAL FACTORS ON GENERATED SURFACE POTENTIALS

MILAN TYŠLER, MÁRIA TIŇOVÁ, JANA KUŽMOVÁ, PETER KNEPPO
Department of Biomeasurements, Institute of Measurement Science,
Slovak Academy of Sciences, Dúbravská cesta 9, 842 19 Bratislava, Czechoslovakia

ABSTRACT
Computer model used for evaluation of selected cardial and extracardial factors on generated surface ecg potentials is presented. In the model realistic geometry of the heart and torso and three types of cardiac generators can be used. Algorithms for computation of heart activation, geometry definition, and simulation of body surface potentials are included. To validate the model, body surface potentials were computed using "normal" heart activation and standard geometrical data and compared with published normal measured and simulated data. In this study qualitative results of body surface potential maps simulations are presented where selected extracardial factors were varied.

1. Introduction

The cardiac electric field measured on the body surface is influenced by the properties of the cardiac generator and the geometrical and electrical parameters of the torso. The detailed relations between the particular factors and the generated potentials are generally not known. Presented computer model enables to simulate changes in the cardiac electric field by changing the anatomical configuration of the torso or by using different equivalent generators (multidipole, uniform double layer, multipole) and changing their parameters. Because of the impossibility to separate individual factor influencing the real data this model can help us to understand the measured potential distribution by simulating patterns obtained in normal cases or in selected pathologies.

2. Method

For modelling of the influence of cardial and extraxardial factors on the generated surface potential a modular program package running on standard personal computer and partially on HP Apollo 720 workstation was developed. It includes selection of heart activation model, torso geometry definition, simulation of surface potential and quantitative data analysis.

2.1. Heart activation

At present 3 models of ventricular depolarization can be used: multidipole, uniform dipole double layer or multipole.

The subject of this study is multidipolar equivalent model generator. Currently a model is used[1] where the ventricular heart surface and cavities are defined analytically by ellipsoidal segments. Ventricular walls and septum consist of isotropic cubic elements of about $1mm^3$, activation propagation is faster on endocardium to simulate the conducting system. Number and position of starting points of the activation can vary. Using this model 28 segmental summary dipoles are computed for each time instant and used as the equivalent generator.

Uniform double layer generator[2] defined on endocardial and epicardial ventricular surfaces was used as the reference model in our study.

Multipolar generator is a point generator and its localization within the heart region and components up to hexadecapole can be defined in our model.

2.2. Geometry definition

Realistic 3-dimensional geometry of inhomogeneous torso and heart is used. Body tissues are treated as isotropic regions with their specific conductivities. All these regions are specified by closed boundary surfaces. Boundary points are digitized from 3-dimensional torso model, from MR images or can be computed analytically. Distance between points can be selected according to the desired accuracy of surface approximation. Boundary surfaces are then triangulated and can be interactively shifted, rotated or scaled to get the desired anatomical torso configuration. The number of defined surfaces is variable, usually heart cavities and epicardium, right and left lungs and torso surface are included.

2.3. Potential simulation.

The potentials are computed on any defined closed surface within torso using boundary element method. Potentials in mapping grids 12x16 or 10x15 points and Frank or McFee-Parungao vectors can be estimated using computed potentials on triangulated torso. The maps and vectors can be compared using relative errors or correlation coefficients.

3. Results and discussion

In this study the multidipole model with analytically defined heart geometry and activation corresponding with the published data[3] was tested. Inhomogeneous torso geometry measured from a normal patient was used, the heart was rotated 45 degrees around the right-left and front-back axes and 90 degrees around its longitudinal axis, as it can be seen in Fig. 1. Simulated body surface potentials during the ventricular depolarization are in Fig. 2. The map patterns were close to real data, maxima and minima were within published normal limits[4] and their

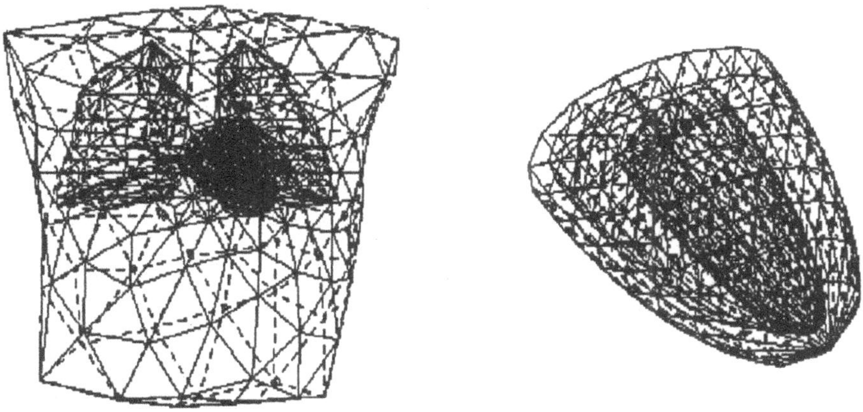

Fig.1. Torso geometry used in this study; left: inhomogogeneous torso with lungs and heart, right: heart ventricles defined using analytical description of epicardium and cavities.

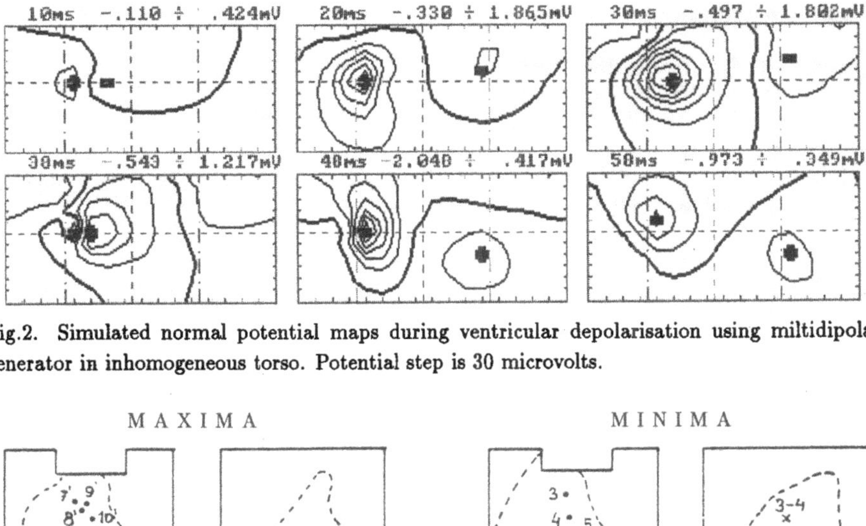

Fig.2. Simulated normal potential maps during ventricular depolarisation using miltidipolar generator in inhomogeneous torso. Potential step is 30 microvolts.

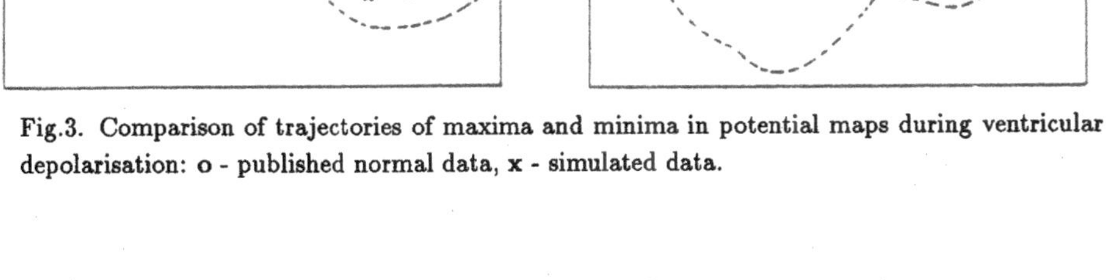

Fig.3. Comparison of trajectories of maxima and minima in potential maps during ventricular depolarisation: **o** - published normal data, **x** - simulated data.

trajectories were also normal as it can be seen in Fig. 3. However, the right ventricular breakthrough was late in this configuration. Comparison with reference model[2] brought similar results.

Similar simulations with homogeneous torso gave different results: the overall map patterns were slightly changed, potential amplitudes were nonlinearly changed (up to 50%, some of the amplitudes were out of normal range) and extremes positions were also changed.

In another simulation the influence of heart position changes was examined. The breathing was simulated by rotating the heart around front-back and longitudinal axes. The effect was relatively strong, the map patterns changed and the extremes in maps significantly moved.

From these first results we conclude, that this model concept seems promising for modelling of cardial and extracardial factors on the generated field: it enables modelling of only selected factors and also comparison of simulated and real data. However, in this study it was not possible to get fully realistic results without changing parameters of heart geometry and activation.

4. Acknowledgements

The authors are grateful to Ass. Prof. I. Ruttkay-Nedecký, Dr. V. Szathmáry and to Prof. A. van Oosterom for their permission to use the multidipole model data and the data and software for implementing the uniform double layer model as reference.

This work was supported by grant GA SAV No. 319/91 from the Slovak Academy of Sciences.

5. References

1. I. Ruttkay-Nedecký, A. Drkošová, V. Szathmáry , in *Advances in Electrocardiology*, ed.P.d' Alché (Publications de l' Université de Caen, 1985).
2. A. van Oosterom, G. Huiskamp, *J. of Electrocardiology* **22** (1989) 53.
3. D. Durrer, R.Th. van Dam, G.E. Freud, M.J. Janse, F.L. Meijler, R.C. Arzbaecher, *Circulation* **41** (1970) 899.
4. D. Stilli, E. Musso, P. Barone, P. Ciarlini, E. Macchi, G. Regoliosi, L.D. Cas, C. Manca, O. Visioli, M. Bo, B. Taccardi, *J. of Electrocardiology* **21** (1988) 1.

MODEL-BASED COMPARISON OF BSPM AND ACTIVATION MAPS BASED ON MULTIPOLAR EXPANSION

PETER KNEPPO, JANA KUŽMOVÁ, MILAN TYŠLER
Department of Biomeasurements, Institute of Measurement Science,
Slovak Academy of Sciences, Dúbravská cesta 9, 842 19 Bratislava, Czechoslovakia

ABSTRACT

The basic aim of this work was study of multipole equivalent generator properties. For inverse solution modified multipole generator transformed into characteristics having an electrophysiological meaning was used. For verification of this approach the forward simulation of the depolarization wave in heart was modeled by uniform double layer in a torso model. Theoretically derivable and in computer model confirmed better possibility of characterizing the real sources by quasiepicardial maps of the *"exposed heart"* when comparing with the *"in situ"* heart was obtained.

1. Introduction

One possible approach to noninvasive identification of cardiac excitation from the body surface measurements is the development of methods for solving the inverse problem in terms of coefficients of cardiac multipolar equivalent generator which are subsequently transformed into characteristics having an electrophysiological meaning. After the hypothetical projection of the depolarization fronts onto the image surface has been found, it is possible to select on this surface regions corresponding to three main electrophysiological states of the ventricular wall, which can be characterized by the instantaneous excitation maps, isochrone maps and maps of delay of the depolarization arrival time[1]. For verification of this method on realistic subjects the forward simulation of the depolarization wave in heart was modeled by uniform double layer spreading through the cardiac muscle located in an inhomogeneous realistically shaped torso model[2]. These body surface potential maps were then used as the input information for verification of the inverse problem solution based on multipolar expansion. The quasiepicardial maps estimated by the inverse solution were finally compared with quasiepicardial maps obtained from forward simulation[3].

2. Method

The electrical field of equivalent generators was computed on a sphere closely surrounding the modeled heart sources and its relation to the field of original quasi realistic generator was studied. For the inverse problem solution a method based on surface integration of body potential maps was used[4]. Equivalent generators describing the ventricles as thin-wall shells with double-layer source were used[5]. The intensity of the double layer is defined by the total dipole moment of the elementary dipole generators, oriented along the normal of the heart wall. If the thickness of the heart wall, as well as the tangential components of the elementary dipoles are decreasing, the apparent generator approaches to the surface equivalent generator, namely the spherical double-layer tightly enveloping the heart. It can be shown that the intensity J of the double layer generator is

$$J(\theta, \psi, t) = J_o(t) + \frac{1}{4\pi} \sum_{n=1}^{\infty} \sum_{m=0}^{n} \frac{2n+1}{nR_H^{n+1}} \{A_{nm}(t).Y_{nm}^{e}(\theta, \psi) + B_{nm}(t).Y_{nm}^{o}(\theta, \psi)\} \quad (1)$$

where R_H is the radius of the double-layer spherical surface and the rest of the notation corresponds to usual multipole expansion with respect to the sphere center. The second term of Eq.1 is proportional to the potential on the surface of a homogeneous sphere with radius R_H including the heart and surrounded by a nonconducting medium; this potential may be considered as the quasiepicardial potential of the so called dry or exposed heart[5].

For computing the potential distribution on torso (and on any surface within the torso) the forward solution based on integral equations was used[2]. Realistic geometry of inhomogeneous torso and heart have been assumed, heart generator was modeled by a uniform double layer spreading through the cardiac muscle.

3. Results

From the body surface potential maps simulated on the torso the equivalent multipolar generator was computed for each time instant of the depolarization. Then the potential distributions were computed on a surface just surrounding the heart or on a spherical surface around the heart. The results were compared with the reference quasiepicardial maps computed from the original heart model.

First the accuracy (estimated by correlation coefficient) of potential distribution computed using multipole generators of different orders and of different localization was calculated. Multipolar generator was located in the origin of coordinates and dipole, dipole+quadrupole or dipole+quadrupole+octupole models were used. The correlations were higher than 0.93 for dipole+quadrupole+octupole model. Then the multipolar generator was located in torso excentrically in so called heart center and dipole or dipole+quadrupole models were used. The correlations were higher than 0.89 for dipole+quadrupole model.

The results of comparison between *"in situ"* and *"exposed heart"* are shown in Fig.1. Epicardial potentials in *"in situ"* experiments are influenced by the surrounding medium and the torso boundary. On the other hand the epicardial potentials on anatomically shaped *"exposed heart"* are theoretically proportional to the intensity of the equivalent double-layer generator on the epicardial surface.

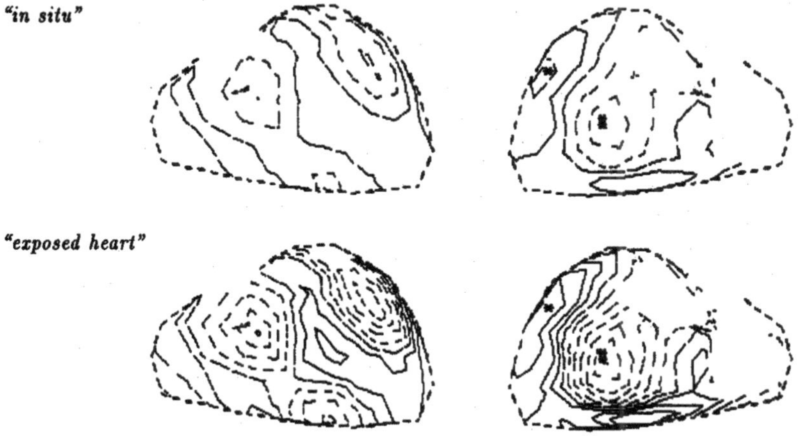

Fig.1. Comparision of epicardial potentials in *"in situ"* and *"exposed heart"* experiments.

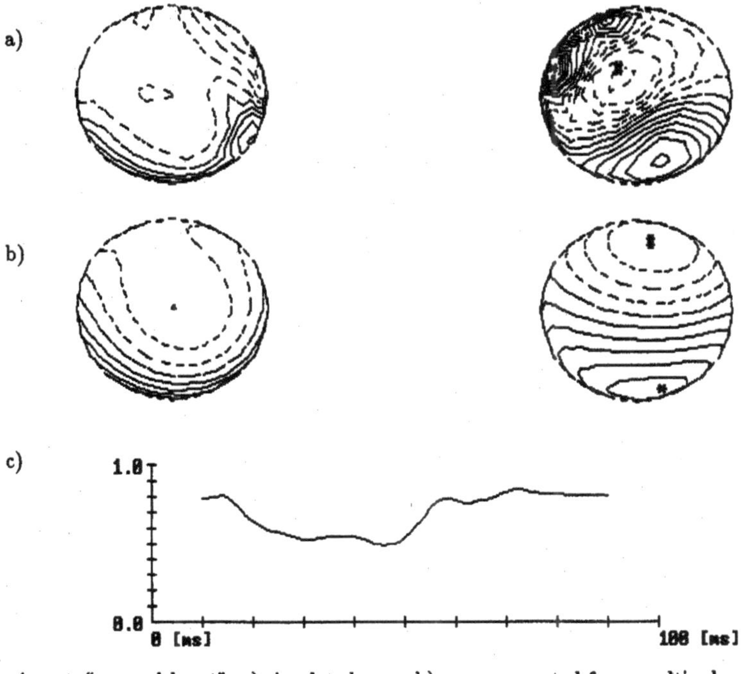

Fig.2. Experiment *"exposed heart"*: a) simulated map, b) map computed from multipolar generator (dipole+quadrupole model) c) correlation coefficients

Then correlations between the potential distributions on a sphere surface (quasi-epicardial map) surrounding the multipolar equivalent generators of different orders and located in so called heart center and potential distributions in bigger distances from the sources were studied. Potential changes dependent on the generator structure in experiments *"in situ"* and *"exposed heart"* were obtained. Comparison of quasiepicardial potential on a sphere surface closely surrounding the heart in experiment *"exposed heart"* is shown in Fig.2.

4. Conclusions

From our results it implies that there is a high correlation between the original (simulated) potential distribution and the potentials computed from equivalent multipolar models for dipole+quadrupole+octupole located in the torso center and dipole+quadrupole located in the heart center.

Theoretically derivable and in computer model confirmed better possibility of characterizing the real sources by quasiepicardial maps of the *"exposed heart"* when comparing with the *"in situ"* heart were obtained. That means higher information contents of of the quasiepicardial maps of the *"exposed heart"*.

The results were influenced by the fact that the forward solution with a double layer generator[2] which was used for model-based verification is only selective simplification of the reality. Some other interesting results from an electrolytic tank experiment of an isolated dog heart were shown in paper[6] .

5. Acknowledgements

The authors are grateful to Prof. A. van Oosterom, Prof. L.I. Titomir and Jana Švehliková for providing them the data and software for implementing the forward and inverse model. This work was supported by grant GA-SAV No.319/91 and in part by grant GA SAV No.242/91 from the Slovak Academy of Sciences.

6. References

1. L.I. Titomir, P. Kneppo, M. Kričfaluši, S. Cagáň, in *Electrocardiology '83*, eds. I. Ruttkay-Nedecký and P. Macfarlane (Excerpta Medica, Amsterdam, 1984).
2. A. Oosterom, *PhD-thesis* (University of Amsterdam, Amsterdam 1978) p.181.
3. P. Kneppo, J. Švehliková, J. Kužmová, M. Tyšler, in *Electrocardiology '91*, ed. J. Jagielski (Excerpta Medica, Amsterdam, 1992).
4. T.C. Pilkington and M.N. Morrow, *CRC Crit. Rev. Biomed. Eng.* **7** (1982) 175.
5. P. Kneppo and L.I. Titomir, *CRC Crit. Rev. Biomed. Eng.* **19 (5)** (1992) 343.
6. Gy. Kozmann, Zs. Cserjes, S. Baruffi, S. Spaggiari, in *Electrocardiology '91*, ed. J. Jagielski (Excerpta Medica, Amsterdam, 1992).

The Analysis of Ventricular Fibrillation Induced by Extra-stimuli on Three Dimensional Computer Heart Model

Osamu Okazaki*
*Nakano National Chest Hospital
3-14-20 Egota, Nakano-ku, Tokyo 165, Japan

and

Daming Wei** and Kenichi Harumi*
**Nihon Kohden Corporation, Tokyo 165, Japan

ABSTRACT

We studied the initiative propagation pattern of ventricular fibrillation (Vf) induced by extra-stimuli using a three-dimensional computer heart model. This heart model was composed of about 50,000 discrete units with spatial resolution of 1.5mm and mounted in a human torso model. The changing rate of action potential duration (APD) in relation at cycle length of extra-stimuli, dynamic coefficient, was determined. The conduction velocity was slowed in near the absolute refractory period with the maximum conduction delay of 3 times of the normal. Five or more successive extra-stimuli could induce a sustained Vf with combined dynamic coefficient and conduction delay. Vf was not induced by 4 or less successive extra-stimuli under the same. At least twice of the conduction delay was necessary for the induction of Vf. Complex irregularity of excitation fronts on the septal region was started during Vf, and then the non-homogeneous irregular excitation front occurred in the endocardium. These results suggest that the reentry in Purkinje and ventricular muscle in high rate would produce non-homogeneous irregular excitation front in the endocardium and might be one of the cause of Vf in the 3-D cardiac model.

BACKGROUND

The two dimensional computer model of fibrillation was introduced by Moe et al in 1964, and this was extended to the idea of vulnerability by Abildskov in 1990. Thakor et al presented the fibrillation by 5 extrastimuli in realistic three dimensional computer heart model, but the cell possessed uniform electrical properties. We attempted to analyze the conditions to induce ventricular fibrillation, and also excitation patterns using the newly developed computer heart model including realistic physiological properties.

METHOD

Three Dimensional Computer Simulation Model (Harumi[1], 1989)

Cross sections of the human heart were collected from the Durrer's model. The heart model was constructed on cubic elements, 1.5mm in diameter with bidirectional conduction. The unit model included sinus node, atrium, A-V node, specialized conduction system, intermediate cells around the Purkinje network and ventricle. A 3-D section of this model with an epicardial pacing site of extra-stimuli. An arrow on the horizontal image indicates the position of successive stimulation. (Fig.1) Action potential duration (APD) and other electrophysiological parameters were assigned to each type of model unit. (Table 1)

Experimental Data

Gettes[2](1964) and our experimental study[3](1989) showed relationship between APD and stimulation coupling interval (CI). This relation was introduced into the model by defining a parameter called dynamic coefficient (DC) as in equation(1).

$$DC = \Delta T / \Delta CI \quad \ldots (1)$$

ΔT: the change in APD result from premature coupling interval
ΔCI: the change in stimulation coupling interval

In addition, the conduction delay during incomplete recovery was also incorporated on the ventriculum.

Condition of Stimulation

Sinus node of the model was paced with cycle length of 500msec. (Table 1) Five successive extra-stimuli were applied to the epicardium of left ventriculum. The stimuli started at 300 msec after the first sinus pacing with 160msec interval. Simulation was performed on a 32-bits workstation (SUN /4).

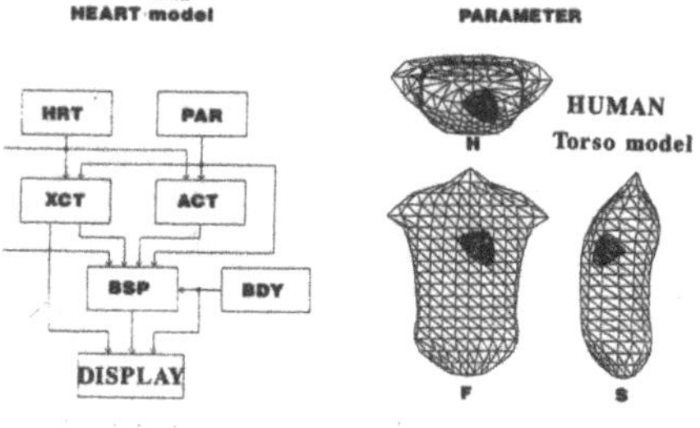

(Fig.1)

ELECTROPHYSIOLOGICAL PARAMETERS

PARAMETER	SN	ATR	AVN	HIS	BB	PKJ	VTR
APD (ms)	255	100	255	255	255	355	255
ARP (ms)	200	80	80	80	80	180	80
FRT (ms)	295	120	295	295	295	395	295
CV (m/s)	0.5	1.0	0.1	2.5	2.5	2.5	0.5
DC (%)	/	/	/	/	/	80	18
〈PACING〉							
Cycle length (ms)	500						
Beat Number	16						
Extra-stimuli							
Starting time (ms)	300						
Cycle length (ms)	160						
Beat Number	5						

(Table 1)

RESULTS

(1) Five or more successive extra-stimuli could induce a sustained Vf with electrophysiologic condition on Table 1. (Fig.2) Vf was not induced by 4 or less successive extra-stimuli under this condition. At least twice of the conduction delay was necessary for the induction of Vf. After 4 sec, the fibrillation rate is significantly longer than that of fibrillation from 2 to 3 sec. Unidirectional block was induced ventricular tachycardia on the septal region.
(2) Complex irregular excitation wavefronts occurred along endocardium and spatially non-uniform wavefronts of excitation could be observed along epicardial region during Vf. (Fig.2) This phenomenon is to be explained theoretically. These figures prove clearly that a dispersion of refractory get ready for Vf on the excitation wavefronts.

Ventricular Fibrillation

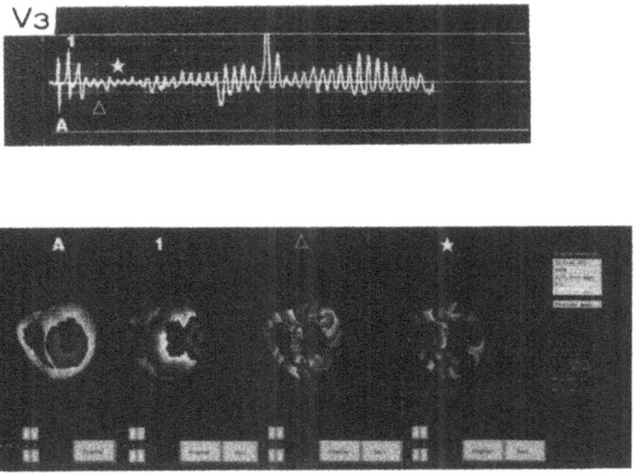

(Fig.2)

DISCUSSION

To explain the mechanism of Vf on 3-D model, we assume that the conditions of unstable cells provide the following:
(1) APD of Purkinje fiber was lower than that of ventricular muscle in the earlier prematurity according to Gettes's and our data. The term "Dynamic Coefficient" can be defined as the effects of cycle length dependent changes consists of APD of Purkinje Fibers and ventricular muscle.
(2) Ventricular gradient of APD was set 5msec by one layer in the ventricular muscle. Ventricular muscle was made up of 10 layers. Conduction velocity in non-refractory ventricular muscle is 0.17 m/s due to 3 times as slow as normal conduction. Even if there is a mismatch of conduction delay on the border of Purkinje and ventriculum, this does not affect the validity of a necessary condition for Vf induced by extra-stimuli. The model has several limitations, as Thakor and Eisenman[4](1989) supposes about isotropic conduction and propagation. I agree with this amount of detail at

the whole-heart level in thinking that to be out of reach of available computing resources.
(3) The first extra-stimulation on the left epicardium propagates as a waveform except Purkinje's rapid conduction. (Fig.3A) During Vf, an analysis of isochronal map proves that the initiation of Vf starts at a distant from the stimulation site in this horizontal separation. (Fig.3B)

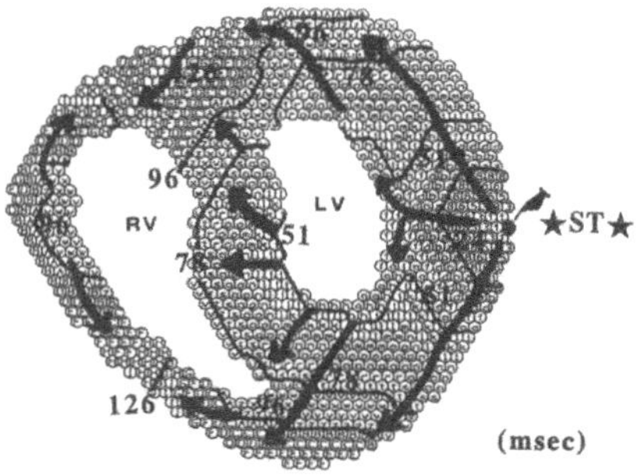

Propagation of Extra-stimulus

(Fig.3A)

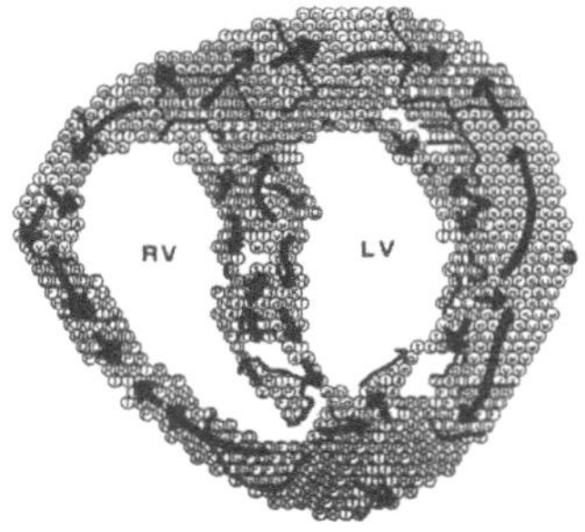

Non-Homogenous Pattern
at The Initiation of Ventricular Fibrillation

(Fig.3B)

CONCLUSIONS

Ventricular fibrillation was simulated with 3-D heart model. The relation of APD of Purkinje fiber and ventricular muscle with coupling interval and conduction delay during incomplete refractory period may play important roles in the induction of Vf. The initiation of Vf starts at a distant from the stimulation site. These results suggested that the reentry in Purkinje fiber and ventricular muscle in high rate would produce non-homogenous irregular excitation fronts in the endocardium and might be one of the cause of Vf in this 3-D cardiac model.

REFERENCES

1) Harumi K, Tsunakawa H, Wei Daming et al: Clinical application of electrocardiographic computer model. J Electrocardiol 22(supple):54-63, 1989
2) Gettes LS, Movehouse N and Surawics B: Effect of premature depolarization on the duration of action potentials in Purkinje and ventricular fibers of the moderator band of the pig heart. Circ Rec 30:66, 1972
3) Harumi K, Tsutsumi T, Sekiya S et al: Classification of anti-arrhythmic drugs based on ventricular fibrillation threshold. Am J Cardiol 64:10J-14J, 1989
4) Thakor NV and Eisenman LN: Three-Dimensional Computer Model of the Heart: Fibrillation Induced by Extrastimulation. Comput and Biomed Rec 22,532-545, 1989

RECONSTRUCTION OF THREE-DIMENSIONAL TOPOGRAPHY OF THE PROCESS OF THE HEART EXCITATION

N.A. ANTONOVA, D.N.SHMAKOV, M.P.ROSHCHEVSKY
Institute of Physiology
of Ural Div. of Acad. Sci. of Russia,
Syktyvkar, Komi Republic, Russian Federation

ABSTRACT

The three-dimensional pattern of excitation wave spread through the heart ventricles was reconstructed on the base of electrocardiograms recorded from several myocardial cross-sections using multipolar needle electrodes. General patterns of excitation of the heart ventricles were simulated between experimental cross-sections of the heart ventricles. Modelling was carried out by method of spline interpolation. Satisfactory conformity was received between experimental and simulating data.

1. Introduction

The purpose of this study is to reconstruct the three-dimensional pattern of the process of distribution of the activation wave in the heart ventricles by a computer analysis of electrocardiograms recorded in the intramural myocard layers.

Earlier we (1) designed a 128-channel minicomputer - CAMAC system. In this work we made an attempt to reconstruct the topography of the process of the depolarization of the free ventricle walls by means of two - dimensional projections of activation process on planes located perpendicular and parallel to long axis of the heart.

2. Material and Method

The experiments have been carried out on adult mongrel dogs. The animals were anaesthetized with sodium thiopental-natrium 30-50 mg/kg body wt. The trachea was intubated and artificial ventilation was instituted by means of a resperator pump. A left thorocotomy was performed through the fourth intercostal space. The multipolar intramural electrodes were introduced in the ventricle myocard perpendicular to the long axis of the heart in several planes.

The arrival of the depolarization wave to the local myocardial points was determined by calculation of the phase displacement between the time reference potential and the first derivative of extracellular potentials recorded from intramural multipolar electrodes.

At the final stage of the experiments the angle and radial co - ordinates of the electrodes, exterior and interior contours of planes were measured. The data conserning time arrival of the activation wave were grouped and geometrical configurations of depolarization wave front were determined by cubic spline in every plane.

Next, a general patterns of excitation of the heart ventricles was simulated between experimental cross-sections of the heart ventricles.

3. Results

Experimental (4, 5) and simulated (4.5) maps of the excitation of the heart ventricles are shown in the fig.1 and fig. 2. Cross-section 4.5 is located in the middle part between 4 and 5 experimental sections. With the aid of simulating it's possible to reconstruct the activation process at anyone distance from experimental cross-sections. It's possible also to reconstruct the pattern of the excitation process in the planes parallel to the long axis of the heart.

Chronotopographic maps of the process of the activation of the heart were presented on a display and as a print copy in every fix time intervals (for example, 2, 4, 5 ms).

Chronotopographic maps of the process of depolarization of the dog heart ventricles compiled on the basis of computer and hand-made analysis were similar. It shows that the program software correctly represents the experimental data.

The value of this model is a in the fact that it gives good information about the sequence of depolarization of the heart ventricles. It provides useful information for physiological interpretation of the results of the measurement of the parameters of the cardioelectric potentials.

The programs and archives of electrophysiological data may be applicable to the study of normal process of excitation of intramural myocard layers and to modelling of heart diseases connected with the disturbances of conductivity and they may be also used for the solution of the problems of genesis of the cardioelectric field.

4. Conclusion

Thus, in the process of these investigations there have been developed:

- methods of registration and analysis of extracellular potentials in the intramural layers of the heart exercised with original electrodes in normal conditions and under pathology;
- a device created on the micro-computer basis allowing to investigate the electric field with the

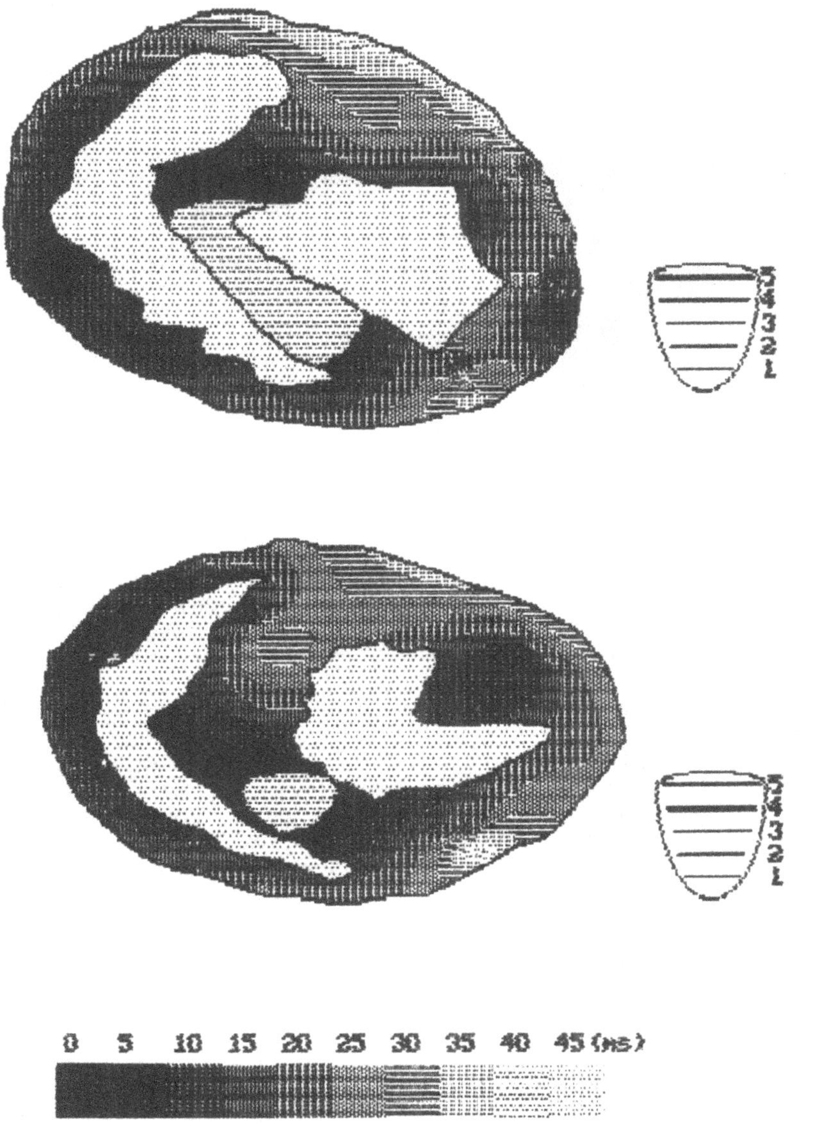

Fig. 1. Experimental chronotopographic maps of depolarization of the heart ventricles in the dog. 4 and 5-cross-sections of heart.

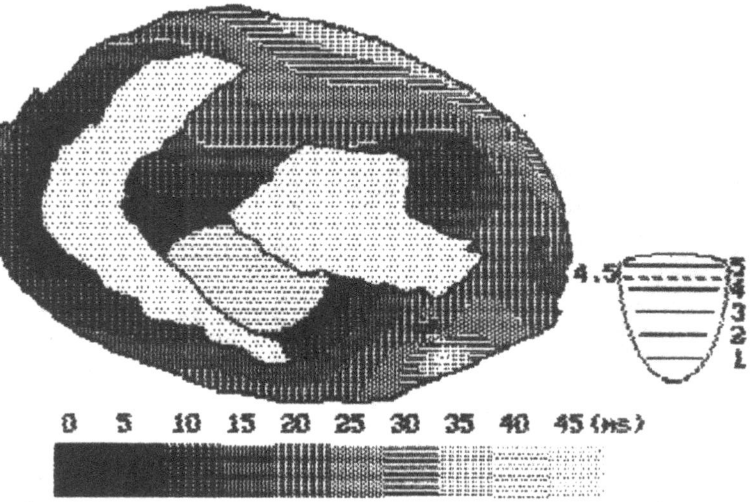

Fig. 2. Culculated chronotopographic map of depolarization of the heart ventricles in the dog.
4.5 - cross-section of heart.

simultaneous registration of a large number of points in the intramural layers of the heart as well as on its surface applying different types of the developed electrodes;

- program software allowing to represent data as maps of the excitation wave distribution, momentous equipotential maps, maps of the distribution of potential forms etc., and also as digital indexes;

- original program support, which on the basis of imitational modelling and dynamic data registration provides a larger volume of information concerning of the activation of the heart ventricles, allows to analyse characteristics of intramural extracellular potentials.

Unfortunately, at present we do not present a three-demensional dynamic pattern of the excitation of the heart ventricles in the whole volume, but we hope that in the near future we shall manage to achieve the goal.

5. Acknowledgements

Authors expresses their gratitude to the firm MERCK SHARP & DOHME I.D.E.A. for the possibility to partipicate in the work of the XIX International Congress on Electrocardiology.

6. References

1. M.P.Roshchevsky et al., Realization of model of an equivalent multipole generator in electrocardiotopography (Acad of Sci. of the USSR, Komi Branch, Syktyvkar,1985) 12p.

PART II

Mapping — Endocardial, Epicardial and Body Surface

MAPPING OF MYOCARDIAL ACTIVATION AT VENTRICULAR PREMATURE BEATS IN DOG

M.P.ROSHCHEVSKY, K.K.MOSTIVENKO, D.N.SHMAKOV, V.A.VITYASEV

Institute of Physiology of Ural Div.of Acad. Sci. of Russia
Syktyvkar, Komi Republic, Russian Federation

ABSTRACT

The excitation sequence in intramural layers and on the epicardial surface of canine heart ventricles was investigated at different sites of ectopic beats in dog. The shortest duration of the ventricle depolarization was observed with stimulation from the subendocard of the middle thirds of the left side of the interventricular septum, the greater duration - from the base of the right ventricle. With stimulation at subepicard the area of the earliest activation on the epicardial surface corresponds to the site of artificial electrical stimulation with more precision, than with the stimulation at subendocard.

The patterns of ventricular excitation are similar in human [1] and canine hearts. Therefore, it is possible to study heart diseases connected with the disturbance of the conductivity on the canine heart.

1. Materials and Methods

The experiments have been carried out on adult mongrel dogs (n = 6). The animals were anaesthetized with sodium thiopentalum-natrium 30-50 mg/kg body wt. The trachea was intubated and artificial ventilation was instituted by means of a respiratory pump. Left thoracotomy was perfomed through the fourth intercostal space. The stimulation multipolar electrodes were introduced perpendicular to interventricular septum and free ventricle walls. Extrasystoles were produced by single rectangular impulses usually at the end of a refractory period. Their amplitude was equal to 0,4-6,0 V and length to - 2 ms. The sequence of the heart ventricle depolarization was carried out during premature ventricular systoles by means of intramural multipolar techniques. Epicardial electrodes were located regularly in the form of a grid containing 8 columns and 8 rows . Sinus rhythm was forced with the interval of 340-360 ms from the base of the right atrial appendage. Unipolar electrograms were recorded in intramural layers successivly with synchronization from 360 points of 45 needles and on the epicard simultaneously from 64 points. Isochronal maps were obtained with a 64-channel mapping system.

2. Results

Electrical stimulation was delivered from the subendocard and from subepicard. With stimulation from the base of the right atrial appendage a chronotopographic map corresponds to the normal distribution potentials on the epicard (fig.1). For premature beats the stimulation points were located at the apex, ventral and dorsal base and at free wall ventricles. As a rule, the earliest time appearance of the excitation wave corresponds to the site of the ectopic beat origin. With the stimulation from the subendocard of the apex of the left ventricle (LV) the movement excitation wave fronts is exercised in several directions to the epicardial surface (fig.2).

It might result from the fact that the excitation wave from the subendocard, wich is abundant in Purkinje fibers, is partly conducted by these fibers. Sometimes, for example in the case of stimulation of ventral base of LV the area of the earliest activation shifts 1-2 sm aside from the site of the ectopic beat origin. This phenomenon was probably due to the fact that the area, where the stimuli were delivered, took place during an absolute refractory period. Besides, it is possible, that the movement of the excitation wave is effected by predominant direction of deep muscle bundles which as is shown by A.Puff in his works [2] in the free wall ventricles run mainly longitudinally and on the apex of the ventricle they are located in cross-direction, especially in the apex of the venricle where they form the so called "curl" of the heart.

With stimulation at the subepicard the successive retrograde distribution of the activation wave into a free wall and along epicardial layers is observed. As a rule, the area of the earliest activation corresponds to the site of artificial electrical stimulation with more precision, than with stimulation at the subendocard.

It was determined that with ventricular extrasystoles the duration of the heart ventricle depolarization process increased by 51-126% as compared with the normal sinus rhythm. The shortest duration of this process was observed from the subendocard of the middle thirds of the left side of the interventricular septum, the greater duration - from the base of the right ventricle [3].

At the normal sinus rhythm the activation wave from

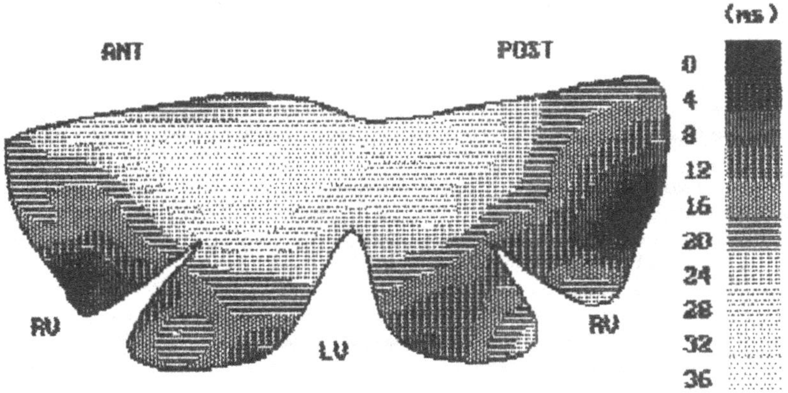

Fig.1.Chronotopographic map of depolarization on the epicard in canine heart at the forced rhythm from the base of the right atrial appendage. RV - right ventricle, LV - left ventricle, ANT - anterior, POST - posterior.

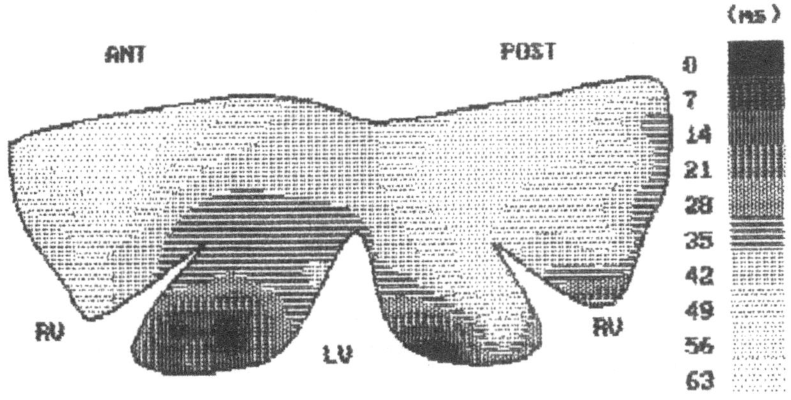

Fig.2.Chronotopographic map of depolarization on the epicard during premature stimulation from apex of left ventricle. Mark are the same as in fig.1.

subendocardial layers of the free walls of the ventricles successively spreads towards their epicard and simultaneously to the apex and the base of the heart. In some areas the depolarization wave first approaches the zones situated deep under the endocard and reversal changes of its direction, especially under the papillary muscles, are observed.

With stimulation at the endocard the successive movement of depolarization wave takes place along endocardial layers and simultaneously to epicard. But as compared to normal heart excitation a uniform course of activation wave is observed.

From ectopic foci of the excitation situated both in epicard and endocard and in intramural myocard layers the depolarization wave is spreading almost identically in all directions with constant speed of 0,3 m/s approximately at a distance of 0,5 - 1,0 sm, while the speed of the excitation wave spread is equal to 1,0 -1,5 m/s for normal sinus beats. Apparently the net of the Purkinje fibers did not take part in the conduction of the excitation in case of artificial electrical stimulation. It is probable, the muscle cells were already repolarized while Purkinje fibers were not yet repolarized in the moment of electrical irritation. That's why, the excitation of the ventricle myocard occured for the main part as muscle conduction in the stimulation zones.

Thus, the application of multipolar technique is useful for the estimation of general peculiarities of spread of the excitation wave in the heart ventricles at ectopic impulses and localization of the site of ectopic foci origin.

3. Acknowledgements

Authors expresses their gratitude to the firm MERCK SHARP & DOHME I.D.E.A. for the possibility to participate in the work of the XIX International Congress on Electrocardiology.

4. References

1. D.Durrer, R. van Dam, G.E.Frend, M.J.Janse, F.L.Meijler, R.C.Arzbaecher / Total excitation of the isolated human heart // Circulation, 1970. -Vol. 41, -N 6. -P. 899-912.

2. A.Puff / Functionelle Bau der Herzkammern// Georg Thieme Verlag, Stuttgart, 1960. -87 s.

3. D.N.Shmakov, M.P.Roshchevsky / Peculiarities of myocard depolarization at experimental disturbances of the heart excitation// Series of preprints "Scientific Reports". Komi Scientific Center of the USSR Acad. Sci., Ural division. 1991. - Issue 267. - 18 p.

THE INITIAL QRS IN SEVERE AORTIC STENOSIS - A BODY SURFACE POTENTIAL MAPPING STUDY

Liebman, J., Thomas, C.W., Rudy, Y., Saltzberg, R.

From the Departments of Pediatrics and Biomedical Engineering - Case Western University and Rainbow Babies and Children's Hospital - Cleveland, OH 44106

Abstract We have previously documented that in severe valvular aortic stenosis (AS), the initial QRS is frequently to the left, usually anterior. BSPM's were performed in 19 consecutive patients going to surgery for severe valvular AS with initial QRS left. In each case the early maximum potential was well to the left, near the left axillary line. Two were posterior to that line. The early minima were always to the right of the maxima. It is hypothesized that the posterior free wall, very hypertrophed in severe valvular AS, is responsible for the observation.

It has been previously observed that the initial QRS is directed to the left in many types of congenital heart disease including various dextrocardias, conduction abnormalities, ventricular inversion, total anomalous pulmonary venous return, hypoplastic left ventricle, severe pulmonic stenosis and severe aortic stenosis (AS)[1-6]. Explanations for these observations are based upon what little is known about normal activation sequences in humans[7-13] and what less is known in the specific pathology. Kulbertus' data add to the knowledge[14-15]. Since the observations have been extremely useful clinically it is an extremely important area to be delineated and expanded.

Putting together what is known from the above we believe that the normal initial QRS to the right anterior and superior is the result of five distinct areas which make up initial activation. Normally, the largest contribution is the rightward anterior vector from stimulation of the left posterior side of the septum half to two-thirds down, by the left posterior branch of the left bundle. (fig. 1a) This branch also stimulates activation of the left ventricular (LV) posterior free wall resulting in a left posterior vector. (fig. 1b) Since the septum at that level has a greater muscle mass than does the LV posterior free wall, the septal vector is larger than the free posterior wall vector. At close to the same time the anterior branch of the left bundle stimulates the septum to cause activation up the septum, resulting in a vector which is superior and slightly to the right. (fig. 1e) The right bundle courses down the right side of the septum to go through the moderator band. From here it gives a small right septal branch causing activation of what is believed to be the right ventricular portion of the septum[16]. The result is a small vector to the left and posterior. (fig. 1c) The right bundle, on going through the moderator band then stimulates the endocardium which, according to Myerberg[16-17] very rapidly causes stimulation of the entire right ventricular endocardium. The result is a prominent anterior vector which should also be to the right. (fig. 1d) Therefore, adding the five vectors that make up initial activation results in a normal initial QRS to the right, anterior and superior (fig. 1).

In our previous studies of AS there was a set of 70 children operated upon (and thus severe) and another set of 71 who had cardiac catheterization (including some of the same patients). All the surgical patients were obviously severe and the stenosis was valvular. Thirty-five of the 70 children had initial QRS to the left and anterior and in the others the magnitude to the right was small. Of the 71 catheterized, 61 were valvular, two supravalvular and eight subvalvular. In the eight with fixed subaortic stenosis, seven had systolic gradients > 50 mmHg and were operated upon. All had initial QRS to the right. Of the other 63, 41 had systolic gradients < 50 mmHg and 37/41 had initial QRS to the right. The other 22 had systolic gradients > 50 mmHg and/or needed surgery. Initial QRS was to the left in 19/22. Thus in valvular AS an initial QRS to the left indicates severity.

In the present study 19 consecutive patients (average age 15 years) with severe valvular AS and initial QRS left and going to surgery had prior body surface potential mapping (BSPM) with our color calibrated and displayed 180 electrode system. In normal children[18] at the onset of ventricular activation there is invariably a maximum (the peak positive potential) over the sternum or slightly to the left and usually superior. The peak negative potential (minimum) is more variable but is usually left anterior or posterior and inferior to the maximum. In the 19 patients with severe valvular AS going to surgery all had initial QRS to the left, with 17 anterior and two posterior on the Frank system VCG (figs. 2a, 3a). In all cases, in the BSPM, the initial maximum was well to the left, near the left axillary line, with two posterior to that line. The early minima were more variable but invariably the overall early negative potentials were to the right of the overall early peak positive potentials. The following BSPM's early in the QRS from two patients clearly demonstrate the data (figs. 3a, 3b).

We can therefore state that the BSPM's are giving evidence for an hypothesis that the initial QRS is to the left in severe valvular AS because the posterior free wall (known to become very hypertrophed in severe aortic stenosis) is now causing a much stronger left posterior vector than in the normal, resulting in the initial QRS being to the left and anterior, (fig. 4) and infrequently even posterior. Obviously since there is no strong hypothesis and certainly no theory as to why a greater cardiac muscle mass causes more voltage on the chest wall, there can only be an hypothesis in this situation as well. However, it stands to reason that the potentials from the very hypertrophed free posterior wall in congenital valvular AS are contributing to the observation. Whether it is doing so by changing the initial QRS vector, by virtue of greater magnitude from the posterior free wall, or by modifying the activation sequence, or other parameter, is not known at this time[19].

Figure 1 **Vector of Initial Activation**

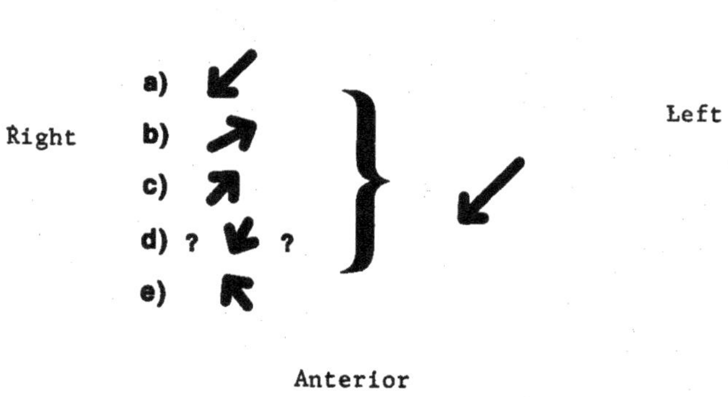

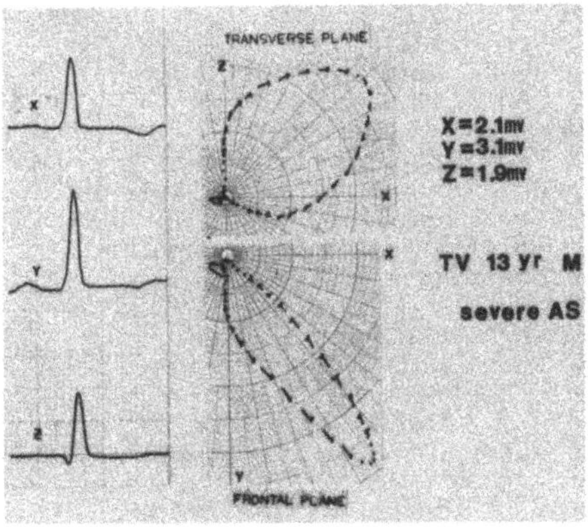

Figure 2a

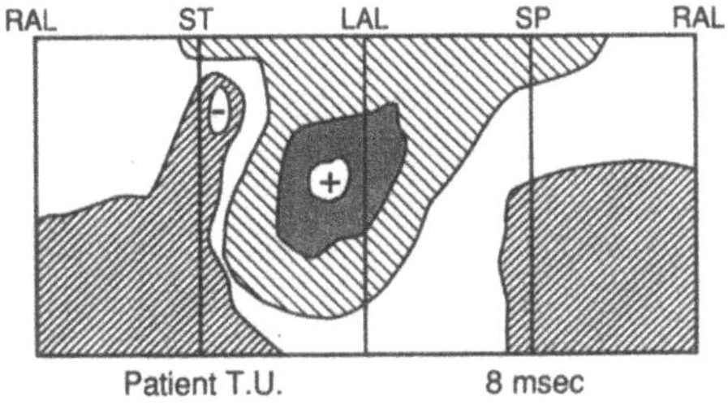

Figure 2b

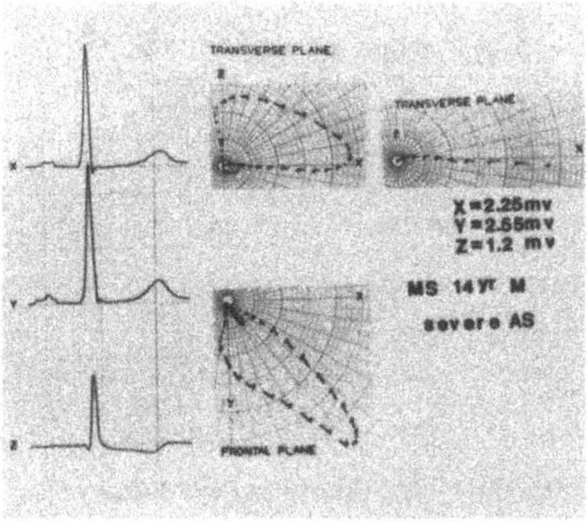

Figure 3a

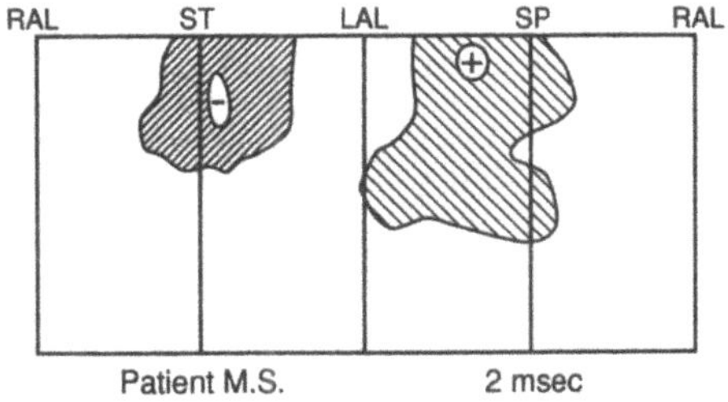

Figure 3b

Figure 4

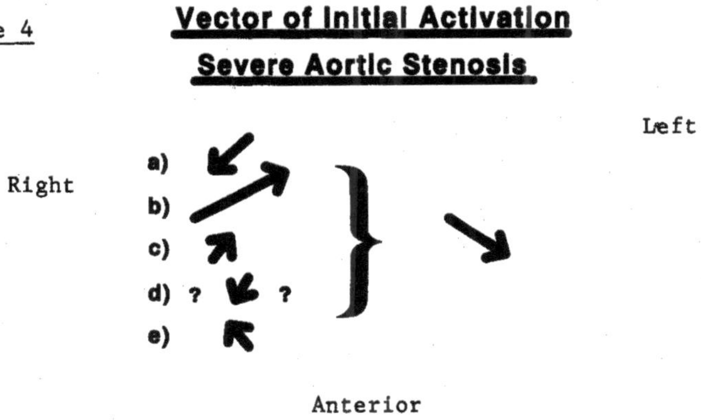

1. Liebman, J., Miller, B.L., Gessner, I.H. The initial QRS vector in children. Vectorcardiograpy 2. Proc. 11th International Symposium on Vectorcardiography. Ed. I. Hoffman, publ. J.B. Lippincott, Philadelphia, 1971, p. 645-648.
2. Mehran-Pour, M., Whitney, A., Liebman, J., Borkat, G. Quantification of the Frank and McFee-Parungao orthogonal electrocardiogram in valvular pulmonic stenosis. Correlations with hemodynamic measurement. J. Electrocardiol. 1979, 12: 69-76.
3. Liebman, J. Electrocardiography in Congenital Heart Disease, Chapter 19 in Comprehensive Electrocardiology (Vol. I), Ed. Macfarlane and Laurie, Pergamon Press, NY 1989 p. 729-798.
4. Liebman, J., Plonsey, R. The initial QRS in ventricular hypertrophy. Proceedings 89th International Congress on Electrocardiology, June 7-11, 1982, Tokyo, p. 315.
5. Liebman, J., Plonsey, R., Ankeney, J.L. The initial QRS in Ventricular Hypertrophy. Japanese Heart J. Vol. 23, (Suppl.) Dec. 1982 p. 480-482.
6. Ankeney, J.L., Tzeng, T.S., Liebman, J. Surgical therapy for congenital aortic valvular stenosis. J. Thoracic and Cardiovasc. Surg. 1983, 85: 41-48.
7. Durrer, D., vanDam, R.Th., Freud, G.E., Janse, M.J., Meijler, F.L. Arzbaecher, R.C. Total excitation of the isolated human heart. Circulation 1970, 41: 899-912.
8. Scher, A.M., Spach, M.S. Cardiac Depolarization and Repolarization and the Electrocardiogram. In Berne, R.M., Sperelakis, N. Geyer, S.R. (Eds): Handbook of Physiology: Circulation, Section 2: The Cardiovascular System. Vol. 1: The Heart. Bethesda, MD, American Physiological Society, 1979, Ch 9.
9. Liebman, J. Anatomy of the Cardiac Conduction System. Chapter 2 in Pediatric Electrocardiography, Ed. Liebman, Plonsey, Gillette. publ. Williams and Wilkins, Baltimore 1989, p. 15-22.
10. Plonsey, R. Activation of the Heart. Chapter 3 in Pediatric Electrocardiography, Ed. Liebman, Plonsey, Gillette, publ. Williams and Wilkins, Baltimore, 1982, p. 23-28.
11. Ruttkay-Nedecky, I. Features of Ventricular Septal Activation in The Cardiac Electric Field, in Electrocardiology '87. Proc. 14th International Congress on Electrocardiology. Berlin. August 17-20, 1987, p. 51-54.
12. Beattie, J.M., Gaffney, F.A., Blomqvist, Transcavitary Conduction and the Mean frontal QRS axis. Electrocardiology '87. Proc. 14th International Congress on Electrocardiology. Berlin. August 17-20, 1987, p. 71-74.
13. VanDam, R. Th. and Janse, M.J. Activation of the Heart. Chapter 4 in Comprehensive Electrocardiology, (Vol. I) Ed. Macfarlane and Laurie publ. Pergamon Press, New York 1989, p. 101-127.
14. Demoulin, J.C., Kulbertus, H.E. Pathological findings in patients with left anterior hemiblock. In Hoffman I and Hamby RI (eds) Vectorcardiography 3. Amsterdam, N. Holland, 1975, 123-127.
15. Kulbertus, H.E. Advances in the understanding of conduction disturbances. Eur. J. Cardiol. 1978, 8: 271-280.
16. Lev, M. Personal Communication
17. Myerberg, R.J., Nilsson, K., Gelband, H. Physiology of the Canine Intraventricular conduction and endocardial excitation. Circ. Res. 1972, 30: 217-243.
18. Liebman, J., Thomas, C.W., Rudy, Y., Plonsey, R. Electrocardiographic body surface potential maps of the QRS of normal children. J. Electrocardiol. 1981, 14: 249-260.
19. Rudy, Y., Plonsey, R., Liebman, J. The effects of variations in conductivity and geometrical parameters in the electrocardiogram, utilizing an eccentric spheres model. Circ. Res. 1979, 44: 104-111.

BODY SURFACE POTENTIAL MAPPING IN PATIENTS WITH ARRHYTHMOGENIC RIGHT VENTRICULAR DISEASE

LUIGI DE AMBROGGI, MARIA S. NEGRONI, CARLO SANTAMBROGIO, MARINA ROVIDA.

Centro E.Malan, Division of Cardiology, San Donato Hospital, University of Milan, 20097 San Donato Milanese, Italy.

ABSTRACT

Maps of the istantaneous potential distributions throughout the QRS and of the integral values of QRST interval were obtained by recording 117 chest leads from 9 patients aged 37±12 years with a mild form of arrhythmogenic right ventricular disease (ARVD) and ventricular arrhythmias. Data were compared with those previously obtained in a control healthy population.

The istantaneous potential maps during QRS exhibited only minor abnormalities, i.e.: 3 pts, in whom magnetic resonance imaging revealed lipomatous infiltration of the right ventricular outflow tract, presented a prominent potential maximum on the upper sternal region during the last 30 msec of the QRS. In 2 patients the QRST integral maps showed a larger than normal negative area on the anterior chest; in 1 of these cases 2 minima were also present in the QRST map. To detect minor disparities of ventricular recovery, ST-T waveforms were analyzed in each patient. By applying principal component analysis, a "similarity index" (SI) was computed: a low value of SI indicates a large variety of ST-T waves, likely to reflect the disparity of ventricular repolarization. The mean value of SI was significantly lower in pts with ARVD than in controls (60±10% vs 77±8%, $p<0.001$); a value <69% (1 SD below the mean for controls) was found in 7 of 9 patients.

These preliminary results show that even in mild forms of ARVD, BSM can reveal abnormalities related to the anatomical substrate and to the susceptibility to ventricular arrhythmias.

The identification of electrical markers of susceptibility to ventricular arrhythmias is an important, but still unsolved problem (1).

In the present study we have considered a condition which is highly arrhythmogenic, that is right ventricular dysplasia (2).

The aim of our study was to analyze body surface potential maps (BSPM) in patients with arrhythmogenic right ventricular dysplasia (ARVD) and to identify possible markers of electrical disparities of the ventricular repolarization.

Study population

BSPM were recorded from 9 patients, 5 males and 4 females, aged 37±12, affected by ARVD, who came to our observation for episodes of sustained ventricular tachycardia (2 pts), nonsustained ventricular tachycardia (6 pts) or frequent premature ventricular beats (1 pt). The diagnosis of ARVD was based mainly on echocardiographic and cardiac magnetic resonance findings. The QRS complexes of the ectopic ventricular beats showed a LBBB pattern. No patient had symptoms or signs of right ventricular failure.

Thirty healthy subjects, 15 males and 15 females, aged 26±7, were also studied as controls.

Methods

117 ECG leads were recorded from the anterior and posterior chest and converted in a digital format with a sample rate of 500 Hz per channel. The data were then processed on a IBM-AT computer.

For each subject the potential distribution every 2 msec during the QRS was examined; moreover the QRST integral map and the "similarity index" were calculated.

The QRST integral maps were obtained by calculating at each lead point the algebric sum of all instantaneous potentials multiplied by the sampling interval (2 msec). The values were transferred to a diagram representing the thoracic surface; then isointegral contour lines were drawn.

The procedure for obtaining the similarity index has been described in previous paper (3). Briefly, in each subject the morphology of the all ST-T waveforms was analyzed. The ST-T wave was divided into successive 20 msec intervals and the mean potential value of each interval was considered. To eliminate the influence of the baseline drift we subtracted the value of the preceding interval from the mean potential value of each interval. Thus, each ST-T wave is represented by a discrete series of 15-20 values. In each subject we performed a principal component analysis (4) of the original 117 sets of values. This analysis allowed the identification of one set of values, corresponding to the first principal component, wich better represents, by mean of appropriate multiplication factors, the majority of the 117 sets of values recorded in that subject. Therefore, we define as "Similarity Index" the ratio between the information content of the first principal component and the total information of the original data. Actually, a high value of SI indicates a great similarity of all waveforms to one fundamental waveform, i.e. a great similarity of all the waveforms to each other. On the contrary, a low value of SI indicates a large variety of ST-T waves, and this is considered a marker of repolarization disparities.

Results

In the ARVD patients visual analysis of the instantaneous potential maps revealed no specific clearcut abnormal patterns. Right ventricular breakthrough occurred at normal time (18 to 48 msec after the onset of QRS). The highest values reached by the potential maximum and minimum were within normal limits. However, it is interesting to note that in 3 patients, in whom magnetic resonance imaging had shown lipomatous infiltration of the infundibulum, a prominent potential maximum was present during the last 30 msec of QRS on the superior sternal region. This finding, wich can be observed also in normal subjects, may suggest a delayed activation of the right ventricular outflow tract.

The mean value of SI was significantly lower in patients wich ARVD than in control subjects (60±10 vs 77±8; $p<0.001$). Considering as cut-off level a value of 69%, that corresponds to the mean value for the control group minus 1 SD, we found that 7 out of 9 patients (78%) had a lower value, whereas only 3 out of 30 controls had a value below this threshold.

As concerns QRST integral maps, in 7 out of 9 patients the distribution of the integral values was within normal limits. In 5 of these patients SI was abnormally low. In 2 patients QRST integral maps showed a larger than normal area of negativity on the anterior thorax. In these two cases SI was lower than normal. In one of these cases the distribution was more complex (Fig. 1): 2 minima were present and the maximum was located more superiorly than normal. This "multipolar" pattern could be considered an expression of repolarization disparities. In this patient the the 12-lead ECG was within normal limits, but the similarity index was definitely low (47%).

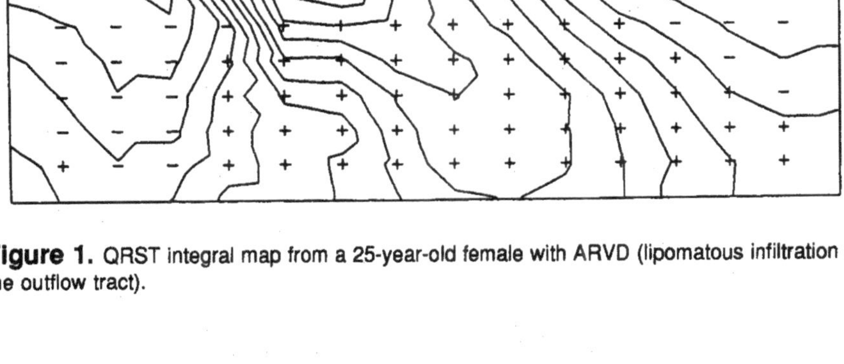

Figure 1. QRST integral map from a 25-year-old female with ARVD (lipomatous infiltration of the outflow tract).

Conclusion

The present study demonstrated that body surface potential maps can reveal, even in mild forms of ARVD, abnormalities related to the anatomical substrate and to susceptibility to ventricular arrhythmias. In particular, the low values of similarity index found in patients with ARVD suggest a greater than normal dispersion of the ventricular recovery times. This condition may enhance the vulnerability to ventricular arrhythmias by favoring the reentry phenomena.

References

1. Abildskov JA, Lux RL: *Distribution of QRST deflection areas in relation to repolarization and arrhythmias.* J Electrocardiol **24**: (1991), 197

2. Marcus FI, Fontaine GH, Guirodon G et al: *Right ventricular dysplasia: a report of 24 adult cases.* Circulation **65**: (1982), 384

3. De Ambroggi L, Negroni MS, Monza E, Bertoni T, Schwartz PJ: *Dispersion of ventricular repolarization in the long QT syndrome.* Am J Cardiol **68** (1991), 614

4. Kleinbaum DG, Kupper LL: *Applied Regression Analysis and Other Multivariable Methods.* (Boston, Duxbury Press, 1978) p. 376

DISTRIBUTION OF QRS SHAPE CORRELATION IN SURFACE POTENTIAL DISTRIBUTION

DRŠKA Z.
Institute of Physiological Regulations of Czechoslovak Academy of Sciences, FN Bulovka, pav.11, 180 85 Prague 8, Czech and Slovak Federal Republic (CSFR)

and

VALOVÁ D., MÁLKOVÁ A., POLÁNKOVÁ M.
Institute of Physiological Regulations of Czechoslovak Academy of Sciences, FN Bulovka, pav.11, 180 85 Prague 8, Czech and Slovak Federal Republic (CSFR)

ABSTRACT

Existence of lines of isomorph ECGs as lines perpendicular to the QRS loop mean plane was demonstrated earlier.In this study we verified the existence of these lines as lines of high value of correlation coefficient, which create smooth continuous line passing over the all chest surface. Correlation values within these lines change their polarity in two (mirror) points, which are also points of intersection of all other lines of high value of correlation coefficient (corresponding to different reference points). The existence of couples of lines, i.e. the line of high value correlation coefficient and the zero value one, and their common intersection in mentioned surface points were demonstrated. Structure of BSPD time succession then corresponds to the family of lines of isomorph ECGs having a couple of (mirror) intersection points placement of which depends on the spatial orientation of QRS (resp. T) loop mean plane.

1. Introduction

From the generally accepted knowledge o BSPD follows the presumption that distribution of surface ECGs shape, expressed as correlation coefficient, exhibits relatively simple structure: values of correlation coefficient within given reference surface ECG and all other surface ECGs are in all directions decreased passing through the zero level to the limit value -1. On the spherical surface the isolines of correl. coef. are to be creating the concentric circular (paralelle) lines.

On the basis of paper of Laufberger[1] and our previous papers[2,3] we realized this study of correlation coefficients distribution structure within the matrix of surface ECGs.

2. Material and Methods

In a group of patients matrix of 5 x 16 surface ECGs was measured by means of multichannel system for BSPD mapping (CARDIG 128.1 developed and made by ZPA Čakovice - ČSFR).

From the matrix of surface ECGs obtained this way the matrix of correlation coefficient was calculated for QRS interval using the individual reference ECG. In this study ECGs from 4th electrodes level were choosen, i.e. ECGs from 15 cm distance caudally from the jugulum.

Data from a group of ramdomly coming patients almost of them exhibiting old myocardial infarction, some of them have prolongation of intraventricular conduction. Any subject with complet RBBB or LBBB was observed in this group.

For methodological reasons, line of maximum values of correlation coefficient were detected as zero values line in reciprocal situation after the determination of maximum value of coefficient at mentioned level of electrodes.

3. Results and Discussion

It was proved that isolines of local maximum values of correlation coefficient within the matrix of surface ECGs have not the concentric character. On the contrary these isolines create continuous ranges. The top edge of them create continuous lines (Rmax) of high level of correlation coefficient.

Moreover, it was found that leads points QRS complexes of which are uncorrelated with choosen reference ECG create analogous continuous lines (Rmin).

Couples of these lines (lines Rmax and Rmin) exhibite two crosspoints, the second, oposite one, having character of mirror point (Fig. 1). Whether these both points are situated in the studied surface is depending on the spatial orientation of electrical field of the heart (EFH).

As it was just mentioned values of correlation coef. are resting on high level within the isolines course. Only in close neighbourhood of point of intersection these values rapidly decrease through the zero level to the high negative values (with the limit value equal to -1). On this high negative level the values of correl. coef. rest up to neighbourhood of the second point of intersection with the line Rmin.

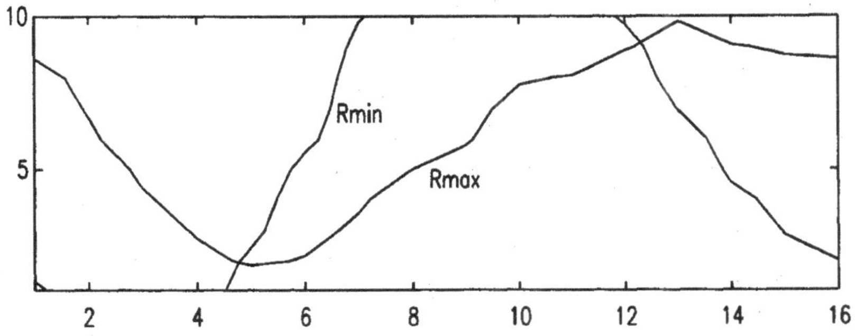

Fig. 1: Couple of lines of local maximum of absolute values of correl. coef. (Rmax) and local minimum absolute values of correl. coef. (Rmin). Orientation of displayed distribution corresponds to the standard orientation of surface maps: lateral margins of unrolled part of the chest surface corresponds to the right medial axillar line.

By repetitional changement of reference point (i.e. the point to which ECG the correlation coef. are calculated) is possible to reach the set of lines Rmax and Rmin (Fig. 2).

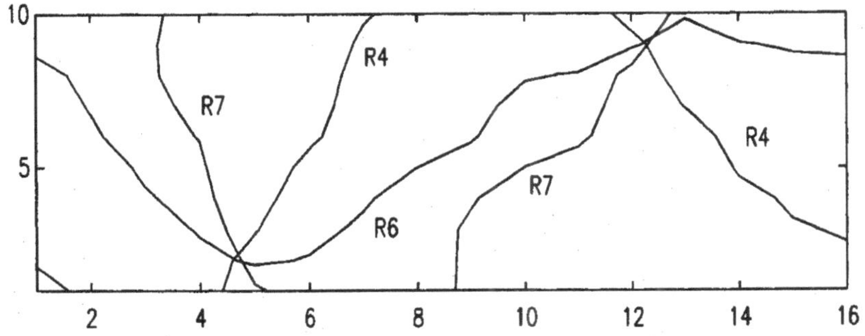

Fig. 2: Family of lines Rmax created by repetitive changement of reference lead point (i.e. reference ECG). In this case both points of intersection are situated within the studied part of the chest surface. Attached numbers represent serial numbers of line determination.

Analogous family of lines is created by lines of zero correlation having the common points of intersection.

By means of this set of lines can be demonstrated that these lines (i.e. Rmax and Rmin) exhibite the common point of intersection and its opposite mirror image point.

Expressing the spatial orientation of EFH by means of polar coordinates, orientation of correlation coef. isolines on the surface depends on the spatial orientation of mean plane of QRS loop (or T loop).

Because of independence of correlation coef. values on the distances from the equivalent source of the field it is reasonable to expect the analogous structure of correlation for example on the spherical surface concentric to the equivalent source of the EFH.

Described results can be kept as a part of basic knowledge of structure of EFH. Contemporary, these findings can be utilized in interpretation of several situation for example in interpretation of non-standard electrocardiographic leads. Discussed findings are also important for interpretation of results of orthogonal expansion procedures.

4. References

1. V. Laufberger, in *Probleme der Raumlichem Vektorkardiographie.* (Verlag der Slowakischen Akademie der Wissenschaften, 1963) p. 15-27.
2. Z. Drška, in *Sources and Surface Representation of the Cardiac Electric Field*, ed. I. Ruttkay-Nedecký, (Sweets and Zeitlinger, Bratislava, SAV - Amsterdam, 1970) p.371.
3. Z. Drška, *Bratisl. lek. Listy*, 86, 6 (1986) p. 612-616.

HOW DOES THE BSPM HELP US IN UNDERSTANDING THE STANDARD ELECTROCARDIOGRAM

Jerome Liebman, M.D.

From the Departments of Pediatrics and Biomedical Engineering - Case Western University and Rainbow Babies and Children's Hospital - Cleveland, OH 44106

Abstract

A 180 electrode electrocardiographic body surface potential mapping system (BSPM) encased in various sized vests and utilizing no electrode paste has been developed. The display is color coded. In a series of projects involving patients with congenital heart disease, the standard ECG has been shown to have missing or inadequate information, clearly evident in the BSPM. In addition misunderstood standard ECG patterns have been clearly explained in the BSPM as well.

The standard 12 lead electrocardiogram (ECG) is the same today as that which was used by Wilson 50 years ago[1-2]. Of the 12 leads, six are limb leads of which only one, aVF, has been shown to be reliable[3-5]. Each chest lead is very complex, is projected on to the chest from the entire heart and the complex volume conductor[6] and is distorted by proximity. Furthermore, the few electrode sites utilized leave large areas of the chest unmeasured, and these areas often contain a critical amount of clinically important information[7].

We have utilized a 180 electrode body surface potential mapping apparatus developed at Case Western Reserve University's departments of Biomedical Engineering and Pediatrics. The acquisition system uses 180 Ag-AgCl passive electrodes with active cable. No electrode paste is necessary. The electrodes are enclosed in a semielastic soft plastic vest secured with velcro. A selection of vest sizes is used to accommodate variations in size and body habitus. Our most recently constructed vest has 135 electrodes anteriorly and 45 electrodes posteriorly. The potentials are displayed on a color video monitor with computer synthesized pseudocolor images in which each color represents a range of potentials[8-11].

In understanding the ECG one event obviously not available is clearly present in high quality multielectrode BSPM's and that is evidence for epicardial right ventricular breakthrough (RVBT)[12-14]. This was first demonstrated by Taccardi in a series of papers and summarized in 1976[15]. In direct epicardial mapping studies of the chimpanzee, correlated with the BSPM[16] and in computer simulations[17], the physiological basis was confirmed. In order for RVBT to be present it is necessary that there be normal excitation in the right ventricle utilizing the normal conduction system, one with endocardial to epicardial excitation. Therefore, in advanced right bundle branch block (RBBB), where activation of the right ventricle results from stimulation across the septum after normal left ventricular activation, there is no evidence for epicardial RVBT. In addition, once the right ventricle is activated it takes an average of 100 ms to complete activation, beginning laterally, extending to the right, then superior and anterior[21]. The very slow terminal rightward anterior superior activation as seen on the surface ECG is thus explained[22]. Advanced and partial RBBB are the only clinical situations where we have **reliably** recognized evidence for epicardial left ventricular breakthrough (LVBT)[23-24]. Analysis of the rsr' complex in the right chest leads (described by Wilson's group as indicating incomplete right bundle branch block) has now been clearly elucidated. The expression should obviously be discarded! The r' or R' in lead V_1 indicates only that the terminal right vector has crossed the projection of the V_1 lead vector. If the terminal vector is not very posterior, it may indicate normality, and if the terminal vector is abnormally far to the right, it may indicate right ventricular hypertrophy (RVH). Although true partial RBBB does indeed occur, it is a difficult diagnosis to be sure of, particularly its differentiation from RVH with terminal right conduction delay. Using BSPM[25], there is always evidence for epicardial RVBT in RVH with terminal right conduction delay as in atrial septal defect, but there is no evidence for RVBT in partial RBBB (post operative children where the moderator band has been partially transected). Obviously there is a spectrum in partial RBBB since there is some normal Purkinje system conduction. But in order to recognize RVBT on the surface ECG even with our highly detailed 180 electrode system, there evidently must be a considerable amount.

In various conduction abnormalities associated with congenital heart disease the BSPM has been very revealing[26]. It is believed that the characteristic ECG associated with endocardial cushion defects, ("the abnormally superior vector[27]") occurs because activation courses <u>down</u> the left posterior bundle, then <u>up</u> the left anterior bundle. In the BSPM, no matter how complex the anatomy, when there is an endocardial cushion defect, the initial maximum potential is always <u>inferior</u> to the initial minimum potential. After that, very soon, there is a sudden change so that the maximum is superior and the minimum is inferior. This characteristic early maximum inferior is consistent with the concept that the left anterior branch causes the initial activation <u>up</u> the septum. The BSPM in the hypoplastic right ventricle syndrome has shown that in all three types, with pulmonary atresia, or tricuspid atresia, with and without transposition, there is evidence for epicardial RVBT. With pulmonary atresia there is no evidence for conduction abnormality, but with tricuspid atresia there is the classical abnormally superior vector because the always present VSD is in the endocardial cushion position. With transposition, the VSD is anterior so that the abnormally superior vector is <u>not</u> present. Thus, the three types of hypoplastic right ventricle appear to be developmentally distinct. Less well understood is that in many patients with tricuspid atresia, the VCG demonstrates an initial QRS vector to the right and <u>posterior</u> before extending left suggesting left anterolateral myocardial infarction. Yet in the BSPM infarction can not definitely be recognized. In the standard ECG, LVH is present because of the hypoplastic right ventricle as well as increased left ventricular volume. However, on the BSPM the amount of LVH is remarkable with maximal positive potentials left often being above 11,000 μv.

Coarctation of the aorta is a lesion of great hemodynamic interest. Furthermore in patients many years after successful surgery the ECG has shown what has often been interpreted as RBBB. However in a series of 24 patients an average of 8.7 years after successful surgery, the BSPM showed definite RVH in 19 with neither RBBB no RVH in the other 5. In only one case was there mild pulmonary hypertension. It is hypothesized that the pathogenesis lies in the capability for hyperplasia in late fetal life and early infancy. The early stimulus to hypertrophy of a larger than normal number of cells may possibly lead to these cells always being electrocardiographically evident.

A QRS to the left (no Q in V_5) is usually abnormal, and is extremely useful in evaluation of various congenital cardiac lesions.

In this conference we have reported on the increased severity of aortic stenosis when initial QRS is to the left with indirect evidence from BSPM that the pathogenesis lies in hypertrophy of the posterior free wall of the left ventricle. Other lesions such as severe pulmonic stenosis, total anomalous pulmonary venous return hypoplastic left ventricle syndrome and ventricular inversion are in the process of being studied with BSPM. Also, elsewhere in the conference we reported on WPW syndrome, having previously demonstrated the BSPM's superiority over electrophysiologic study in precisely identifying the area of ventricular insertion of the accessory connection (the standard ECG being of little use). The BSPM can now accurately guide the electrophysiologists to successful and more rapid radiofrequency ablation.

1. Wilson, FN, Johnston, FD, Macleod, AG, Barker, PS. Electrocardiograms that represent the potential variations of a single electrode. Am. Heart J. 1934; 9:447-458.

2. Wislon, FN, Johnston, FD, Rosenbaum, FF. The precordial electrocardiogram. Am. Heart J. 1944; 27:19-85.

3. Buyer HC, van Milaan, JB. Heart-vector and leads, Part I Br. Heart J. 1946; 8:157-161, Part II Br. Heart J. 1947; 9:154-160, Part III (Geometrical Representation) Br. Heart J. 1948; 10:229-233.

4. Brody, DA, Atzbaecher, RC. A comparative analysis of several corrected vectorcardiographic leads. Circulation 1964; 29:533-545.

5. Plonsey, R. Electrocardiographic Lead Theory and Lead Systems - Chapter 4 in Pediatric Electrocardiography, ed. Liebman, Plonsey, Gillette, publ. Williams and Wilkins, 1982; p 29-39.

6. Rudy, Y, Plonsey, R, Liebman, J. The effects of variations in conductivity and geometrical parameters in the electrocardiogram, utilizing an eccentric spheres model. Circ. Res. 1979;44:104-111.

7. Kornreich, F, and Rautaharju, P. The missing waveform and diagnostic information in the standard 12 lead electrocardiogram. J. Electrocardiol. 1981; 14:341-350.

8. Kavuru, MS, Vesselle, H, Thomas, CW. Advances in body surface potential mapping (BSPM): Instrumentation Ch 15 In Liebman, J, Plonsey, R, Rudy, Y, (eds): Pediatric and Fundamental Electrocardiography. Martinus Nijhoff, The Netherlands, 1987, 315-327.

9. Huebner, W, Thomas, CW, Rudy, Y, Liebman, J. An improved pseudoeolar scale for the display of body surface potential maps. Proc. 13th International Congress on Electrocardiology. Washington, D.C. (1986) Sept. 10-12, p. 9.

10. Thomas, CW, Lee, D. Methodology in constructing body surface potential maps Chapter 16. In Liebman, J., Plonsey, R., Rudy, Y. (eds): Pediatric and Fundamental Electrocardiography. Martinus, Nijhoff. The Netherlands 1987, 329-345.

11. Lee, D, Thomas, CW, Rudy, Y, Liebman, J. A knowledge-based approach in generating body surface potential maps. Proc. 13th International Congress on Electrocardiography, Washington, D.C. (1986) Sept. 10-12, p. 17.

12. Liebman, J, Thomas, CW, Rudy, Y, Fraenkel, R. Electrocardiographic body surface potential maps of the QRS of normal children. J. Electrocardiol. 1981; 14:249-260.

13. Liebman, J, Thomas, CW, Salamone, R, Rudy, Y, Plonsey, R. Electrocardiographic body surface potential maps of the QRS and T of normal children. Qualitative description and selected quantitations chapter 19. In Liebman, J, Plonsey, R, Rudy, Y (eds): Pediatric and Fundamental Electrocardiography, Martinus Nijhoff, The Netherlands, 1987 381-388.

14. Widman, LE, Liebman, J, Thomas CW, Fraenkel, R, Rudy, Y. Electrocardiographic body surface potential maps of the QRS of normal young men. Qualitative description and selected quantifications. J. Electrocardiol. 1988; 21:121-136.

15. Taccardi, B, DeAmbroggi, L, Viganotti, C. Body Surface Mapping of Heart Potentials in Nelson, CV, Geselowitz, DB (eds): Theoretical Basis of Electrocardiography, Clerandon Press, Oxford, 1976, 436-466.

16. Spach, MS, Barr, RC, Lanning, CR et al. Origin of body surface QRS and T wave potentials from epicardial potential distributions in the intact chimpanzee. Circulation 1977; 55:268-278.

17. Miller, WT, Geselowitz, DB. Simulation studies of the electrocardiogram I. The normal heart. Circ. Res 1978; 43:301-

18. Myerburg, RJ, Nilsson, K, Gelband, H. Physiology of the canine intra-ventricular conduction and endocardial excitation. Circ. Res. 1972; 30:217-243.

19. Myerburg, RJ, Gelband, H, Nilsson, K. et al: The role of canine superficial ventricular muscle fibers in endocardial impulse distribution. Circ. Res. 1978; 42:27-

20. Nagao, K, Toyama, J, Kodema, I. et al Role of the conduction system in the endocardial excitation spread in the right ventricle. Am. J. Cardiol. 1981; 48:864-870.

21. Liebman, J, Rudy, Y, Diaz, PV, Thomas, CW, Plonsey, R. The spectrum of right bundle branch block as manifested in electrocardiographic body surface potential maps. J. Electrocardiol. 1984; 17:329-346.

22. Liebman, J. Interpretation of Conduction Abnormalities, Chapter 12, in, Liebman, Plonsey, Gillette (eds) Pediatric Electrocardiography, publ. Williams and Wilkins. Baltimore 1982; p 172-191.

23. Sugenoya, J, Sugiyama, S, Wada, M. et al: Body surface potential distribution following the production of right bundle branch block in dogs. Circulation 1977; 55:49-54.

24. Toyama, J, Tabato, O. Recognition of the epicardial breakthrough in body surface maps. Jpn Circ. J. 1981; 45:1172-

25. Liebman, J, Rudy, Y, Thomas, CW, Plonsey, R. RVH with terminal right conduction delay various partial right bundle branch block (utilizing body surface potential maps), in Pediatric and Fundamental Electrocardiography Ed Liebman, Plonsey, Rudy, publ. Martinus Nijhoff 1987; p 389-398.

26. Liebman, J, Thomas, CW, Rudy, Y. Body surface potential mapping in conduction abnormalities (with particular reference to congenital heart disease. Chapter 12, in Mirvis D (ed): Body Surface Potential Mapping publ. Martinus Nihjhoff 1988; p 153-166.

27. Liebman, J, Nadas, AS. An Abnormally Superior Vector (formerly called left axis deviation). Am. J. Cardiol. 1971; 27:577-580.

THE NON-DIPOLAR BODY SURFACE POTENTIAL MAPS IN RIGHT BUNDLE BRANCH BLOCKS

ZOLTáN ANTALóCZY and MIHáLY MEDVEGY

Postgraduate Medical University, 2nd Medical Clinic
Budapest, XIII. Szabolcs street 35.
P.O.Box: 112. H-1389, Hungary

Abstract

Non-dipolar body surface potential map based upon a new method representing the non-dipolar electric forces of the heart in each of the measured instants. This map is a resultant of the substraction of the calculated single moving dipole's potentials from the ptentials measured over the body surface. Body surface potentials were constructed using the 32 unipolar lead system, whereas for the determination of the dipolar parameters - the method of multipolar expansion introduced by *Geselowitz* was used. According to our current experiments the non-dipolar map may discover the minor electrical events hidden by the dipolar electrical forces. The non-dipolar map also contributes to the better understanding of the activation sequence of the right ventricle in the presence of right bundle branch block. The right-sided terminal depolarization maximum splits only rarely into two parts on the measured body surface potential maps /lateral and superior/ in contrast to the non-dipolar maps which are always showing these two maxima.

The single moving resultant dipole /magnitude, direction, location/ determination /using *Geselowitz's* multipolar expansion method (3), the 192 *Lux* leads derivated from the 32 measured potentials (6) and an IBM PC based forward program package (1)/ provides possibility to calculate a theoretic dipolar body surface potential map /middle map on the figures/. Comparison of this map to the measured real surface map /upper map on the figures/ results another theoretic maptype: the difference map /lower map on the figures/, which shows the non-dipolar content of the heart (7). The evaluation of this new electric examination method in the clinical practice is presented in right bundle branch block cases.

We analysed the characteristics of the non-dipolar maps in 8 RBBB cases in adults during depolarization according to the 4 *Liebman's* phases (4) /1-4 figures/, then we compared the position and extension of maximum-minimum areas to those that are seen on the "traditional" body surface potential map (5) - 16 cases.

Results

During the initial period of the depolarization /*Liebman's* 1st phase/ the non-dipolar maximum can be found in front, in the middle, a little below. However a separated positivity of less value appears also at the back side. The minimum area can be seen in front, in the middle, above /1st figure - upper map/. During this same period an extensive maximum is in the centre, but higher up in comparison to the non-dipolar map on the dipolar /middle map/ and the measured body surface potential map /lower map/, at the same time the negativity extends to the whole back. This initial potential distribution does not differ from the picture of normal cases not even from that of left bundle branch block.

Later maxima move to the left, downwards on all the three maps, and in the period of maximal left ventricular activation /2nd figure/ /a cursor shows the time on the leading V_3 lead/ all three types of maps are quite similar. Also a maximum of the frontal-upper right side often appears on the non-dipolar map already at this time /2nd figure - lower map/.

The third temporary phase takes the shortest time and this shows us the most varied picture. In some cases the already extant positivity of right frontal upper side further increases on the non-dipolar map, but in most cases the whole frontal part of the chest and left part of the back are occupied in middling height by a large positive area. Positivity of the left side gradually disappiers and the frontal one falls apart: positivity of the right side and that of upper one. During this same period the extensive maximum on the measured body surface potential map is divided into two parts. Dividing negativity may arrive from above - as in the upper map of the 3rd figure - or from below. /Also *Liebman* mentioned both possibility (5)./ Left part removes backwards, later on it disappears while the right part gets more and more forwards, to the middle and rightwards, later it gets a bit upwards and rightwards. This removal of the maximum takes a few /4-10/ msecs. At the same time the location of maximum-minimum is changing very rapidly /in 1-2 msecs/ on the dipolar maps, but at that time its amplitude value is very small, 0.1 - 0.2 mV altogether. This "turn over of time" corresponds exactly to the minimum point of spatial magnitude curve and this time the dipolar content is the less, too.

However varied the 3rd phase may be, all the more homogeneous is the following *Liebman's* 4th phase belonging to the right ventricular activation. This period takes the longest time. The maximum-minimum values first increase, at 60-70 msec after the QRS onset they reach their highest amplitude later they decrease. Pictures of different cases are very similar to one another, not even an associated left ventricular necrosis will change them. On the non-dipolar map 2 positive areas can be seen all the time: the one on the right side, the other in front-above, a bit to the left /4th figure, lower map/. On the measured body surface map the only

Figures

Three types of body surface potential map: upper the real measured, in the middle the calculated dipolar map, lower the difference of the two above mentioned maps: the non-dipolar map. On the V_3 ECG lead a cursor shows the time instants in Liebman's four phases, in right bundle branch block.

1. Initial or septal activation
2. Second, rapid phase during the left ventricular activation
3. Third, short phase - beginning of right ventricular activation
4. Fourth, slow phase - activation of the right ventricle

1

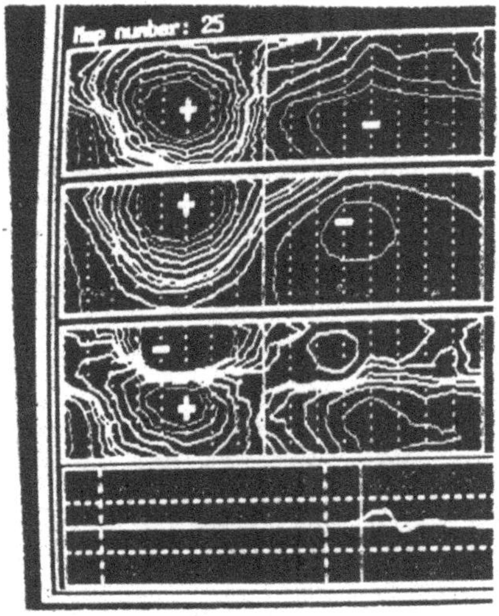

2

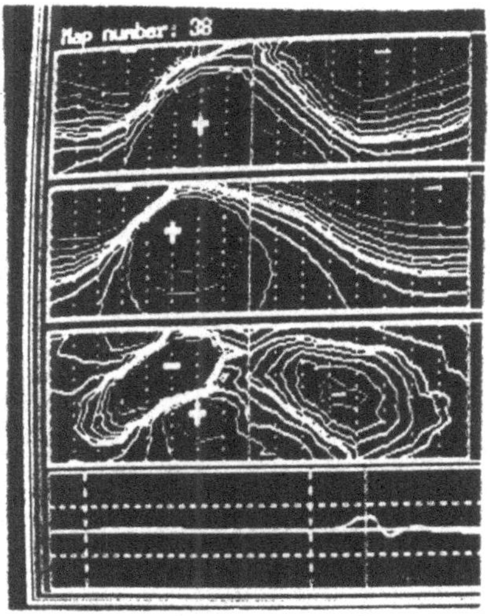

3

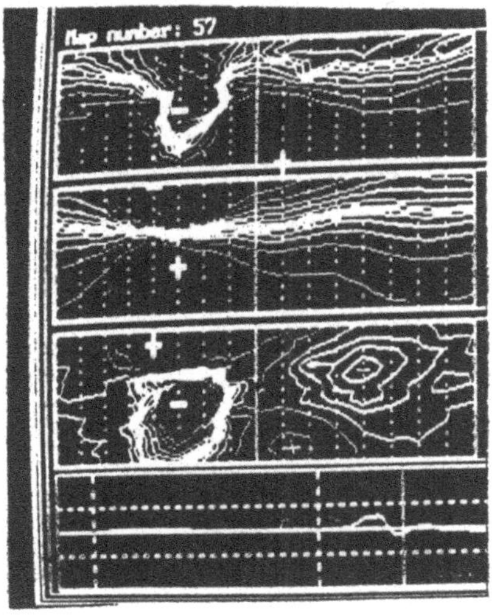

4

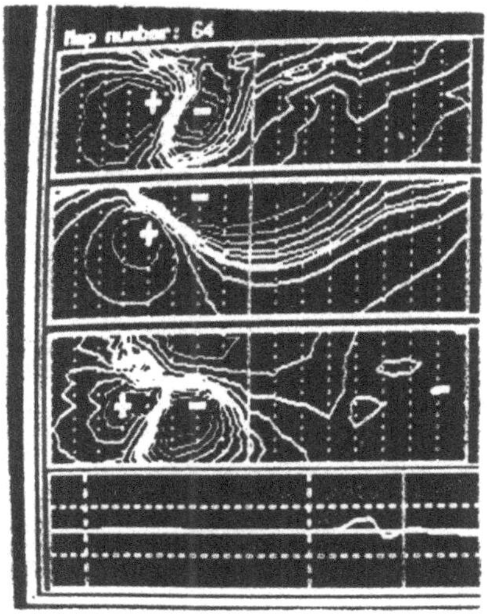

positivity fills the whole right side /4th figure, upper map/, as it is given by *Liebman*, too (5).

Discussion

There are consistent differences between the non-dipolar and the measured body surface potential maps in two phases: in the first and in the fourth. In the first phase the positivity of the non-dipolar map on the back may correspond to the posterior septal activation. The positivity in front-above next to the right sided one in the 4th phase can always be seen on the non-dipolar map, but only rarely on the measured body surface potential map (2,8). The anatomical bases of the two positivity may be the free wall of the right ventricle and the right outflow tract. The picture of the right outflow tract activation just the posterior septal activation in the first phase are usually covered by the dipolar forces on the measured body surface maps, but they are visible on the non-dipolar maps.

Studiing the non-dipolar maps helped us in better understanding above the activation in right bundle branch block as we presented it, but this method can be useful to study other ECG anomalies, too.

References

1. Cserjés,Zs, Doktori disszertáció, (Budapest 1990)
2. vanDam,R, in: *Conduction System of the Heart*, eds.: Wellens,H.J.J., Lie,K.I., Janse,M.J., (Stenfert Kroese, Leiden, 1976) pp: 377-384
3. Geselowitz,D.B., *Proc. IRE* **D48** (1960) pp: 75-98
4. Liebman,J., Rudy,Y., Diaz,P., Thomas,C.W., Plonsey,R., in: *Advances in Body Surface Potencial Mapping,* eds: Yamada,K., Musha,T., Harumi,K., (Univ. Nagoya Press, Nagoya 1983) pp: 217-225
5. Liebman,J., Rudy,Y., Diaz,P., Thomas,C.W., Plonsey,R., *J Electrocardiol.* **D17** (1984) pp: 329-346
6. Lux,R.L., Smith,C.R., Wyatt,R.F., Abildskov,J.A., *IEEE Trans.Biomed.Eng.* **D25** (1983) pp: 270-283
7. Medvegy,M., Antalóczy,Z., Cserjés,Zs., *Card.Hung.* (in print, 1992)
8. Wennemark,J.R., Blake,D.F., Kazdi,P., Lev,M.,*Circ.Res.* **D11** (1962) pp: 904-908

MAPPING OF ACTIVATION AND RECOVERY TIMES IN HUMAN HEART IN SITU

D'ALCHÉ P., MOREL M., GAUTHIER V.
Laboratory of Physiology, University of Caen
14000 Caen, France

and

KHAYAT A., ROSSI A., BABATASI G., KAPADIA N.
Department of Cardiovascular Surgery, University of Caen
14000 Caen, France

ABSTRACT

Peroperative epicardial mapping of activation, recovery and activation-recovery intervals in human heart have been performed in a group of 12 patients. These patients had a coronary disease but electrocardiograms with normal characteristics. For this mapping, 240 unipolar electrograms were simultaneously recorded with the system SATAPEC built in our Laboratory. The results confirm the classical data obtained on the dog heart. In particular, it was well established that the durations of activation corresponding to activation-recovery intervals are shorter at the base than at the apex of the posterior surface of heart. With SATAPEC it is very easy to obtain in a few minutes the epicardial mapping of the electrical activity during open heart surgery.

1. Introduction

The aim of this work is to make a mapping of epicardial electrical activity in human heart during cardiac surgery for several reasons :

- few results exist concerning activation, particularly recovery and activation-recovery intervals in human normal or pathological hearts in situ,
- previous results have been obtained from a number of electrograms inferior to one hundred generally not simultaneously recorded,
- some discrepancies exist between the results given by DURRER and col [1] in isolated human heart, WYNDHAM and col. [2] in human heart in situ or ABILDSKOV [3] in dog heart.

2. Material and Methods

It is obviously impossible to have patients without cardiac diseases but a homogeneous group of 12 patients having a coronary disease without previous myocardial infarction, ventricular hypertrophy or conduction defects has been chosen. All patients have electrocardiograms with normal characteristics without ST segment displacement and a duration of QRS complex inferior or equal to 0.1 s.

240 unipolar electrograms were simultaneously recorded with an epicardial mesh connected to the automatic mapping system SATAPEC built in our Laboratory [4]. The reference potential was taken at WILSON'S terminal.

Activation times, recovery times and activation-recovery intervals have been computed on the 240 electrograms in the following manner :

- local activation time corresponds to the time of the most negative derivative during the QRS complex,
- local recovery time corresponds to the time of the most positive derivative during the T wave,
- local activation-recovery intervals correspond to the difference between recovery and activation times.

After a necessary normalization of times due to the difference in cardiac frequency and display of tracings for control and if necessary corrections, the maps were visualized and a statistical analysis performed with a mapping of means, standard deviations (SD) and standard errors of the means (SE).

3. Results

3.1. Mean epicardial activation (Fig.1)

Total duration of activation is inferior to 40 ms. The activation starts near the apex of the right ventricle on the anterior surface with a small dispersion of values (about 5 ms) in this area. The activation ends at the base of the left ventricle, but an abnormal delay is observed at the base of the right ventricle due to an ischemic area observed in 9 patients, giving 20 ms of SD. Except in the anterior base area, SE does not exceed 5 ms.

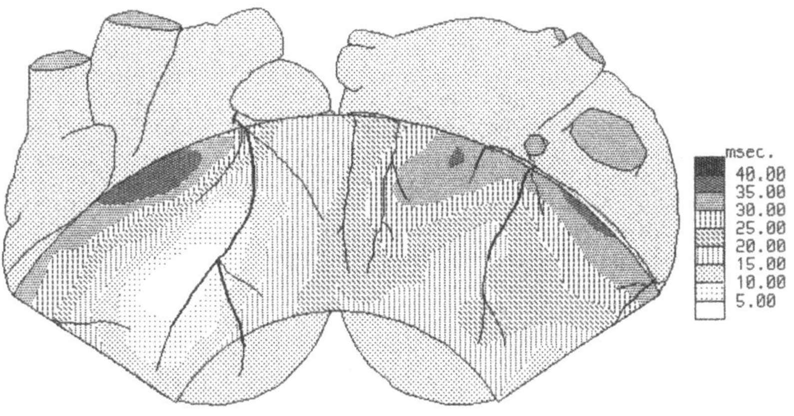

Fig.1. Map of mean epicardial activation

3.2. Mean epicardial recovery (Fig 2)

Total duration of recovery is about 50 ms. On the anterior cardiac surface, the shape of recovery map is similar to activation one. On the posterior cardiac surface, the first area of recovery is located at the base of the left ventricle and the latest area of recovery at the left ventricular apex. However this result observed in the mean map is mainly due to 2 patients. The other individual maps have a pattern quite similar to the activation one. These important variations of recovery give great values of SD (about 30 ms) and SE (inferior to 20 ms).

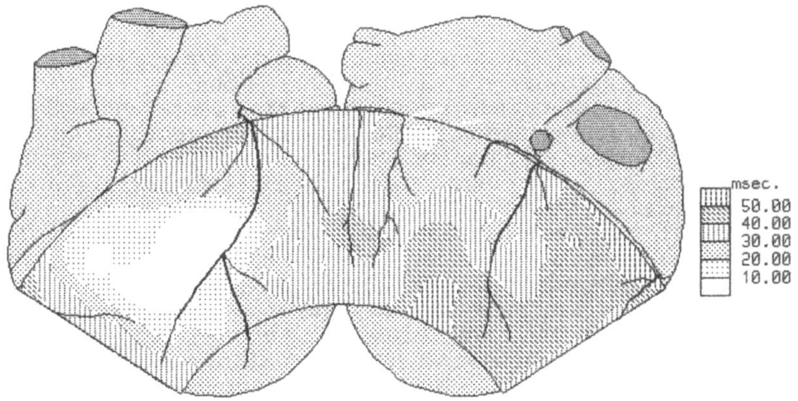

Fig.2. Map of mean epicardial recovery

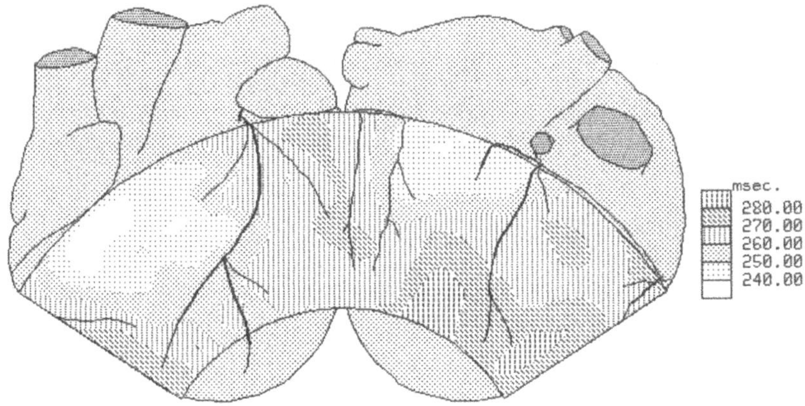

Fig.3. Map of mean epicardial activation-recovery intervals

3.3. Mean epicardial activation- recovery intervals (Fig.3)

This map gives the durations of activation at the epicardial surface which are included between 230 and 280 ms (that is to say a difference of 50 ms). The lowest durations are located at the anterior surface and at the base of posterior surface of the left ventricle. The highest durations are observed at the apex of the posterior surface. The values of SD are high (10 to 30 ms for a total duration of 50 ms), proof of dispersion of individual maps. The SE values, inferior to 10 ms at the posterior surface and 20 ms at the anterior surface, are regularly distributed.

4. Discussion

The values of activation and recovery times are in good concordance with those generally observed in identical conditions.

The propagation of activation from apex to base of epicardial surface shows a good homogeneous results in contrary to those obtained by WYNDHAM and col.[2] on human heart in situ in a group of patients with a similar pathology. For instance, 42 sites of epicardial breakthrough in 11 patients were noted by WYNDHAM and col., but they explored only 54 to 70 epicardial ventricular sites in each heart with a hand-held probe. The delay we have observed anteriorly in the conus region of 9 patients is probably due to the presence of an ischemic area.

Till now the sequence of ventricular recovery of excitability stems almost exclusively from measurements of dog heart.

The durations of activation are shorter at the base than at the apex. The latter finding corresponds to the results reported by ABILDSKOV[3] on dog heart. However a possible influence of coronary disease is not negligible.

5. Conclusion

The great facility of epicardial mapping during open heart surgery with our system SATAPEC makes feasible its use as a tool for a best evaluation of the cardiac ischemic zones, the areas of conduction delay or the location of periinfarctus zones causing ventricular arrhythmias.

6. References

1. D. Durrer, R. Van Dam, G. Freud, M. Janse,F. Meijler and R. Arzbaecher, *Circulation*, 41 (1970) 899.
2. C. Wyndham, M. Meeran, T. Smith, A. Saxena, R. Engelman, S. Levitsky and K. Rosen, *Circulation*, 59 (1979) 161.
3. J. A. Abildskov, *Circulation*, 52 (1975) 442
4. P. d'Alché, M.Morel and V.Gauthier, *Innov. Tech. Biol. Med.*,11 (1990) 183.

CORRELATION OF MEASURED AND SIMULATED EPICARDIAL ACTIVATION MAPS: AN APPLICATION OF A MULTIPOLAR HEART MODEL

ZS. CSERJES, GY. KOZMANN
Central Research Institute for Physics of Hungarian Academy of Sciences, Budapest, P.O.Box 49., 1525, Hungary

and

S. BARUFFI, S. SPAGGIARI, E. MACCHI
Department of Biology and Physiology of University of Parma, Viale delle Science, 43100 Parma, Italy

ABSTRACT

In this paper an inverse procedure is proposed based on the identification of a multipolar generator set to compute epicardial activation maps (EAM–s) from body surface potentials. EAM–s were calculated in infinite medium, because the conducting media surrounding the heart does not affect the EAM–s (L.S. Green at al.[1]). The simulated EAM–s preserve the main features of the measured ones, so, the typical events, as e.g. the major ventricular breakthroughs, can be detected, in spite of the rather low value ($\leq$0.852) of the correlation coefficient of the measured and simulated EAM–s.

1. Introduction

Multipolar expansion is a method for characterizing the potential field of the (real) cardiac electric generators with an infinite set of equivalent multipolar sources, located in the region of a suitably chosen coordinate system inside of the heart[2]. The field of equivalent multipolar sources is convergent everywhere outside of a sphere enclosing all the cardiac electric generators. In practical computations only the first few terms can be estimated. Because the convergency properties of such truncated multipolar expansions are not explored enough, in this study the field representation accuracy of truncated multipolar expansions is assessed with the aim of simulating EAM–s.

2. Method

The experimental data were collected in isolated dog heart experiments, performed at the University of Parma[3]. The dog heart was immersed in a cylindrical bath, and was perfused with blood drawn from the carotid artery of a donor dog. 12 comb–shaped electrode supports were placed in the bath. The potentials were recorded from the tank wall and from the near epicardial surface simultaneously. In the analysis 120 electrodes close to the heart surface supplied reference data on the epicardial signals, while 108 tank wall ECG–s were used for estimating the equivalent multipolar sources throughout the cardiac cycle in each 2 msec.

The following steps were performed for 6 dog data sets: The first task was to solve the forward problem for the tank wall geometry, for unit strength multipolar components placed in an origin inside the heart. Truncated multipolar expansion was carried out up to 4 terms, that is up to 24 (dipolar, quarupolar, octupolar and hexadecapolar) components. The origin of the multipolar expansion was placed in the approximate center of the heart[4].

The second step was to determine the equivalent 24 multipolar components of the measured tank wall potential distribution, in each time instant of the QRS complex. The computation of the equivalent multipolar components was carried out by the least–squares approximation method using singular value decomposition technique[5].

In the next step near epicardial potential distribution was computed assuming infinite and homogeneous conducting medium, in the time instants of the QRS interval. This calculation was performed in 16 cases for each dog. The calculation was carried out not only for the real epicardium, but for 3 heart–shaped surfaces too, 1, 2, and 3 cm from the heart surface (Figure 1).

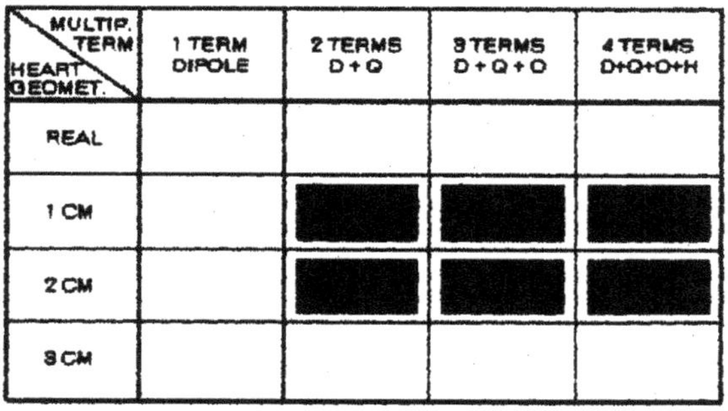

Figure 1. The 4×4=16 examined cases, and the 6 cases (black) after the investigation (see text).

Finally the simulation of epicardial activation maps was performed, in the 16 cases mentioned above, and the computation of epicardial activation map based on the measured near–epicardial potentials. The time of activation was defined as the instant of the most negative time derivative.

To characterize the quality of the simulation the correlation coefficients (CC–s) of the measured and calculated EAM–s were calculated in the 16 cases.

3. Results and Discussion

The best CC–s of calculated and measured epicardial activation maps can be seen in Figure 2 for the 6 dog data sets. In 4 cases we got the best CC 1 cm from the real epicardium (dog number 2, 3, 4, and 6), and in 2 cases 2 cm from it (dog number 1 and 5).

For the number of multipolar terms the result is the following: to get the best CC in 3 cases only 2 multipolar terms were required, in 2 cases 4 multipolar terms, and in 1 case 3 mult. terms were necessary. From these results it can be concluded that taking into account more and more terms does not increase necessarily the value of the CC.

As we have never got the best CC using only 1 multipolar term, and we have never got one on the real heart surface or 3 cm from the epicardium, we can state, that in further investigations we can leave 10 cases from the originally examined 16 variants (Figure 1).

A normalized noise parameter was calculated for each dog data set. We expected that the higher CC would belong to a lower noise parameter. This expectation is true in tendency but there isn't a one–to–one relationship between them.

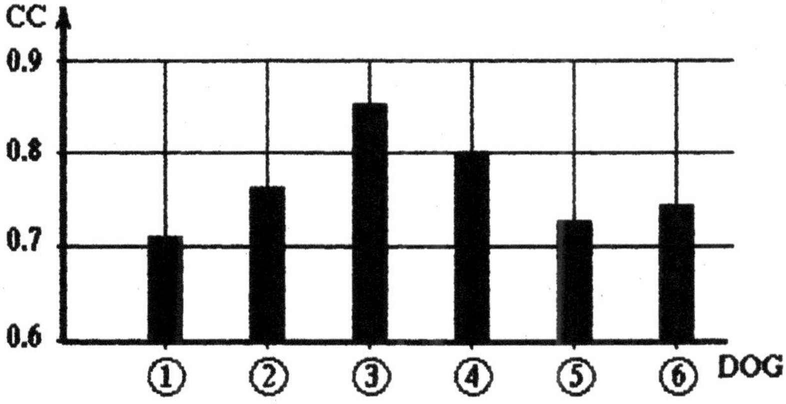

Figure 2. The best CC–s of measured and simulated EAM–s for the 6 dog data sets.

The best simulated epicardial activation map is shown in the Figure 3. The upper part of the figure shows the measured epicardial activation map, while the lower part the simulated one. The value of CC is 0.852. Comparing the measured and simulated EAM–s it can be concluded, that the main features of epicardial isochrone pattern could be detected, e.g. the ventricular breakthroughs, as it can be seen on the left isochrone maps (the most inner isochrone lines).

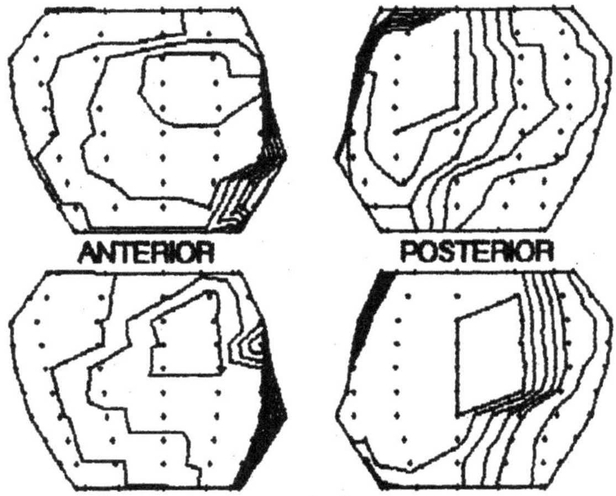

Figure 3. Measured (upper) and simulated (lower) EAM–s. This dog (No.3.) was paced in the right ventricle. The step between two isochrone lines is 7 msec. The value of CC is 0.852.

4. Acknowledgements

The authors should like to thank prof. L. Guerri, prof. P. Colli Franzone and Dr. C. Viganotti for valuable discussions on the topic.

5. References

1. L.S. Green, B. Taccardi, P.R. Ershler, R.L. Lux, *Circulation*, **84**, (1991) p. 2513.
2. B. Taccardi, E. Musso, L. De Ambroggi, in *The Electrical Field of the Heart*, Ed. P. Rijlant (Presses Academiques Europeennes, Bruxelles, 1972), p. 566.
3. D.B. Geselowitz, *The theoretical basis of electrocardiology*, Ed. C.V. Nelson, D.B. Geselowitz, (Clarendon Press, Oxford, 1976).
4. Zs. Cserjes, *PhD. Thesis*, Ch. 4, (Budapest, 1990).
5. T.F. Chan, *ACM TOMS*, **8**, (1982), p. 84.

Body Surface Potential Mapping Predicts Radiofrequency Catheter Ablation Site

Mark D. Carlson, M.D., M.A.
Department of Medicine
Case Western Reserve University
University Hospitals of Cleveland
2074 Abington Road
Cleveland, OH 44106 U.S.A.

Jerome Liebman, M.D.
Department of Pediatrics
Case Western Reserve University
Rainbow Babies & Children's Hospital
Cleveland, OH 44106 U.S.A.

Abstract

We determined the utility of the body surface potential map (BSPM) in 27 patients prior to radiofrequency catheter ablation of an atrioventricular accessory pathway. A surface 12 lead electrocardiogram and BSPM were performed in each patient prior to the procedure. The BSPM was performed during sinus rhythm using 180 dry Ag-AgCl transthoracic electrodes, and the accessory pathway site was determined by examining both positive and negative QRS complex potentials. Accessory pathway location was also determined by examining the polarity of the initial 40 ms of the delta wave on the 12 lead electrocardiogram. Accessory pathways were mapped during sinus rhythm and ablated with a large tip (4 mm) quadripolar electrode catheter with 2 mm interelectrode spacing. The 27 patients had 29 atrioventricular accessory pathways; 2 patients had 2 accessory pathways. The BSPM localized accessory pathways to within 1 Guiraudon grid site in each of the 27 patients. The 12 lead electrocardiogram localized the accessory pathway to within 1 Guiraudon grid site in 12 patients, missed the accessory pathway location by > 1 Guiraudon grid site in 13 patients and was indeterminate in 2 patients. Neither the BSPM nor the 12 lead electrocardiogram detected second accessory pathways that were present in 2 patients. The BSPM predicted the side of the heart from which 9 of the 10 posterior paraseptal accessory pathways could be ablated. The BSPM did not detect 1 left posterior paraseptal accessory pathway in a patient with 2 accessory pathways. The 12 lead electrocardiogram discriminated between right and left in 3 of 6 patients with right sided accessory pathways and none of the 4 patients with left sided accessory pathways. Thus, the BSPM predicted the ablation site more accurately than the 12 lead electrocardiogram. The BSPM was particularly useful in predicting the ablation site in patients with posterior paraseptal atrioventricular accessory pathways and thus may decrease the time required for radiofrequency ablation.

Introduction

We previously reported on the use of body surface potential mapping to predict atrioventricular accessory pathway site in patients undergoing surgical ablation[1]. We hypothesized that noninvasive tests that accurately localize atrioventricular accessory pathways would also facilitate radiofrequency catheter ablation of these pathways. Therefore, we determined the utility of the body surface potential map in 27 patients with the Wolff-Parkinson-White syndrome prior to radiofrequency catheter ablation of an atrioventricular accessory pathway.

Methods

A surface 12 lead electrocardiogram and body surface potential map were performed in each patient prior to the procedure. The body surface potential map was performed during sinus rhythm using 180 dry Ag-AgCl transthoracic electrodes. The ventricular insertion of the accessory pathway was determined by examining both positive and negative QRS complex potentials as described previously.[1] The maps were examined when the negative potentials of the delta wave reached negative 150 μV at a time when both the positive and negative potentials had reached a stable position (usually between 15 and 18 ms after the beginning of ventricular activation). Accessory pathway locations were classified according to the Guiraudon grid. Representative body surface potential maps and their corresponding site on the Guiraudon grid are shown in Figure 1.

Figure 1

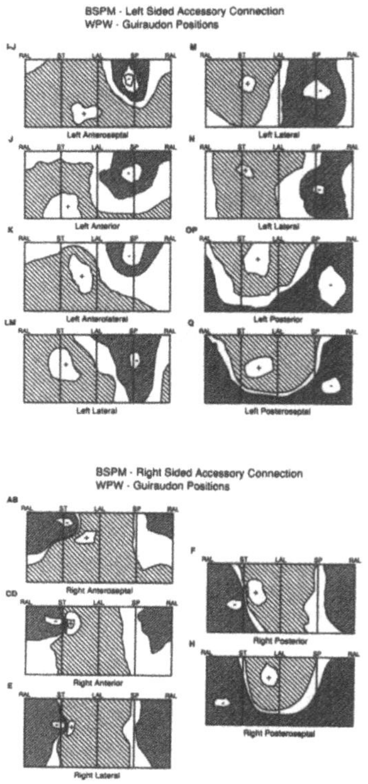

The 12 lead electrocardiogram was performed using standard techniques. Delta wave polarity during the initial 40 ms of the QRS complex was determined in each lead. Accessory pathway location was classified according to the Gallagher map and correlated with locations on the Guiraudon grid.

Catheter mapping of the accessory pathways was performed during sinus rhythm. Accessory pathways were mapped and ablated with a large tip (4 mm) quadripolar electrode catheter with 2 mm interelectrode spacing. Ablations were performed at the site of earliest ventricular activation. Right sided accessory pathways were ablated from above the tricuspid valve. Left sided accessory pathways were ablated from below the mitral valve. Accessory pathways were localized radiographically in the left anterior oblique position and assigned to the corresponding position on the Guiraudon grid.

Results

Twenty seven patients (19 males and 8 females) had 12 lead electrocardiograms and body surface potential maps performed prior to radiofrequency catheter ablation. The mean age of the patients was 37 ± 3 years. None of the patients were taking antiarrhythmic drugs at the time of the electrocardiogram, the body surface potential map, or the catheter ablation. The 27 patients had 29 atrioventricular accessory pathways; 2 patients had 2 accessory pathways.

The body surface potential map localized accessory pathways to within 1 Guiraudon grid site in each of the 27 patients. The 12 lead electrocardiogram localized the accessory pathway to within 1 Guiraudon grid site in 12 patients. The 12 lead electrocardiogram missed the accessory pathway location by > 1 Guiraudon grid site in 13 patients and was indeterminate due to minimal ventricular preexcitation in 2 patients. Neither the body surface potential map nor the 12 lead electrocardiogram detected second accessory pathways that were present in 2 patients.

There were 10 posterior paraseptal accessory pathways; 6 were ablated from the right side, 4 were ablated from the left side. The body surface potential map correctly localized and predicted the side of the heart from which 9 of the 10 could be ablated. Accessory pathways between sites P and H (6) could be ablated from the right; those to the left of site P (4) could only be ablated from the left side. Accessory pathways at site Q, although designated as left posterior paraseptal for surgical ablation, could be ablated using a catheter from the right side. The body surface potential map did not detect 1 left posterior paraseptal accessory pathway in a patient with 2 accessory pathways. The 12 lead electrocardiogram discriminated between right and left in 3 of 6 patients with right sided accessory pathways and none of the 4 patients with left sided accessory pathways. Thus, the body surface potential map was particularly useful in patients with paraseptal accessory pathways, allowing us to avoid inserting an arterial introducer and left ventricular catheter in 6 patients.

Conclusions

The body surface potential map predicted the radiofrequency catheter ablation site more accurately than the 12 lead electrocardiogram. Neither the body surface potential map nor the 12 lead electrocardiogram detected the presence of multiple atrioventricular accessory pathways. The body surface potential map was particularly useful in predicting the ablation site in patients with posterior paraseptal atrioventricular accessory pathways and thus may decrease the time required for radiofrequency ablation.

Reference

1. J. Liebman, J.A. Zeno, B. Olshansky, A.S. Geha, C.W. Thomas, Y. Rudy, R.W. Henthorn, M. Cohen and A.W. Waldo, *Circulation* **83** (1881) 886.

SURFACE CARDIOELECTRIC FIELD IN HYPERTENSIVE PATIENTS WITH MYOCARDIAL INFARCTION

SLAVOMÍRA FILIPOVÁ, STANISLAV CAGÁŇ
Department of Internal Medicine IV, School of Medicine, Comenius University
Bezručova 5, 815 26 Bratislava, Czechoslovakia

and

PETER KNEPPO, MILAN TYŠLER
Department of Biomeasurements, Institute of Measurement Science, Slovak Academy of Sciences
Dúbravská cesta 9, 842 19 Bratislava, Czechoslovakia

ABSTRACT

QRS integral maps (I-maps) have been useful in detecting depolarization abnormalities in patients with myocardial infarction. The aim of the study was to compare the signs of cardioelectric field in patients with anterior myocardial infarction (aMI) and left ventricular hypertrophy (LVH) and aMI patients without the hypertensive syndrome. I-maps were constructed and compared in control group (I), hypertensive persons (II), patients with aMI without LVH (III) and patients with aMI+LVH (IV). It is possible to differ the group III from IV according to maps QoJ (MAX, $p<0.05$) and I-maps QoRm (MIN, $p<0.01$, and SUM, $p< 0.01$). Our findings suggest that I-maps of QRS can manifest the characteristics of hypertrophic and non-hypertrophic myocardium despite of the aMI, masking the standard ECG and VCG criteria of LVH.

1. Introduction

The development of ischemic heart disease (IHD) exerts influence upon the ECG criteria of left ventricular hypertrophy (LVH) in the surface cardioelectric field (CEF). Myocardial infarction especially acts on the distribution and the intensity of CEF as the intensive factor. The purpose of the study was to compare the characteristic signs of CEF in anterior myocardial infarction (aMI) patients with/without LVH according to ECG surface mapping[1].

2. Study population and Methods

Patients comprised the following 4 groups: Group I (n=32) control subjects; group II (n=35) patients with arterial hypertension without IHD; group III (n=28) patients with aMI without LVH; group IV (n=30) hypertensive patients with LVH and aMI.

ECGs were recorded to construct surface integral (I) and isopotential (P) maps using the equipment CardioPC[2]. Unipolar ECGs were recorded simultaneously

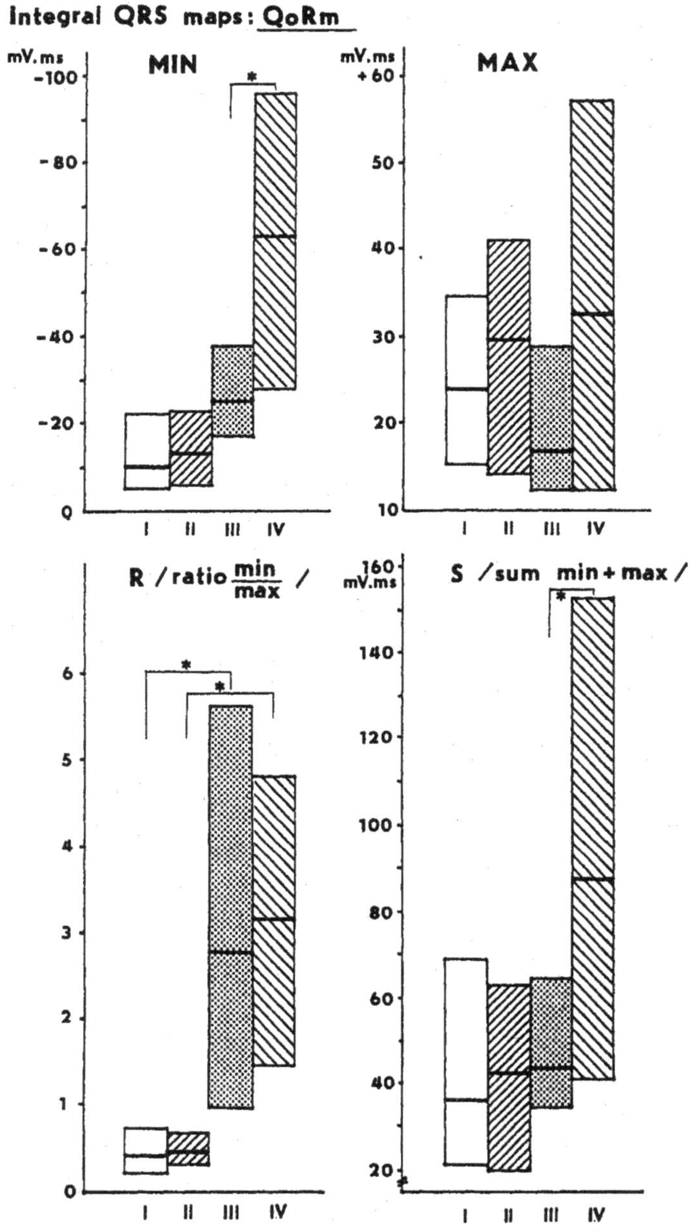

Fig.1. Integral QoRm maps: mean values and 95 percentile ranges of quantitative parameters for the groups I-IV.

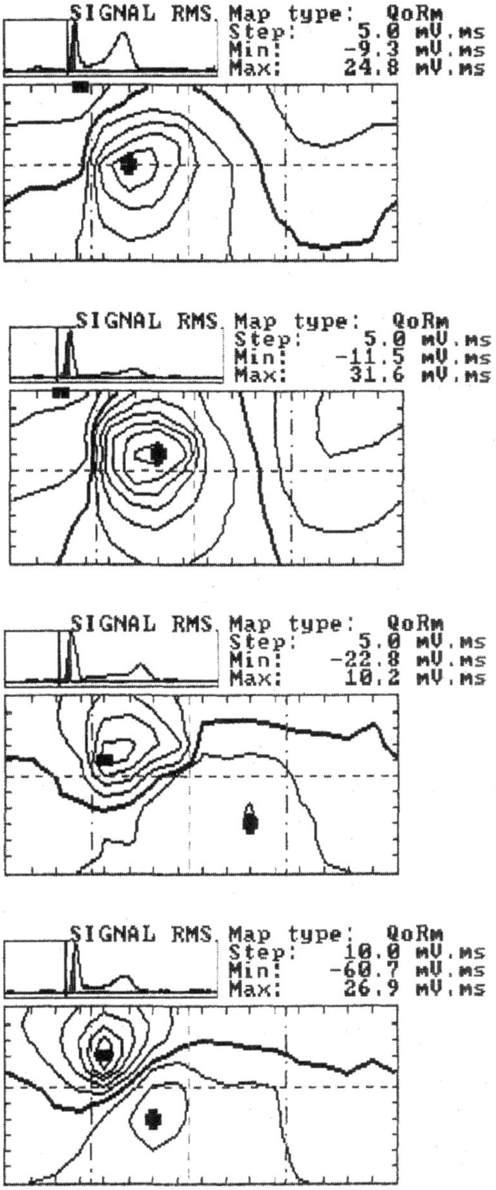

Group I

R: 0.375
S: 34.1 mV.ms

Group II

R: 0.364
S: 43.1 mV.ms

Group III

R: 2.235
S: 33.0 mV.ms

Group IV

R: 2.257
S: 87.6 mV.ms

Fig.2. Integral QoRm maps characteristic for the groups I-IV.

from 32-lead points on torso surface[3]. QRS integral maps (I-maps) were constructed in various intervals (QoJ: from QRS onset to J point; QoRm: from QRS onset to peak RMS; QoQ3: from QRS onset to 30 ms of QRS). Quantitative parameters of I-maps were calculated and compared (MIN; MAX; R = MIN/MAX; $S = |MIN| + |MAX|$). Also 12-lead ECG, VCG and echocardiography were performed in all subjects.

3. Results

The quantitative analysis of I-maps QoJ, QoRm, QoQ3 in all groups and statistical analysis (Student's t-test, values were expressed as mean and 95 percentiles) showed:

a) significant differences between the groups I-II and III-IV in I-maps QoJ (parameter R) and I-maps QoRm (parameter R, $p < 0.01$) [Fig.1];

b) significant differences between the group III and IV in I-maps QoJ (parameter MAX, $p < 0.05$) and in I-maps QoRm (parameter MIN, $p < 0.01$; parameter S, $p < 0.01$) [Fig.1].

In Fig.2 the characteristic I-maps QoRm in the groups I - IV are shown.

4. Conclusions

1. P-maps of QRS cannot differ significantly the LVH as the ischemic heart disease is present.

2. Results of the study indicate that analysis of I-maps, especially QoJ and QoRm maps, provide information about the presence/absence of LVH after the aMI. This fact is an important information in patients with aMI without the history of hypertension or LVH, as the LVH represents the significant risk factor of cardiac sudden death and changes the patient's prognosis significantly.

5. Acknowledgement

This work was supported in part by grant GA-SAV No. 319/91 from the Slovak Academy of Sciences.

6. References

1. F. Kornreich, T.J. Montague et al., *Am. J. Cardiol.* **63** (1989) 610.
2. M. Tyšler, V. Rosik, P. Krakovský, M. Turzová, *Cardiac Electrical Field, its Measurement, Modelling and Interpretation* (Symposium Stará Lesná, Czechoslovakia, 1990).
3. R.L. Lux, M.J.Burgess, R.F. Wyatt, A.K. Evans, G.M. Vincent, J.A. Abildskov, *Circulation* **59** (1979) 356.

BODY SURFACE MAPPING DURING VENTRICULAR REPOLARIZATION OF THE RAT AND GUINEA PIG

I.M. ROSHCHEVSKAYA
Institute of Physiology
of Ural Div. of Acad. Sci. of Russia,
Syktyvkar, Komi Republic, Russian federation

ABSTRACT

Comparative investigations of the cardioelectric field on the body surface of guinea pig and rat in the period of ventricles repolarization showed their differences resulted from cellular electrogenesis peculiarities.

The comparative studies of cardioelectric fields on the body surface of the rat and guinea pig during ventricular repolarization was conducted. Thise animals are applaid to the rodents, but have a great difference in the form of intracellular action potential in the pattern of ventricular action potential and ECG in the standart limb leads (1).

1. Materials and Methods

The cardioelectric fields on the body surface of 105 adult Wistar rats and 15 adult Guinea pigs in supine and abdominal position were studied. The animals were anaesthetized with the soduim solution of thiopentalum-natrium. Unipolar ECG were simultaneously recorded from 64 subcutaneos needle electrodes, distributed regularly around the body. The first ECG limb lead was used as control. The data were recorded with the multichannel computer system with the time discretization of 1 ms. The date were analized by a personal computer.

2. Results

On the equipotentional momentous maps (Fig. 1A) on the body surface of a guinea pig during the isopotential S-T interval on the ECG in the standart leads the stable positive and negative zones with the extrema with the low amplitude (0,1-0,15 mB) were formed. At the beginning of the T-wave the positive extremum displacement was similar to the same at the end of ventricular depolarization process. During the first part of the T-wave on the ECG in

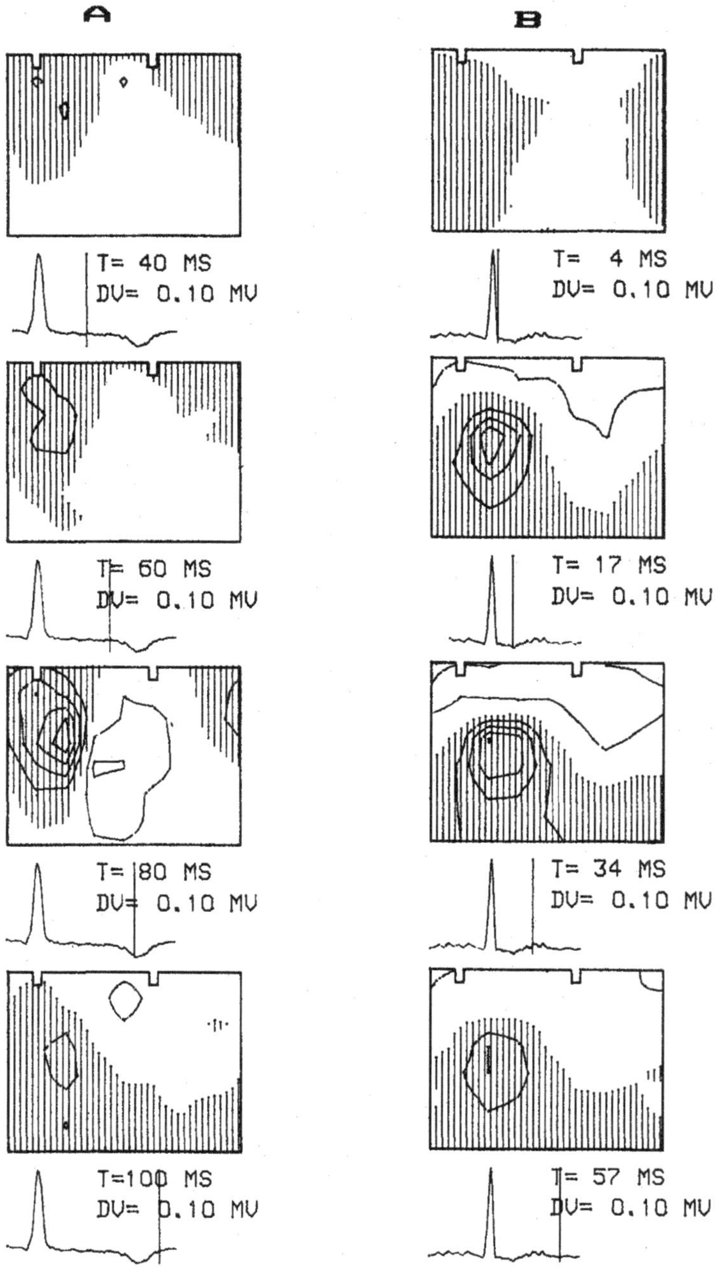

Fig. 1. Equipotential momentous maps on the body surface of rat (B) and guinea pig (A).

the standard leads the increase of amplitude of positive and negative extrema was noted. Displacement of extrema during this process is practically invariably. The 0-line, separates the zone of positive and negative potentials under ventricular repolarization shift at the left-lateral surface of the chest in the cranial direction, at the right-lateral surface of chest - in the caudal direction. The distance of the 0-line shifting in this period of time is greater, than the shifting of extrema. Change of the place of positive and negative zones in the beginning of the period of ventricular repolarization is vivid, than the displacement and shifting of extrema reflection of the development of process of ventricular repolarization . During repolarization the positive extremum reached 0,4-0,5 mV and negative -0,15-0,2 mV.

On the equipotentional momentous maps on the body surface of a guinea pig during T-wave the positive extremum is formed on the zone of the projection of the right ventricle of the heart on the ventral surface of chest. The negative extremum with the lower amplitude is located in the zone of the projection of the left ventricle of the heart on the ventral surface of heart.

The negative extremum shifted from the area of the right ventricle projection up to the left shoulder. The positive extremum shifted in the medial direction - from the area of the right ventricle projection to the sternum. The duration of the process of repolarization noted on equipotential momentous maps was from 40 to 50 msec. The duration of T-wave on the ECG in second standart limb leads was 25-30 ms.

The reflection of the process of ventricular repolarization on the body surface of guinea pig is influenced the position of an animal under the record of bioelectrical activity. If the guinea pig during the experiment is in the abdominal position,the equipotentional momentous maps notes the greater shift of the negative extremum on the ventral surface of the chest.

Since action potential of the rat ventricle cells has no plate, ECG in the standart leads doen't show isopotential S-T period. While studying cardioelectric field on equipotential momentous maps on the body surface of the rat it is possible to distinguish an extremely (1-2 ms) period, characterized by potentials with a low amplitude (less than 0,05 mV).

In the process of rat ventricular repolarization the positive extremum (Fig.1B) is located in the zone of right ventricle projection on the ventral surface of chest. In 6 ms after the R-wave peak in the control lead a positive extremum with the amplitude of 0,12-0,2 mV appears on the body surface approximately in the zone of a positive extremum formation at the beginning of ventricle depolarization. Positive extremum shifts in the cranio-medial direction. The location of the positive extremum at ventricles repolarization is similar to the one at their depolarization. The negative extremum is formed in the initial period of ventricular repolarization on the ventral-lateral surface of the chest in the area of the right shoulder, right clavicular in some animals it shifts to the right shoulder-blade.

Earlier we showed (2) the similarity of the process of ventricles depolarization of the hearts of a guinea pig and rat. Investigations of the electrical field on the body surface of guinea pig and rat in the period of ventricles repolarization showed their differences resulted from cellular electrogenesis peculiarities.

Our comparative investigation of the cardioelectric fields of rat and guinea pig , and another rodents on the body and heart ventricular surfaces, in the intramural and endocardial layers make it possible to use this animals as a model and in the pharmacology.

3. Acknowledgements

Authors expresses their gratitude to the firm MERCK SHARP & DOHME I. D. E. A. for the possibility to participate in the work of the XIX International Congress on Electrocardiology.

4. References

1. The rat electrocardiogram in pharmacology and toxicology, ed. R.Budden, D.K.Detweiler, G.Zbinden (Pergamon Press, Oxford, 1981)

2. I.M.Roshchevskya, in *Abstract book of the XVII International Congress on Electrocardiology* (O.I.C. Medical Press, 1990) p. 129

RELATIONSHIP BETWEEN CALCULATED AND EXPERIMENTAL CARDIOELECTRIC FIELDS ON EPICARDIAL AND BODY SURFACE IN RAT

I.M. ROSHCHEVSKAYA, N.V. YEVSTIFEEVA
Institute of Physiology
of Ural Div. of Acad. Sci. of Russia,
Syktyvkar, Komi Republic, Russian federation

ABSTRACT

The cardioelectric field during ventricular depolarization over the surface, close to the real torso of a Wistar rat was simulated on the base of the potentials measured from the heart ventricles epicardium of the same animal and compared directly with the corresponding experimental data. It was found that the torso surface potentials simulated from the real epicardial distribution were in good agreement with the experimental ones.

The agreement of real reflection of epicardial cardioelectrical potentials onto the body surface to the model connecting potentials on the heart ventricles epicardium and on the body surface was studied.

1. Materials and Methods

The cardioelectric field on the body and heart ventricles surface of 20 adult Wistar rats in supine position was studied. The animals were anaesthesized with the soduim of thiopentalum-natrium. Unipolar ECG were simultaneously recorded from 64 subcutaneos needle electrodes, distributed regularly around the body. After that the chest of the same animal was open and the cardioelectric potentials were simultaneously measured from 64 subepicardial electrodes. Time discretization was 1 ms. Cardioelectrical potentials from the surfaces of body and of the heart ventricles were synchronized according to ECG in the I limb lead.

The forward solution was obtained by means of the model which was used (1) to solve the inverse problem. This model connecting epicardial and body surface potentials on the base of geometry of torso and heart takes the form of an integral equation of the first kind in which the kernel is interpreted as a 'Green's function. The computing of the inverse solution using this equation requires a complete regularization procedure while the solving of the forward problem isn't attended by any mathematical difficulties.In the model heart surface was considered as a sphere mounted in an infinite homogeneous medium. The spatial location of all the epicardial and body surface lead points was accurately measured and included into the formulation.

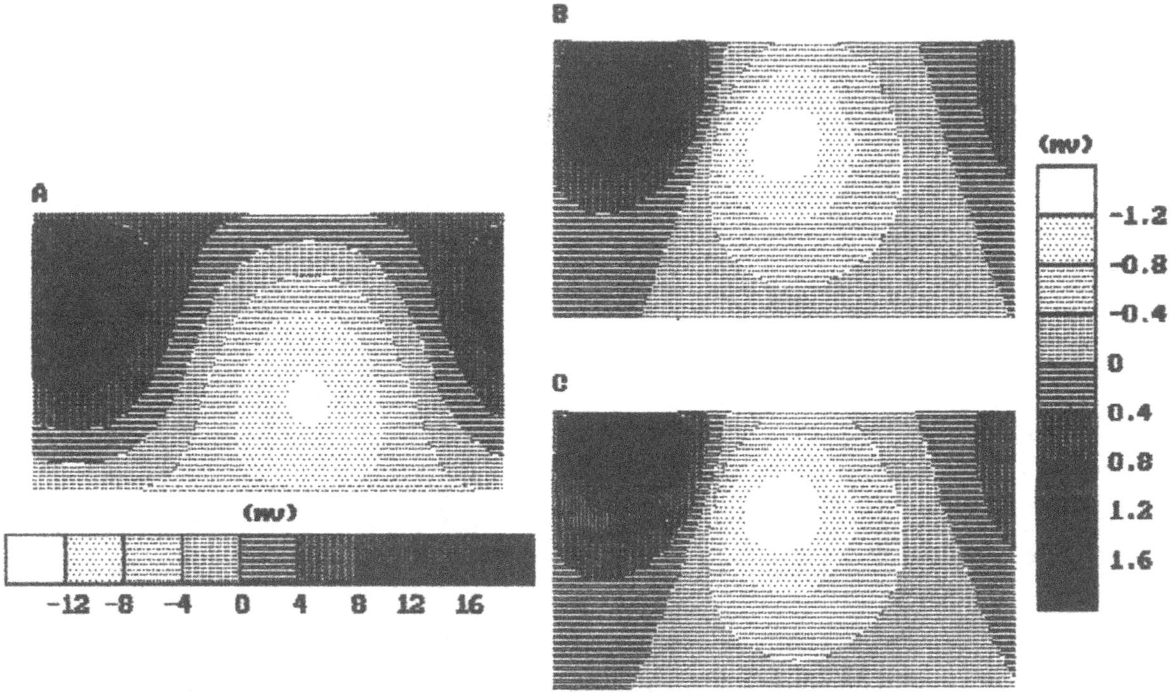

Fig. 1. The results of the model studies.
A – equipotential map over a sphere computed from a dipole; B – simulated potential map over the surface of a cylinder containing the sphere; C – analagous map computed analytically.

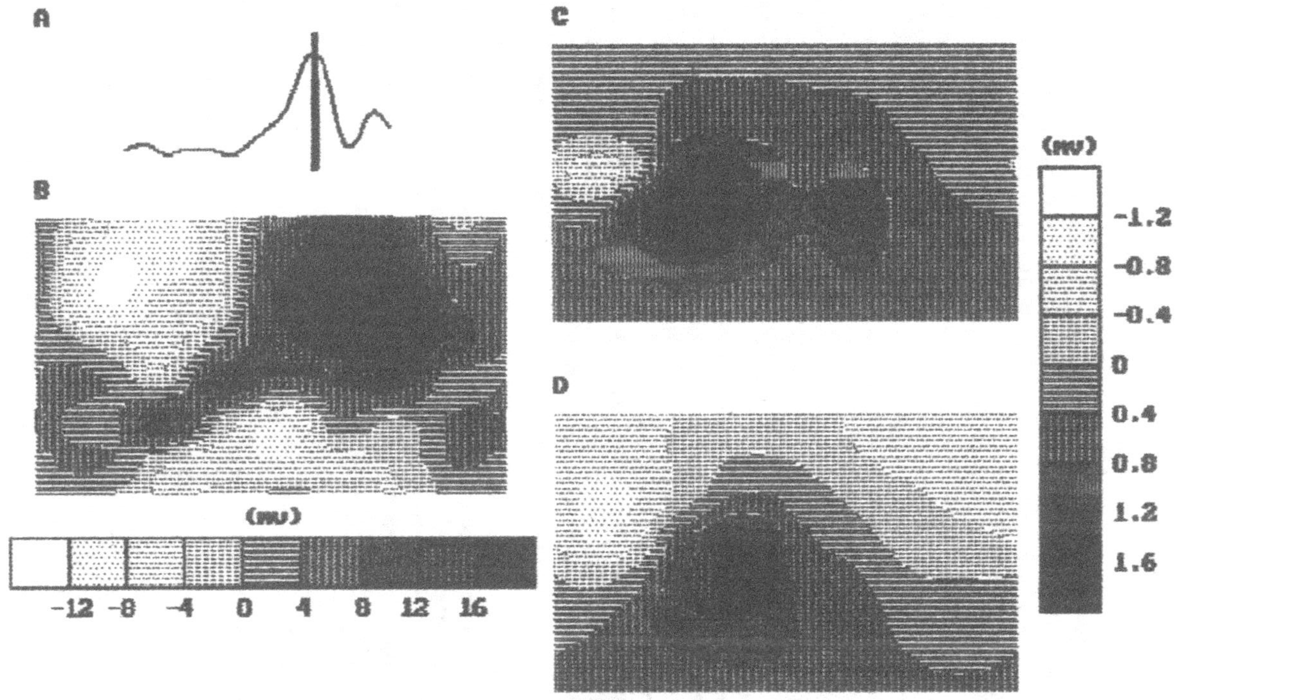

Fig. 2. The results of simulation based on the real data measured from a rat. A – ECG in the I limb lead with a time marker; B – real epicardial equipotential map; C – simulated body surface potential map over a surface close to the real surface of body; D – experimental body surface potential map.

2. Results

First the feasibility of the model in the sense of solving the forward problem was investigated using an ideal electrical generator -a single dipole mounted in the centre of the heart sphere. On the base of the analytically calculated equipotentional map on the sphere (Fig.1A), the simulated equipotentional map on the cylindrical surface (Fig. 1B) was modelled and compared with the same map computed directly from the dipole (Fig. 1C). Both maps on the cylindrical surface were just the same. It was also found that even when the epicardial potentials were perturbed with a significant amount of random noise, the cylindrical surface potentials simulated by means of the model were in good agreement with the analytically computed solution.

Then the potentials over the surface close to the surface of the real torso were computed from the experimentally measured epicardial potentials for several moments of the cardiocycle (Fig. 2A) and compared with real body surface potentials measured from the same animal.

As it was shown by experimental measurements in Wistar rats (2), the wave of depolarization breaks through the surface of the heart ventricles in two regions (Fig. 2B). First the equipotentional maps of the subepicardium of the ventricles show one zone of negative potential located in the basal part of the right ventricle free wall. In 2-3 ms the second zone of electronegativity arises on the ventral surface of the apex of the left ventricle. But due to the smoothing effect of the torso volume conductor only one negative and one positive extrema are reflected on the body surface (Fig. 2C).

The surface equipotentional map modelled from experimental epicardial potentials (Fig. 2D) also showed one positive and one negative extrema located close to the real ones. At the same time the magnitudes of the negative potentials and the size of the negative zone on the simulated surface equipotentional map were less than those on the experimental map while the positive zone on the simulated map was larger. But in spite of this difference which can be explained by the simplicity of the model used, both real and simulated equipotentional maps were similar and reflected the general direction of the excitation wave spread through the ventricles. So the present model makes it possible to compute a feasible distribution of body surface potentials on the base of epicardial ones.

3. Acknowledgements

Authors expresses their gratitude to the firm MERCK SHARP & DOHME I. D. E. A. for the possibility to participate in the work of the XIX International Congress on Electrocardiology.

4. References

1. R.O. Martin and T.C.Pilkington, *IEEE Trans. on Biomed. Eng.* ***BME-19, N 4 (1972) 276.***
2. I.M.Roshchevskaya, *J. Electrocardiology,* ***V. 22, N.3*** (1989) 247.

EFFECTS OF AGING ON CARDIAC ELECTRICAL ACTIVITY IN A RAT MODEL. A LONGITUDINAL STUDY

Aimi B., Stilli D., Sgoifo A., Manghi M., Musso E.

Dipartimento di Biologia e Fisiologia Generali, Università di Parma, Italy

ABSTRACT

In a longitudinal study aimed at detecting new electrical signs of presbycardia, we analyzed body surface distribution of heart potentials of 17 normal male rats at 6, 12 and 18 months of age. In each animal, a 3 minute continuous recording of 44 simultaneous chest ECGs was performed. Approximately 50 (N) beats belonging to the expiratory pause were selected and used for computing: a) an average beat and the related QRST instantaneous potential maps, b) N QRST integral maps. From both sets of maps we derived 134 variables regarding: 1) instantaneous location and magnitude of potential extrema at every tenth of QRS and T wave, 2) duration of ECG intervals, 3) orientation of the zero equipotential line during QRS and 4) beat to beat variability of QRST integral maps. By submitting the variables to stepwise discriminant analysis, 4 classifiers were selected to produce a model for differentiating the 3 classes of age. The Jacknife option enabled us to separate the 18 month group (88% of the cases) from 6 and 12 month groups which instead partially overlapped. The discriminant function was preliminarily applied to human data with comparable results.

1. Introduction

In all aging studies, the differentiation between changes associated with specific pathological events and those related to the aging process itself is often difficult[1]. The present investigation was aimed at detecting new reliable criteria of presbycardia in the normal rat, by analyzing body surface potential maps in a longitudinal study. The analysis regarded topographical and voltage related aspects of instantaneous potential maps and beat to beat variability of QRST integral maps (BBV-IM). BBV-IM analysis was used on account of the ability of QRST integral maps to provide information on local disparity of ventricular repolarization which in turn is markedly affected by changes of the autonomic input to the heart. Thus, the procedure might constitute a powerful tool for evaluating the effect of aging on the modulatory action of the autonomic tone on ventricular recovery properties.

2. Method

We studied 17 normal Wistar male rats, at 6, 12 and 18 months of age. All animals had normal systolic blood pressure and no evidence of rhythm disturbances and respiratory diseases. In each animal under anesthesia (Leptofen Farmitalia-Carlo Erba 0,5 ml/Kg i.m.), we performed a 3 minute continuous recording of 44 simultaneous unipolar ECGs from as many electrodes regularly distributed on the anterior and posterior aspects of the chest. The signals were amplified, multiplexed (1 kHz) and A/D converted. The digital data were stored on disk and then automatically processed.

2.1 Analysis of QRST instantaneous potential maps.

Approximately fifty (N) beats belonging to the expiratory phase were selected and used for computing an average beat and the related instantaneous potential maps throughout QRST. From maps we derived the following variables: coordinates and magnitude of the absolute potential maximum and minimum at every tenth (subinterval) of QRS and T wave; orientation of the zero equipotential line at the instant of the highest QRS potential difference on the chest, taken as index of the cardiac electrical axis; duration of the ECG intervals. The variables obtained were 133.

2.2 Analysis of BBV-IM.

QRST integral maps of the N selected beats were computed and BBV-IM was evaluated by means of a statistical method[2] which makes it possible to establish whether the differences between two maps are related to the following parameters: 1) magnitude of the signals (scale differences), 2) spatial shift (shift differences), 3) other factors independent of magnitude and shift (arbitrarily defined as shape differences). Among the N beats we randomly selected 10 (reference beats) and compared each of them with all the remaining (N-1) beats. In each comparison, the number (n) of beats significantly differing from the reference beat for at least one parameter was expressed as percentage of N. The average value of the ten percentages was taken as index of BBV-IM of the animal (BBV-IM index).

2.3 Statistical analysis.

The 133 variables derived from instantaneous potential maps and the BBV-IM index were submitted to stepwise discriminant analysis to produce a model for separating the 3 classes of age. The results were validated by means of the Jacknife procedure. A preliminary attempt was also made to establish whether the discriminant function could be successfully applied to human data, by using a population of 10 normal young males (20-30 years) and 6 normal old subjects (50-60 years).

3. Results

3.1 QRST instantaneous potential maps.

Significant differences among groups were found by comparing the 18 month animals with those belonging to the two remaining groups. At QRS subintervals 3 to 6, in the 18 month animals we observed a lower magnitude of the chest potentials, a leftward shift of the Mx and an earlier appearance of the Mn on the anterior chest. The null equipotential line was oriented more vertically (Fig. 1). The magnitude of the Mn was lower at subintervals 2 and 5 to 7 of the T wave.

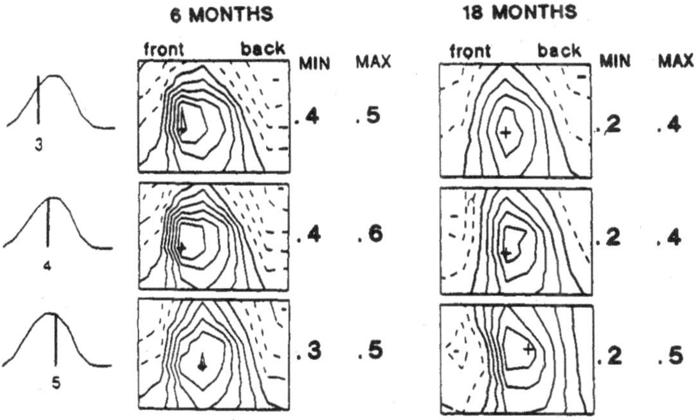

Figure 1. Average instantaneous maps relating to 6 month animals (left column) and 18 month animals (right column) at 3 QRS subintervals with significant differences between groups. In each map the light solid lines, the heavy solid line and the dashed lines indicate the positive, zero and negative equipotential lines, respectively. The symbols + and - indicate the location of the potential Mx and Mn whose values are reported on the right of each map, in millivolts. The step between equipotential lines is 100 µV.

3.2 BBV-IM

In all animals QRST integral maps showed a considerable variability due to scale and shape differences. However, BBV-IM index measured at 6, 12 and 18 months was respectively equal to 32%±21, 43%±10 and 32%±20, with no significant difference among groups.

3.3 Statistical analysis.

The following 4 classifiers were selected by stepwise discriminant analysis at the 0.01 significance level: location of the highest positive potential during QRS; location of the potential Mn at the fifth and seventh subintervals of QRS;

magnitude of the potential Mn at the seventh subinterval of the T wave. By using the Jacknife option, the model enabled us to separate 88% of the 18 month animals from the two younger groups which instead partially overlapped (Tab. 1).
By applying the discriminant function to human data a correct classification of more than 80% of old people was obtained (Tab. 1).

RATS

GROUPS	6 MONTHS	12 MONTHS	18 MONTHS	TOT
6 MONTHS	12(71%)	4(23%)	1(6%)	17
12 MONTHS	8(47%)	8(47%)	1(6%)	17
18 MONTHS	1(6%)	1(6%)	15(88%)	17

HUMANS

GROUPS	YOUNG (20-30 YEARS)	OLD (50-60 YEARS)	TOT
YOUNG	7(70%)	3(30%)	10
OLD	1(17%)	5(83%)	6

Table 1. Classification of study populations.

4. Discussion

Our data might be interpreted by considering that aging provokes a significant loss of myocytes in the left ventricle and a compensatory hypertrophy of the remaining cells. These events are generally associated with the appearance of small areas of interstitial and replacement fibrosis, mostly at the subendocardial level[3] . The altered myocardial substrate may partially explain the changes of topographical and voltage related aspects of maps, observed with increasing age. Conversely, the finding that BBV-IM did not significantly differ among groups suggests that, in our experimental conditions, the modulating action of the autonomic tone on ventricular recovery properties was not affected by aging. The discriminant model obtained by linearly combining 4 classifiers derived from maps enabled us to characterize rat presbycardia. Preliminary results indicate that similar variables might be used for describing the normal aging of human heart.

5. References

1. M.L. Weisfeldt, The Aging Heart (Raven Press, New York, 1980) 1.
2. P. Barone, P. Ciarlini, E. Musso, D. Stilli, Comparison of electrocardiografic data (P Waves): tests of a shape-based approach, Comput. Biomed. Res. 22 (1989) 215.
3. P. Anversa, B. Hiler, R. Ricci, G. Guideri, G. Olivetti, Myocyte cell loss and myocyte hypertrophy in the aging rat heart, JACC 8 (1986) 1441.

PART III

Cardiac Arrhythmias

THE ANALYSIS OF MULTIFOCALIS RHYTHM DISTURBANCES FROM BODY SURFACE POTENTIALS MAPPING

M.Górnicki, J.Jagielski

Department of Pathophysiology Medical Academy of Wrocław
Marcinkowskiego 1, 50-368 Wrocław, Poland.

INTRODUCTION

The analysis of cardiac potentials maps is regarded as a highly useful method for locating the site of ectopic generation of stimuli, especially coming from small local focuses and abnormal conduction paths in WPW syndrome (1,2,3). The rewealed heterogeneity of the maps: nodes, pseudopodia, irregular courses of their lines and, above all, the occurrance of several extrema, juxtaposes with the occurrence of abnormal depolarization sequence in patients with ventricular rhythm disturbances. This is also confirmed by maps of isomagnetic lines (4).

This paper is aimed at evaluating usability of cardiac sinus rhythm mapping analysis in patients exibiting additional activations of diversified etiogenesis in order to find and locate areas that generate these rhythm disturbances.

MATERIALS AND METHODS

The research included 12 patients, aged 36-74 (average X = 56.8, SD = 12.9) with clinical diagnosis of cardiac ischaemia and documented and/or present premature ventricular and supraventricular activation. The patients were followed up by the Cardiology Clinic Wrocław Medical Academy. The cardiac potentials maps were recorded and analysed in an 87-electrode HPM -7100 Fukuda Denshi system. The electrocardiograms are recorded simultaneously, referred to a Wilson-type central terminal and sampled at a frequency of 1000 samples /sec.

The isopotential and isointegral maps were computed for chosen cardiac sinus cycles for the depolarization and repolarization periods. In case an premature beat was detected in a record, drawn were maps of sinus evolution and extrasystolia coupled thereto. The results were referred to mean mapping values from a group of clinically healthy individuals. Computed was departure maps correlation coefficient for the tested cardiac cycles (CC) for an area corresponding to QRS complex, ST segment and T-wave, compared to the reference group.

RESULTS

In 9 of the patients examined detected were, in different moments of the depolarization period, irregular courses of isopotential lines, the irregularities generating an extra local extreme. 3 patients, who had exibited additional ventricular activations before, had a normal image of the maps, the course being regular.

Fig.1 plots exemple of changed morphology of isopotential maps from patient after anterior myocardial infarction and multifoculis ventricular arrhythmias. Maps display irregularity of depolarization propagation with two extremas: E-2,F-4 and abnormal small area of additional potential in the vicinity of electrodes H,I-1,2.
The isointegral maps for the analysed sinus cycles, corresponding to the summed - up area of the entire QRS, in 9 cases displayed additional extremes of the functional potential.

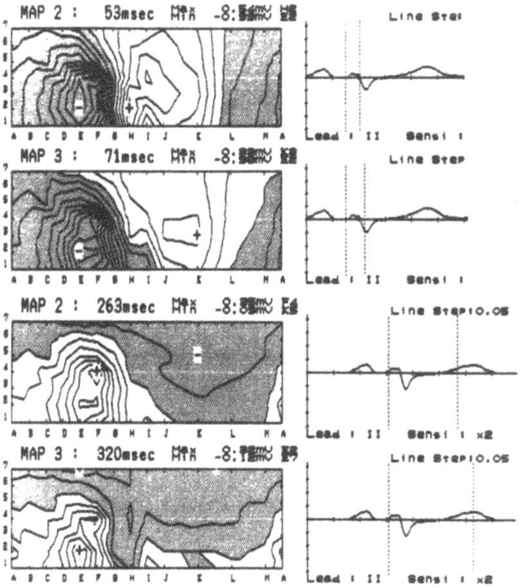

Fig.1 Isopotential maps from a patient with ventricular arrhythmias.

For 5 of the patients, plotted were detailed maps taking into account sinus activation and that of an additional beat.

Fig.2 maps T deflection of sinus activation and the onset of R wave of ectopic beats recorded from the patient. The T maps exibit very similar image corresponding to the arm of the occurring R deflection of the additional activation.

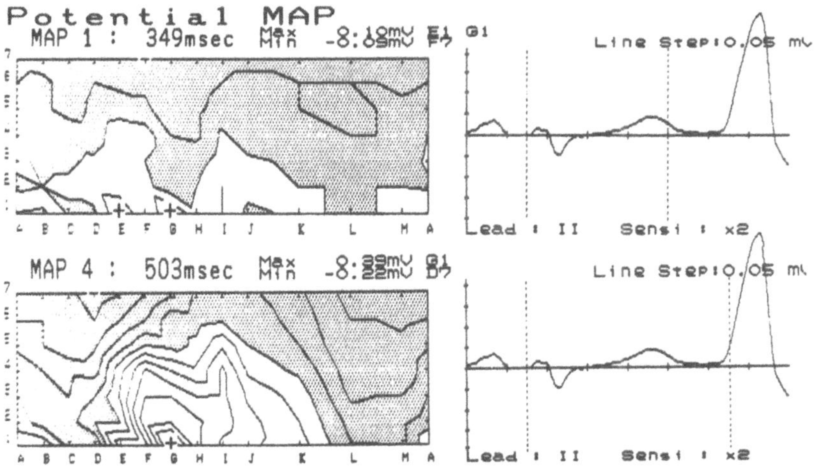

Fig.2 Additional beat created by abnormal repolarization period during sinus cycle.

The propagation of the persistent potential coming from ventricular repolarization period, which suggests the the source of the ectopic activation. In order to determine the irregularity degree of the maps in question, applied was the measurement of the correlation coefficient for QRS complex, ST,T period and the sum of this,i.e. according to Wilson, ventricular gradient.The subject to determination was the correlation of the maps investigated into as compared to mean values taken from the reference group.
The correlation coefficients, for 6 patients, display differences if compared to the reference group in respect to ventricular depolarization time. In 4 cases, especially marked is such a difference for the repolarization period: the correlation coefficient negative or smaller then 0,5.

DISCUSSION

The analysis of the cardiac potentials maps for ventricular depolarization and repolarization displays a heterogeneity of the electric field of the heart in patients with rhythm disturbances. Such a heterogeneity is referred to some authors as maps nondipolarity (4,5).

It also seems to correspond to cardiac micropotentials recorded from the body surface, especially late potentials. The recorded areas of disturbed activation in the heart, can be located as reffered to heart anatomy and one can determine within which time of ventricular activation they occur. These areas heterogeneously and with a delay conduct the activation during ventricular depolarization, whereas during repolarization they seem to be the source of persistent potential.

CONCLUSIONS

1.Isopotential and isointegral maps of the sinus cycle of the heart, taken from the body surface of the patients with cardiac rhythm disturbances, display characteristic aberrations.

2.The irregularities in body surface potential mapping courses manifest themselves as activation heterogeneity, often as additional extremes that prove multipolarity of the source.

3.The analysis of the maps, within the range from the outset of T deflection of sinus activation up to the onset of the additional beat may reveal the mechanism of rhythm disturbances and its location.

REFERENCES

1.Spach M.,Barr R.,Lannig C.,Tucek P.: Origin of body surface QRS and T wave potentials from epicardial distributions in the intact chimpanzee. Circulation,1977,55:268. 2.Taccardi B.:Body surface mapping and cardiac electric sources.J.Electrocardiology,1991,23 suppl.150. 3. Liebman J.Body surface mapping in conduction abnormalities.Martinus Nijhoff Publishers.1986,77-5. 4.Stroink G.,Lant J., Elliot Ph.,Charlebois P.,Gardner M.:Discrimination between myocardial infarct and ventricular tachycardia patients using magnetocadiographic trajectory plots and isointegral maps. J.Electrocardiology, 1992, 25, 129. 5.Gardner M., 8.Montague T.,Armnstrong C.,Horacek B.,Smith E.:Vulnerability to ventricular arrhythmia. Circulation,1986,73.

ATRIAL FIBRILLATION IN WOLFF-PARKINSON-WHITE SYNDROME. REVERSAL OF ISOPROTERENOL EFFECTS BY SOTALOL

Madrid AH, Moro C, Mestre JL, Marín Huerta E, Novo L. Lafuente C. Arrhythmia Unit. Ramón y Cajal hospital.C/ Colmenar Viejo Km 9,100. 28034 Madrid, Spain.

ABSTRACT

Sotalol has class II and III antiarrhythmic effects. Its efficacy and safety in the treatment of atrial fibrillation in patients with Wolff-Parkinson-White syndrome is controversial. We evaluated the effect of isoproterenol and simultaneous IV sotalol (1.5 mg/kg in 10 min) and Isoproterenol over the antegrade conduction through the AV node and accessory pathway. Atrial fibrillation was induced in 22 patients with WPW (13 M, 9F, 36 ± 16 years old). Both AV node and accessory pathway conduction were enhanced by isoproterenol, although with a greater effect on the AV node.

The percent of preexcited QRS complexes was not significatively modified because changes in the ventricular preexcitation results from a balance between the relative effects on refractoriness of accessory pathway and AV node in anterograde and retrograde concealed conduction. There was no serious adverse effects. Reversion to sinus rhythm was documented in 12 patients (60%).

Sotalol reversed all the effects of isoproterenol during atrial fibrillation. Sotalol has a balanced class II and III effects and therefore is a safe and effective drug for the treatment of patients with WPW and atrial fibrillation.

INTRODUCTION

We studied the efficcacy and safety of intravenous sotalol, an antiarrhythmic drug with non selective beta-blocking effects and and that also prolongs the duration of repolarization, in both slowing the ventricular response and terminating sustained induced atrial fibrillation in WPW. Previous studies have reported that catecholamines may reverse the effects of antiarrhythmic drugs (1,2).

MATERIAL AND METHODS

The study consisted of 22 patients (pt) (13 male and 9 female) aged 36 ± 16 years. All pt presented manifest anterograde ventricular preexcitation on the surface electrocardiogram. They were symptomatic because of palpitations (15, 68%), syncope (5, 23%) or cardiac arrest (2, 9%). Clinical atrial fibrillation had been documented in 11 pt (50%) before the study, and atrioventricular reciprocating tachycardia in 14 (63%). Two Pt had been resuscited for ventricular fibrillation. No Pt had associated heart disease.

ELECTROPHYSIOLOGIC STUDY

After informed consent all patients underwent electrophysiological study, in the non sedated and postabsorptive state. No patient was on antiarrhythmic drug during the study (discontinued al least 5 half-lives before study).

Under fluoroscopic guidance, 3 quadripolar catheters (6 Fr) were positioned in the high right atrium, right ventricular apex and coronary sinus, for local electrical stimulation and recording; a tripolar catheter with interelectrode distance of 10 mm was used for recording of the His bundle electrogram. Intracardiac electrograms and surface ECG leads DI, VF, V1 and V6, were displayed on an oscilloscope and recorded on paper (speed 100 and 25 mm/sec). Atrial and ventricular stimulation were performed at twice diastolic threshold (pulse width 2 ms). Refractory periods of the atrium, atrioventricular node and accessory pathway were determined. Induction of atrioventricular reentrant tachycardia was also attempted. Atrial fibrillation was induced by rapid atrial pacing, if it did not occur during the study. Atrial fibrillation was defined as sustained only if it persisted for > 5 min.

STATISTICAL ANALYSIS

Data are presented as mean values ± standard deviation. The student's t test was used to determine the significance between two continuous variables (baseline and postsotalol study). Analysis of variance was used to compare changes in shortest RR intervals, during atrial fibrillation.

RESULTS

The mean sinus cycle length was 720 ± 102 mseg during the control study. Atrioventricular reentrant tachycardia could be induced in 11 patients, the mean cycle length was 350 ± 75 ms. Refractory effective periods of atrium, atrioventricular node and accessory pathway were:

220 ± 22 ms, 240 ± 30 ms, 265 ± 35 ms, respectively. However, because of the presence of preexcitation changes in AV nodal conduction could not be assessed in all cases.

ATRIAL FIBRILLATION

The percent of preexcited QRS complexes was 68 ± 43 % at baseline, 57 ± 40 % after isoproterenol, 65 ± 41 % after isoproterenol plus sotalol and 62 ± 41% with sotalol exclusively. This parameter was not significatively modified in any way.

EFFECTS OF SOTALOL

After sotalol infusion mean cycle length significantly increased, from 720 to 830 ± 135 ms ($p < 0,05$).

No patient presented anterograde conduction block of the accessory pathway after sotalol infusion, during sinus rhythm.

The anterograde effective refractory period of the atrium, accessory pathway, and atrioventricular node increased from previous data to 254 ± 40 ms, 290 ± 62 ms, and 315 ± 42 ms, respectively after sotalol administration.

Orthodromic atrioventricular reciprocating tachycardia was induced in 11 patients at the baseline study. After sotalol treatment the tachycardia was still inducible in 5 patients, inducible, non sustained in 3, and non inducible in 3. Its rate was significantly slowed (mean cycle lenght from 350 to 394 ± 30 ms), only the AH interval was significatively prolonged. QRS complex duration, HV and VA intervals did not show significative modifications. the interruption of the tachycardia occurred in the anterograde limb of the circuit (the AV node).

REVERSAL TO SINUS RHYTHM

During the simultaneous infusion of isoproterenol and sotalol 4 Pt reversed to sinus rhythm (22%). 7 pt more reversed to sinus rhythm in 30 min after starting the infusion of sotalol. 8 pt (40%) did not reverse to sinus rhythm.

DISCUSSION

Sotalol may acomplish the goal of treatment in WPW syndrome, 1.- to prevent inducibility of the reciprocating tachycardia 2.- prolong anterograde refractory period of the AP 3.- suppress atrial and ventricular premature beats 4.- Sotalol may have antifibrilatory effect, modifying the electrophysiological characteristics of atrial tissue 5.- slowinq of the reciprocating tachycardia may prevent AF, because AF often arises during a paroxysm of fast reciprocating tachycardia (3).

The combination of beta blocker effects and class III effects of sotalol may be useful in these patients, preventing not only a rapid ventricular response but also a spontaneous clinical recurrence of atrial fibrillation or reciprocating tachycardia (4,5).

Sotalol reversed the effects of isoproterenol during atrial fibrillation. Sotalol has a balanced class II and II effects and is a safe drug in patients with Wolff-Parkinson-White syndrome and atrial fibrillation. Our data support the use of sotalol for the inmediate treatment of atrial fibrillation associated with WPW syndrome, before cardioversion, unless the latter is urgently neccessary. The data also suggest that sotalol may be a safe and effective drug for preventing atrial fibrillation or reciprocating tachycardia in patients wit WPW syndrome.

REFERENCES

1.-**Swerdlow CD, Peterson J, Liem B.** Effect of flestolol on ventricular rate during atrial fibrillation in Wolff-Parkinson-White syndrome. Am J Cardiol 1988; 62: 78-82.
2.-**Helmy I, Scheinmann M, Herre J, Sharkey H, Griffin J.** Electrophysiologic effects of isoproterenol in patients with atrioventricular reentrant tachycardia treated with flecainide. J Am Coll Cardiol 1990; 16: 1649-1655.
3.-**Madrid AH, Moro C, Rayo I, Marín-Huerta E.** Efectos electrofisiológicos de sotalol sobre la aurícula y la unión aurículoventricular en pacientes con síndrome de WPW. Rev Esp Cardiol 1991; 44 (suppl): 151.
4.-**Marcus F.** The hazards of using type Ic antiarrhythmic drugs for the treatment of paroxysmal atrial fibrillation. Am J Cardiol 1990; 66: 366-367.
5.-**Feld GK.** Atrial fibrillation. Is there a safe and highly effective pharmacological treatment?. Circulation 1990; 82: 1932-1939.

FLECAINIDE VERSUS PROCAINAMIDE FOR THE TREATMENT OF PAROXYSMAL ATRIAL FIBRILLATION

Madrid A.H., Moro C., Marín-Huerta E. Novo L., Mestre J.L., Costa A. Arrhythmia Unit. Ramón y Cajal Hospital. Ctra de Colmenar Viejo Km 9,100. 28034 - MADRID (SPAIN).

ABSTRACT

In this prospective randomized crossover study 80 patients (Pt) (30F, 50M, mean age: 55 ± 14 years) were included. Pt entered into the study if they had atrial fibrillation of recent onset (<24 hours) with a ventricular rate > 100 b/min at rest and aged < 75 years. Exclusion criteria were any sign of heart failure, conduction disturbances, sick sinus syndrome or acute ischemic events. Ramdomly 40 pt received flecainide and 40 procainamide as the first treatment. There were no significant clinical difference between both groups. Procainamide dose was 1 gr infused in 30 min, and followed by infusion of 2 mg/min for 1 h. Flecainide dose was 1.5 mg/Kg in 15 min followed by infusion of 1.5 mg/kg for 1 h. Drug infusion was continued until maximal dose, intolerance or reversion to sinus rhythm. After 1 hour of wash out patients remaining in atrial fibrillation started treatment with the second drug. Left atrial size was measured by echo. Serum levels of drug and atrial size were not different between pt in sinus rhythm or those remaining in atrial fibrillation.

Conversion to sinus rhythm was achieved in 37 (92%) of the 40 pt treated with flecainide and 25 (65%) treated with procainamide ($p<0.001$). The time required for reversion to sinus rhythm was similar between both groups.

INTRODUCTION

Paroxysmal atrial fibrillation is an extremely frequent clinical arrhythmia, with disabling symptoms. The conventional treatment of atrial fibrillation was rapid intravenous digitalization, but it takes several hours to achieve control of the ventricular response, and the aim is not the conversion to sinus rhythm. This treatment has lost importance after new safe and effective antiarrhythmic drugs have been developed.

MATERIAL AND METHODS

PATIENTS

During a 24-month period, eighty patients (50 men and 30 women), aged 55±14 years were included. Patients were admitted in this prospective study if they had paroxysmal atrial fibrillation lasting < 24 hours, aged less than 75 years. Patients with a slow ventricular rate (<100 beats/min) were excluded. The criteria to define the time onset of the arrhythmia was an abrupt, well-defined onset of palpitations.

Exclusion criteria were any sign of acute heart failure, conduction disturbances, known sick sinus syndrome, severe hypoxemia (oxigen partial prssure < 55 mm Hg) acute ischemic events, acute myocardial infarction or electrolyte alterations. Patients with atrial flutter were excluded of this study, as well as those currently receiving antiarrhythmic drugs.

PROTOCOL

A complete medical history, physical examination, 12-lead electrocardiogram and chest X-ray were performed in all the patients before entering this study. Criteria for exclusion were any sign of heart failure on pulmonary auscultation, physical examination or cardiomegaly on chest X-Ray. This protocol was approved by the ethical committe board of the hospital. Informed consent of the patient was obtained. After that, they were randomly assigned to receive procainamide or flecainide.

Flecainide was administered at a dose of 1.5 mg/Kg body weight in 15 minutes, followed by 1.5 mg/kg in 45 minutes. Procainamide was administered at a dose of 1 g in 30 minutes and followed by an infusion of 2 mg/min until 1 hour. The treatment with a drug was considered successful if conversion to sinus rhythm occurred within 1 hour after starting the infusion.

Patients who did not convert to sinus rhythm after one hour of infusion waited for one hour of washing-out before being treated with the alternative drug. During this time they were monitored for conversion to sinus rhythm.

Plasma samples were collected just at the time of conversion to sinus rhythm, or after 5 minutes of the end of the infusion if the patient persisted in atrial fibrillation after one hour.

RESULTS

PATIENTS

The clinical characteristics of the patients were similar in the flecainide and procainamide groups (Table I). There were no statistically significant difference in age (54 ± 15 in F group and 55 ± 13 in P group), sex (66% men in F group and 59% in P group), heart rate (140 ± 18 in F group and 147 ± 24 in P group), mean duration of the atrial fibrillation before starting the treatment (5.9 ± 5.5 in F group and 8.9 ± 8.1 in P group), incidence of heart disease and frequency of episodes of atrial fibrillation / year between F and P groups.

CONVERSION TO SINUS RHYTHM

Following Flecainide therapy conversion to sinus rhythm was achieved in 37 (92,5%) of 40 patients, and in 25 (62,5%) following treatment with procainamide (see Figure 1, management tree). The time required for conversion to sinus rhythm in the F group was 34 ± 33 min and 31 ± 17 in the P group, if we consider only the first treatment. If we added the time to conversion of those patients after the crossing over, the data are very similar, with a mean time of 31 ± 17 min for the procainamide group and 32 ± 31 min for flecainide group.

LEFT ATRIAL SIZE

The mean left atrial size on 2D-echocardiogram was 38 ± 52 mm in patients with successful treatment and 39 ± 10.6 mm in those who did not convert to sinus rhythm; this difference was not significative.

ADVERSE EFFECTS

A significant decrease in systolic blood pressure was observed in one patient treated with procainamide and in two treated with flecainide. After flecainide one patient developed dizzines and other nausea. One patient after flecainide presented sinus bradicardia and posteriorly atrioventricular block and hypotension. Overall the adverse effects were observed in 5 of 55 patients receiving flecainide and 1 of 42 receiving procainamide. All the patients did well after intravenous fluids.

DISCUSSION

Amiodarone has been used for conversion of ventricular and supraventricular arrhythmias to sinus rhythm (TABLE 2). Its efficacy for termination of atrial fibrillation is low, with an overall success rate of 71% of patients with a duration of the arrhythmia less than 48 hours or 80% within 24 hours (1,2). Verapamil is a drug of choice for slowing the ventricular rate in atrial fibrillation, although is useless to terminate atrial fibrillation (3,4). Propafenone seems less effective in converting atrial fibrillation of recent onset to sinus rhythm with an overall succes rate of 57 to 71% (5). Procainamide had a reported success of 43 to 88%, it depends on the duration of the arrhythmia, the dose employed or the time considered to be the end-point to reversion (for some authors even a day) (6,7). Intravenous flecainide its a safe drug, with only mild side-effects, its efficacy vary from 82 to 93%, depending on end-point or mean duration of the arrhythmia (8,9). All of these drugs are of course superior to digoxin to convert atrial fibrillation to sinus rhythm.

Our results show that flecainide is superior to procainamide for the acute conversion to sinus rhythm, and is the drug of choice because is faster, had a higher incidence of reversion and a similar low incidence of adverse effects.

REFERENCES

1.- Negrini M, Gibelli G, De ponti C. Confronto tra amiodarone e chinidina nella conversione a ritmo sinusale della fibrilazione atriale di recente insorgenza. G Ital Cardiol 1990; 20: 207-214.
2.- Suttorp M, Kingma J, Lie-A-Huen L, Gijs E. Intravenous flecainide versus verapamil for acute conversion of paroxysmal atrial fibrillation or flutter to sinus rhythm. Am J Cardiol 1989; 63: 693-696.
3.- Noc M, Stajer D, Horvat M. Intravenous amiodarone versus verapamil for acute conversion of paroxysmal atrial fibrillation to sinus rhythm. Am J Cardiol 1990; 65: 679-680.
4.- Bianconi L, Boccadamo R, Papalardo A, Gentil C, Pistolese M. Efectiveness of intravenous propafenone for conversion of atrial fibrillation and flutter of recent onset. Am J Cardiol 1989; 64: 335-338.
5.- Halpern SW, Ellrodt G, Singh BN, Mandel WJ. Efficacy of intravenous procainamide infusion in converting atrial fibrillation to sinus rhythm. Relation to left atrial size. Br Heart J 1980; 44: 589-595.
6.- Fenster P, Comess K, Marsh R, Katzenberg C, Hager W. Conversion of atrial fibrillation to sinus rhythm by acute intravenous procainamide infusion. Am Heart J 1983; 106: 501- 504.
7.- Borgeat A, Goy JJ, Maendly R, Kaufmann U, Gorbic M, Sigwart U. Flecainide versus quinidine for conversion of atrial fibrillation to sinus rhythm. Am J Cardiol 1986; 58: 496-498.
8.- Cohen Solal A, Juliard JM, Jaeger P, et al. Réduction des fibrillations et tachycardies auriculaires par le flécainide intravenieux. Arch Mal Coeur 1987; 8: 1290-1296.
9.- Crozier I, Ikram H, Kenealy M, Levy L. Flecainide acetate for conversion of acute supraventricular tachycardia to sinus rhythm. Am J Cardiol 1987; 59: 607-609.

INITIAL CLINICAL EXPERIENCE WITH A THIRD GENERATION IMPLANTABLE CARDIAC DEFIBRILLATOR

L. Chiodi[*], D. Rossi[*], A. Fazi[*], E. Lebrun[#], C. Gremigni[*]
G. Calamai[°], M Vaccari[°], R. Vergassola[*]

[*]UO Cardiologia, Ospedale S.M. Annunziata, USL 10/H, Florence Italy
[#]Cardiomedica, Telectronics, Rome, Italy
[°]Cardiochirurgia, Policlinico Careggi, U.S.L. 10/D, Florence, Italy

INTRODUCTION

The aim of our study was to evaluate the effectiveness of a third generation implantable cardioverter defibrillator (ICD), i.e., a device complete with an antitachycardia pacing device (ATP), and to evaluate the clinical and diagnostic utility of its features.
We began our study in 1991 with the Guardian 4210 Telectronics, multiprogrammable ICD which has all the features of the earlier models as well as the following advantages:
1) it provides multiple treatments according to automatic classification of the arrythmia in response to programmed parameters (antibradycardia support, ATP, low and high energy shocks);
2) it is capable of distinguishing sinus and ventricular tachycardia (VT) using an onset detection algorithm;
3) it has an advanced system for storing diagnostic information (DATA LOG);
4) it is capable of inducing arrythmias telemetrically for non-invasive electrophysiological studies (SEF);
5) the automatic condenser regenerator makes it possible to extend the time interval between follow-ups.

MATERIALS AND METHODS

The survey comprised 15 patients (13 males and 2 females) ranging from 53 to 77 years of age (mean 66.2). Twelve patients had post-infarctual ischemic heart disease and 3 had dilatative cardiomyopathy. The mean ejection fraction was 29.2% (range 20-40).
Four patients had survived cardiac arrest from ventricular fibrillation (VF) the remaining 11 had had VT of which 4 were high frequency (180 bpm), 3 an onset with syncope and the remaining 4 sustained VT at a lower frequency (160 bpm) but accompanied by rapid hemodynamic deterioration.

SEF at baseline and after loading with amiodarone (15 mg/kg per os for 10-15 days) with reinduction of clinical arrythmia was done on 11 patients. In the remaining 4 patients ICD implantation was decided on the basis of clinical findings (recurring VT and/or VF notwithstanding adequate chronic amiodarone treatment).
During the SEF an ATP was capable of cardioverting the VT in 5 patients. However, in one patient during pre-discharge SEF the ATP always caused the VT to degenerate into VF and therefore, this function was not activated.
The implant was performed with epicardial electrodes via median sternotomy in all the patients.

RESULTS AND DISCUSSION

The mean follow-up period was 5.1 months (range 1-10) with a 1/15 mortality rate (perioperative death on the seventh day; the patient had undergone a contemporaneous coronary revascularization; this was the only death among the 28 patients who received ICD implants done by our team).
Eleven patients (73%) received shocks (from a minimum of 1 to a maximum of 23 per patient). The total number of activations came to 11389, and spontaneous conversions to sinus rhythm came to 10368.
This high number is due mainly to two patients (3593 and 6579 activations and 3580 and 5806 immediate spontaneous restorations of sinus rhythm, respectively). Thus the recognition algorithm was changed for 8 events out of 10 in the VT recognition window, in 14 out of 16 to prevent ICD activation on unsustained VT.
There were 65 delayed reconversions to sinus rhythm, that is with already loaded condensers. In fact, the Guardian 4210 is a non-committed ICD and performs a double reconfirmation of the VT and/or VF and in the second case, as we have mentioned, with the condensers already loaded, just before emitting the shock.
This prerogative, of considerable importance, made it possible to avoid emitting 65 inappropriate shocks in our study, that is in those cases in which the arrythmia that caused the condensers to load had ceased and the ICD internally dissipated the accumulated energy. There were no inappropriate shocks emitted in our 15 patients and there were only 2 patients who received doubtful shocks (one each) that occurred during sleep and therefore were not preceded by any significant symptoms. In 2 cases we could not verify the events in the DATA LOG, these were

the patients with numerous activations and the DATA LOG only stores the last 25 events.
The ATP was activated and went into operation in four patients (26% of the total). The algorithm used was the PASAR-ORTODROMICO that is capable of effecting an autodecremental pacing. Impulse trains ranged from a minimum of 1 to a maximum of 5, each of which consisted of not less than 5 and not more than 7 impulses with a maximum VT cycle interval of 90% and a minimum coupling interval of 65%.
The number of effective ATPS came to 886 out of a total of 914 (in the 4 patients, 12, 27, 101 and 746, respectively). In 3 patients it did not cause any effect on 25 occasions (in the 3 patients , 4 ineffective out of 16, 14/41, 7/753, respectively) and in one patient it increased VT by more than 50 msec twice and once it caused the VT to degenerate into VF (that is, it worsened the situation 3 times out of 104).
Each time the ATP was ineffective or worsened the situation, one shock was sufficient to restore sinus rhythm.

CONCLUSIONS

Notwithstanding the limited number of patients and the relatively short follow-up, our results confirm the effectiveness of ICD treatment.
The onset detection algorithm that distinguishes sinus tachycardia from VT and the double riconfirmation prior to emitting the shock are effective mechanisms for reducing the number of inappropriate shocks.
The ATP which must be supported by pre- and post-operative SEF markedly reduces the number of shocks emitted, thus avoiding the discomfort that they cause and at the same helps conserve energy. One drawback is that it can only be used in a limited number of selected patients. On the other hand, we do not consider it better to perform antitachycardia pacing for VT without the support of a shock in the event--rare but ever present among these patients-that the ATP can cause the arrythmia to degenerate.

PECULIAR HOLTER PATTERN IN HEALTHY ALCOHOL ABUSERS SUFFERING ACUTE ATRIAL FIBRILLATION

DONI F.
Cardiology Department, Policlinico S.Pietro, Bergamo, Italy

and

PERNPRUNER S., KHEIR A., MANFREDI M., NEGRINI P., STAFFIERE E., RIMONDINI A.
Cardiology Department, Policlinico S.Pietro, Bergamo, Italy

ABSTRACT

We investigated by means of Holter monitoring parameters the possible arrhythmogenic role of cronic alcohol intake in 48 patients without detectable heart disease, suffering for a recent episode of acute atrial fibrillation.
The study population was divided in two groups on the basis of an alcohol consumption of at least 100 gr a day (group A - 25 patients) or not (group B - 23 patients).
The two groups were not significantly different in age, sex, intracavitary cardiac sizes but showed significant differences ($p<0.01$) in plasma levels of GGT and MCV.
The 24 hour Holter monitoring recorded during hospitalization at the resuming of sinus rhythm showed statistically significant differences in the mean heart rate (70 ± 9 vs 64 ± 9; $p<0.05$) and in PQ mean duration (180 ± 29 vs 159 ± 26 msec; $p<0.02$).
The difference in the number of supraventricular ectopic beats (803 ± 798 vs 73 ± 51; $p<0.001$) was the most statistically impressive factor.
These data may suggest an homogeneous electrophysiologic pattern alcohol induced with increased automaticity and refractory dispersion, facilitating, in absence of anatomical difference, atrial fibrillation induction.
A further follow up will investigate whether these Holter monitoring parameters may be considered as an early marker of a concealed alcoholic cardiomiopathy.

Alcohol consumption has been associated with the genesis of supraventricular tachyarrhthmias[1;2].
To indicate the alcohol-related arrhythmias appearing around weekends the term "Holiday heart" syndrome has been coined[3].
Recent observation have indicated that acute and chronic alcohol ingestion may induce changes in cardiac conduction and automaticity[4].
In the absence of an overt cardiomiopathy the specific role of excessive alcohol intake in inducing arrhythmias is still not well understood.
We investigated the possible arrhythmogenic effect of alcohol in a group of patients suffering for acute atrial fibrillation, without any detectable heart disease, by means of 24 hour Holter monitoring at the resuming of sinus rhythm.

Methods

We studied 48 patients (28 men and 20 woman) admitted to our hospital for symptomatic atrial fibrillation.
The diagnosis of the arrhythmia was based on a 12 lead electrocardiogram taken on admission.
All the patients underwent chest x ray, laboratory tests with regard to GGT and MCV levels, a complete echocardiographic examination and a exercise stress test.
A 24 hour Holter monitoring was performed in each patient at the resuming of sinus rhythm. Mean heart rate and PQ duration were measured. The total number of supraventricular ectopic beats was calculated.
The alcoholic drinks consumed each day by every patient during the six months preceding the arrhythmia were calculated as grams of absolute ethanol and the study population was divided on the basis of an alcohol consumption of at least 100 grams a day (group A - 25 patients) or less (group B - 23 patients).
Comparison between these two groups were made utilizing Student's t test for unpaired data; $p<0.02$ was considered significant.

Results

The two groups considered were not significantly different in sex and age (53±4 vs 52±5 years).

The patients of group A had an history of at least 15 years of ethanol consuption; all of them were wine drinkers.
The two groups did not show differences in time of spontaneous resolution of the arrhythmia.
No significant differences were found in glycemia, cholesterol, urea, bicarbonate plasma levels. Plasma potassium was normal in all the patients.
Group A showed significant differences in plasma levels of GGT (75±24 vs 24±16; $p<0.001$) and MCV (94±8 vs 88±5; $p<0.01$), as espected on the basis of history.
Electrocardiograms recorded at the resuming of sinus rhythm were fully normal in all the 48 patients.
The chest x rays indicated a normal cardiopulmonary situation in all patients. Intracardiac size measured by means of echocardiographic examination were normal. Exercise stress test did not disclose signs of ischaemic heart disease.
The results of the 24 hour Holter monitoring are summarized in the table below:

	group A	group B	
Mean heart rate (beats per minute)	70±9	64±9	$p<0.05$
Mean PQ interval (mseconds)	180±29	159±26	$p<0.02$
Supraventricular ectopic beats (total number)	803±798	73±51	$p<0.001$

Discussion

Our study shows significant differences, in the absence of anatomical dissimilarity, in the two groups concerning the results of 24 hour Holter monitoring.
These differences in mean heart rate, in PQ duration and in the total number of supraventricular ectopic beats are concordant with the described alcohol electrophysiologic effects.
Ethanol and acetaldehyde, its first metabolic product, induce conduction abnormalities, especially conduction delays with refractory dispersion[4].

Laboratory investigations have shown chronic conduction abnormalities, especially HV prolongation, in otherwise healthy and well nourished dogs fed with large quantity of ethyl alcohol for more than one year[3].
Ethanol and acetaldehyde induce release of catehecolamines with increase of automaticity as documented by laboratory measurement of reduction of the sinus node recovery time[5].
Considering these electrophysiologic effects the Holter pattern observed in the group of chronic drinkers may be considered as expression of a situation facilitating atrial fibrillation onset.
The 48 patients considered in our study did not show evidence of organic heart disease. Atrial fibrillation developing in this situation is usually considered to be "idiopathic".
Still, the peculiar pattern showed by the Holter monitoring observed in group A, may be considered as an early marker of a subclinical alcohol cardiomiopathy.
We suggest that a preclinical cardiomiopathy, whose only evident signs are so far the occurrence of paroxismal atrial fibrillation and described holter pattern, be present in these patients and that a follow up may describe the transition to an overt cardiomiopathy.
If our hypothesis is correct then such a simple method as Holter monitoring might become a valuable mean to screen alcohol abusers.

We gratefully aknowledge the secretariat services rendered by Ms. S. Beretta.

References

1. Anonymous , *Alcohol and atrial fibrillation*, Lancet 1985; 1:1374
2. Lowenstein SR., Gabow PA., Cramer J., Oliva PB., Ratner K, *The role of alcohol in new onset atrial fibrillation*, Arch Intern Med 1983; 143:1882- 1885.
3. Ettinger PO., Wu CF., De La Cruz C., Weisse AB., Ahmed SS., Regan TJ, *Arrhythmias and the "Holiday Heart2 alcohol related cardiac rhythm disorders*, Am Heart J 1978; 95:555-562.
4. Thornton JR, *Atrial fibrillation in healthy non alcoholic people after an alcoholic binge*, Lancet 1984; 2:1013-1014.
5. Greenspon AJ and Schaal SF, *The "Holiday Heart": electrophysiologic studies of alcohol effects in alcoholics*, Ann Itern Med 1983; 1:816-818.

MS-551, A NOVEL CLASS III ANTIARRHYTHMIC AGENT.

1. ITS SAFETY, PHARMACOKINETICS AND PHARMACODYNAMICS AT INTRAVENOUS ADMINISTRATION IN HEALTHY SUBJECTS

T. KATOH, H. ATARASHI, T. INO, S. KUROKI, S. KAMEI, Y. ENDOH, H. HAYAKAWA, K. MABUCHI*,

The 1st Department of Internal Medicine, Nippon Medical School, 1-1-5 Sendagi Bunkyo-ku, Tokyo 113, Japan and * Institute of Biological Science, Mitsui Pharmaceuticals, Inc., Chiba, Japan

ABSTRACT

This phase I clinical study was designed to evaluate the safety, pharmacokinetics (PK) and pharmacodynamics (PD) at intravenous administration of MS-551, which is newly synthesized class III antiarrhythmic agent with selective inhibition of a time-dependent outward K^+ current.

MS-551 was administered by 5 min intravenous injection to healthy volunteers at doses from 0.003 to 0.4 mg/kg. Plasma concentrations of MS-551 were measured by HPLC.

QT interval was significantly prolonged after the administration of 0.1mg/kg or more of MS-551 with the dose-dependent manner. Peak QT prolongations were usually reached by the end of injection, indicating a rapid equilibrium between plasma and myocardium. The highest dose of 0.4 mg/kg produced prolongation in QT of 26.5±2.7% (mean±S.D., n=5) from baseline value. The changes of QT interval were almost completely abolished by 60 min after the end of injection. PK was best fitted to a 2-compartment model, and elimination half-lives(T1/2α and β) were 3.6 min and 1.7hr respectively. Linear relationship between doses and plasma concentrations (both Cp0 and AUC0-∞) was observed. And a significant positive correlation between plasma concentrations and the degree of QT prolongations was observed. MS-551 has generally been well tolerated. No adverse effects other than the QT (QTc) interval have been observed.

It is concluded that intravenous MS-551 excerts highly selective class III action in man and merits further clinical studies as a novel antiarrhythmic agent.

1. Introduction

Recently, the Cardiac Arrhythmia Suppression Trial (CAST) indicated that Class Ic antiarrhythmic drugs increased the mortality in postmyocardial infarction patients[1]. In this setting, more attention has been focused on Class III antiarrhythmic drugs which may prevent the development of lethal arrhythmia more efficiently than Class I drugs[2].

MS-551(1,3-dimethyl-6-{(2-[N-(2-hydroxyethyl)-3-(4-nitrophenyl) propylamino]ethylamino}-2,4(1H,3H)-pyrimidinedione hydrochloride, Figure 1) is a new Class III antiarrhythmic agent devoid of beta-adrenergic blocking action which inhibits the delayed rectifier outward potassium current (personal communication; T. Iijima and N. Taira). In an in vitro study[3], MS-551 at concentrations above 1μM selectively prolonged the cardiac action potential duration and the effective refractory period (ERP) of canine Purkinje fibers without a significant influence on the resting potential and the maximum upstroke velocity of phase 0 depolarization even at 100 μM. In an in vivo study[4,5], MS-551 (range 0.1 - 10mg/kg, i.v.) decreased the heart rate accompanied by QTc prolongation and increased atrial and ventricular ERP in a dose-dependent manner and suppressed ventricular fibrillation and reentrant ventricular tachycardia induced by electrical stimuli in anaesthetized or conscious dogs following intravenous or oral administration.

The aim of this study was to evaluate the safety, pharmacokinetic and pharmacodynamic characteristics at intravenous doses of MS-551 to healthy Japanese volunteers.

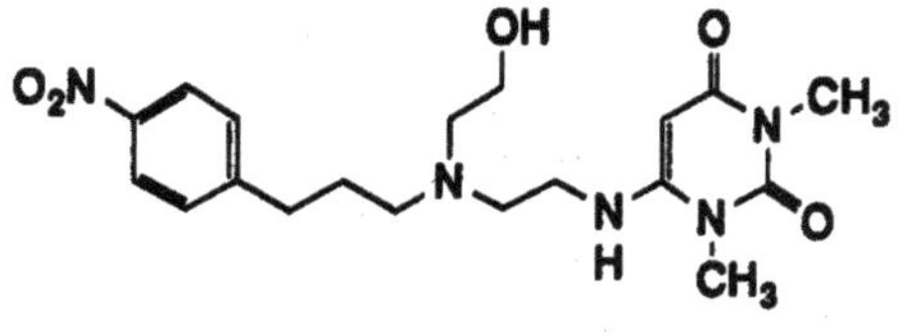

Figure 1. Chemical structure of MS-551

2. Methods

2.1. Objectives and test articles

Seventeen healthy male volunteers were recruited: the age was 30.2±6.3 (mean ± S.D.) years, and the weight was 63.5 ± 6.8 kg.

The study was designed as a double-blind, placebo-controlled method as shown in Table 1.

Lyophilized MS-551 in a vial was dissolved in saline to make solutions of 0.03 mg/ml - 4.0 mg/ml. A weight-adjusted dose (0.1 ml/kg) of MS-551 or placebo administered by slow intravenous injection for 5 min. Each individual subjects received higher dose of drug only if there were no concerns about safety, and in particular no evidence of arrhythmogenicity from electrocardiographic aspects.

Table 1.
Trial design for intravenous MS-551

step	dose (mg/kg)	n		
1	0.003	4	(MS-551 3,	placebo 1)
2	0.01	4	(MS-551 3,	placebo 1)
3	0.033	4	(MS-551 3,	placebo 1)
4	0.1	7	(MS-551 6,	placebo 1)
5	0.2	7	(MS-551 6,	placebo 1)
6	0.3	7	(MS-551 6,	placebo 1)
7	0.4	7	(MS-551 5,	placebo 2)

2.2 Pharmacokinetics

Plasma concentration of MS-551 were measured with venous blood samples which were collected at immediately before the drug administration and then successively at 0 (end of injection), 5, 10, 15, 30 min. 1, 2, 4, 7, 10 and 24 hr after each dose. Blood samples were subsequently analyzed for plasma MS-551 concentration by HPLC. The lower limit of assay sensitivity was 5 ng/ml. The most fitted pharmacokinetic model was selected upon the basis of application of general linear test. From the fitted parameters the pharmacokinetic values were derived.

2.3. *Electrocardiographic aspects and vital signs*

ECG parameters including RR interval, PR interval, QRS width, QT interval and QTc were obtained from lead II ECG at immediately before drug and 1, 1.5, 2, 2.5, 3, 3.5, 4, 4.5 min after the start of injection and 0 (end of injection), 5, 10, 15, 30 min, 1, 1.5 and 2 hr after dosing. Subjects also undertook 24 hr Holter ambulatory ECG monitoring on each study day.

Blood pressure, heart rate, respiratory rate and oral body temperature were measured successively before and after the drug administration.

2.4. *Clinical conditions*

The clinical condition of each volunteer was carefully monitored throughout the study periods.

2.5. *Statistical analysis*

Statistical analysis was done by analysis of variance and paired t tests. $P<0.05$ was considered as the level of significance.

3. Results

3.1. *Pharmacokinetics*

Plasma concentration of MS-551 in each doses declined in a biphasic mode after the end of administration as shown in Figure 2. Changes of plasma concentrations and derived pharmacokinetic parameters demonstrated that the pharmacokinetics of MS-551 in man were approximately linear within the range of doses studied (Table2).

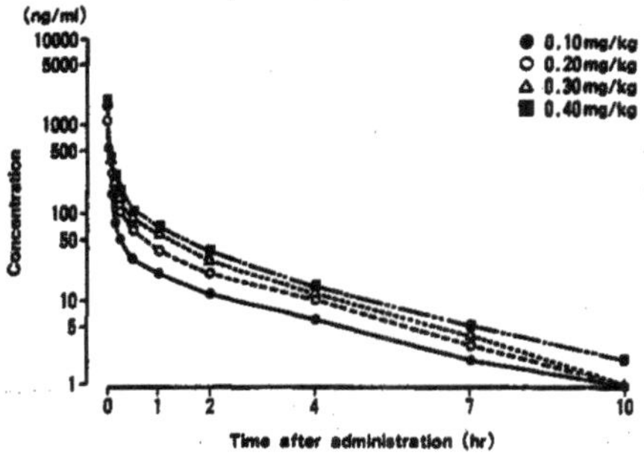

Figure 2.
Plasma concentration of MS-551 following intravenous administration.

Table 2.
Pharmacokinetic parameters for MS-551

Dose (mg/kg)	Cp0 (ng/ml)	T1/2α (min)	T1/2β (hr)	AUC0-∞ (ng·hr/ml)
0.10	564±134	3.3±0.8	2.1±0.4	137±35
0.20	1141±373	3.3±0.3	1.7±0.3	228±48
0.30	1695±170	2.9±0.3	1.5±0.2	321±37
0.40	1948±710	3.6±1.3	1.7±0.2	382±51

mean ± S.D.
Cp0:plasma concentration immediately after administration

3.2 *Electrocardiographic aspects and vital signs*

A dose-dependent prolongation in QT interval was observed following 0.1mg/kg and above. QT intervals prolonged as a function of time during an 5 min injection and then returned to baseline by 60 min after dosing (Figure 3). A significant positive correlation was observed between % changes of QT interval and the plasma concentrations of MS-551 as shown in Figure 4. RR interval, PR interval and QRS width did not change significantly in any subject throughout the study period.

No clinically significant changes were seen in blood pressure, heart rate, respiratory rate or body temperature.

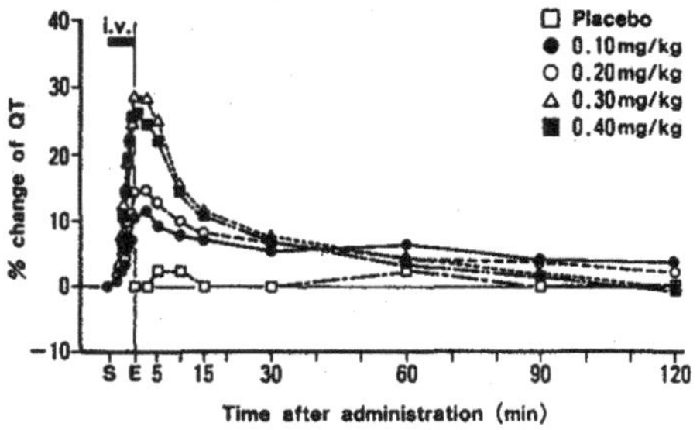

Figure 3.
Changes in QT interval following intravenous administration of MS-551

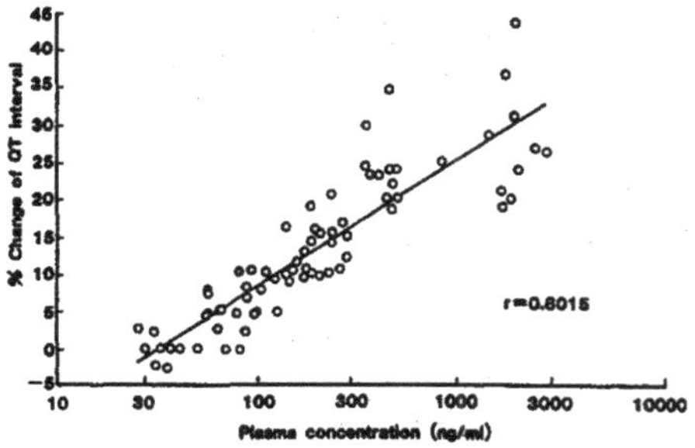

Figure 4.
Correlation between % changes of QT interval and plasma concentrations of MS-551

3.3. Adverse effects

No side effects were observed in any subjects and the haematological and biochemical tests showed no abnormal changes after the administration of MS-551.

4. Discussion

This study showed that intravenous MS-551, with a dose of 0.1 mg/kg and above, selectively prolonged the QT interval on ECG, without influencing the RR interval, PR interval or QRS width. These effects on ECG were considered to be consistent with selective Class III antiarrhythmic activity.
In two subjects who had long QT interval over 440 msec before the administration of MS-551, the QT interval exceeded 600 msec after the drug. However, the QT prolongation was almost dependent to the any clinical symptoms including the provocation of new arrhythmias were not observed.

The pharmacokinetic analysis indicates that MS-551 has relatively short half life, and is eliminated shortly after single intravenous dosing. The lack of a significant effects on vital signs, together with the absence of adverse events suggests that MS-551 can be used safely within the doses tested also in the clinical setting.

In conclusion, this study has shown that MS-551 excerts pure Class III antiarrhythmic actions in man by single intravenous administration and MS-551 is considered to be fairly stable in man from the pharmacokinetic and pharmacodynamic points of view.

5. References

1. The CAST Investigators, *N. Engl. J. Med.* 321 (1989) 406.
2. T. J. Colatsky and C. H. Follmer, *Cardiovasc. Drugs Rev.* 7 (1989) 199.
3. K. Hashimoto, M. Ishii and J. Kamiya, *Eur. J. Pharmacol.* 183 (1990) 1164.
4. J. Kamiya, H. Banno, M. Ishii and T. Katakami, *Eur. J. Pharmacol.* 183 (1990)1776.
5. J. Kamiya, M. Ishii and T. Katakami, *Japan. J. Pharmacol.* 58 (1992) 107.

MS-551, A NOVEL CLASS III ANTIARRHYTHMIC AGENT. 2. ITS SAFETY, PHARMACOKINETICS AND PHARMACODYNAMICS AT ORAL ADMINISTRATION IN HEALTHY SUBJECTS

Katoh T, Atarashi H, Ino T, Kuroki S, Kamei S, Endoh Y, Hayakawa H, Mabuchi K*

The lst Dept. of Medicine, Nippon Medical School, Tokyo 113, Japan
and *Inst. Biol. Sci., Mitsui Pharmaceuticals, Inc., Chiba 297, Japan

ABSTRACT

MS-551 is a newly developed antiarrhythmic agent, which inhibits the time-dependent outward K^+ current in isolated cardiac tissue. This clinical study was designed to evaluate the safety, pharmacokinetics and pharmacodynamics of MS-551 at oral administration in man.

In the single dose study, MS-551 of 100mg and 150mg significantly prolonged the QT interval about 20% from baseline value. Maximum prolongation of hte QT interval wa observed approximately 40min after the administration of the drug and lasted about 4 hours. Cmax and AUC increased with a dose-dependent manner. Cmax was reached at around 45 min after hte administration in the fasting subjects, while it delayed to around 100 min in the food-intake subjects. Pharmacokinetic parameters were calculated by fitting to a one-compartment model. Mean elimination half-lives were almost fixed to 1.4 hours.

In the 7-days repeated administration study, signifiant QT prolongation were repeatedly observed 1.5-2 hours after each drug administration. No cumulative effects on the QT interval were observed throughout the study. Pharmacokinetic parameters at the final dosing on 8th day were very close to those obtained at single dose study.

MS-551 has generally been well tolerated in man by oral administration. No adverse effects on vital signs and ECG parameters except QT prolongation have been observed during the entire study.

It is concluded that MS-551 is safe and pharmacologically stable compound, which exerts a pure class III antiarrhythmic action in man.

1. Introduction

MS-551, 1,3-dimethyl-6-{(2-[N-(2-hydroxyethyl)-3-(4-nitrophenyl)propylamino] ethylamino}2,4(1H,3H)-pyrymidinedione hydrochloride, is a newly synthesized class III antiarrhythmic agent, which inhibits the time-dependent outward K^+ current in isolated cardiac tissue. The electrophysiological properties of MS-551 are similar to sotalol, but is devoid of beta-adrenergic blocking action[1].

This phase I clinical study was designed to evaluate the safety, pharmacokinetics and pharmacodynamics of MS-551 at oral administration in healthy volunteers.

2. Subjects and Methods

2.1. Single Dose Study

Forty four healthy volunteers, young male adults with the age of 20-26 years, were assigned to dose ranging protocol (single oral dose of MS-551 with 10, 25, 50, 100, 150mg or placebo with double blind fashion as shown in Table 1). At step 3, eight volunteers were divided into two subgroups to investigate the influences of meal to pharmacokinetics of the drug by cross-over method.

Table 1. Dose Ranging Protocol of Single Dose Study

Step 1	: 10mg, n=7	(test drug 6, placebo 1)
Step 2	: 25mg, n=7	(test drug 6, placebo 1)
Step 3-1:	50mg, n=8	(A-group: given during fasting; test drug 3, placebo 1)
		(B-group: given after meal; test drug 3, placebo 1)
Step 3-2:	50mg, n=8	(A-group: given after meal; test drug 3, placebo 1)
		(B-group: given during fasting; test drug 3, placebo 1)
Step 4	: 100mg, n=7	(test drug 6, placebo 1)
Step 5	: 150mg, n=7	(test drug 6, placebo 1)

Subjective and objective symptoms, vital signs including blood pressure and heart rate, electrocardiogram including telemeter ECG, standard 12 leads ECG and Holter ECG, laboratory tests and serum concentration of MS-551 were checked or recorded successively after the administration of the drug for 24 hours.

Pharmacokinetic parameters were obtained by fitting each time-concentration curve to a one-compartment model.

2.2. 7-days Repeated Administration Study

Eight healthy volunteers participated in this 7-days repeated administration study. 100mg of MS-551 tablets were administered orally three times a day (at 9:00, 15:00, 21:00 which were 30 min after each meal) for 7 days. Two subjects were given placebo with double blind fashion.

Almost same parameters as single dose study were checked successively throughout the repeated administration study. In addition, echocardiogram was recorded on the 7th day to evaluate the negative inotropic action of the drug.

2.3. Statistical Analysis

Data were expressed as the mean±SD. Statistical analysis was done by the analysis of variance and the paired t test. And the p value less than 0.05 was thought to be statistically significant.

3. Results

3.1. Single Dose Study

Significant prolongation of the QT interval occurred at the dose of 100mg or more. Maximum prolongation was observed approximately 40 min after the administration of the drug and lasted about 4 hours. Maximum rate of prolongation reached to about 20% from baseline value as shown in Figure 1. No effects on RR,

PR and QRS were observed throughout the study.

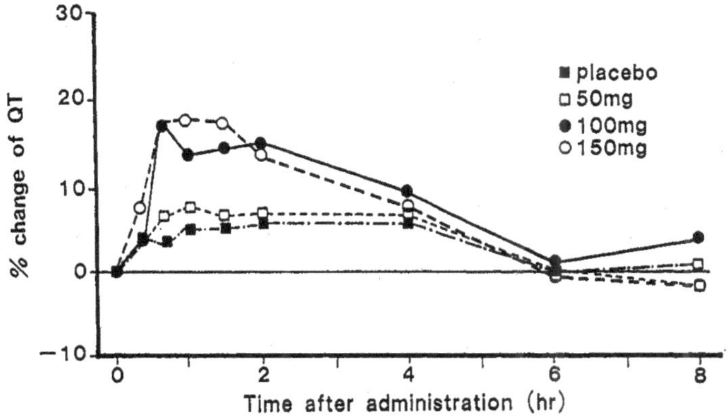

Figure 1. Time Course of Prolongation Rate of QT Interval

Cmax and AUC increased with a dose-dependent manner and a significant linear correlation was found between doses and plasma concentrations of MS-551 as shown in Table 2. Tmax was around 45min after the administration in the fasting subjects, while it delayed to about 100min in the food-intake subjects. However, Cmax and AUC have not been affected by meal. Mean elimination half-lives were almost fixed to about 1.4 hours at the higher range of doses.

No significant changes were seen on vital signs including HR and BP and laboratory examinations.

Table 2. Pharmacokinetic Parameters of Unchanged Form of MS-551

Step	Dose (mg)	Cmax (ng/ml)	Tmax (hr)	$AUC_{0-\infty}$ (ng·hr/ml)	$T_{1/2}$ (hr)	Cl/F (l/hr)
1	10	13±4	0.67±0.13	26±10	1.63±1.09	469±230
2	25	26±12	0.88±0.49	87±38	1.95±1.04	355±137
3	50	91±43	0.83±0.34	234±64	1.49±0.20	245±51
4	100	365±136	0.67±0.20	665±202	1.37±0.20	187±55
5	150	452±279	0.63±0.14	840±267	1.36±0.24	197±59

3.2. 7-days Repeated Administration Study

Significant QT prolongations were repeatedly observed approximately 1.5-2 hours after each dosing. The prolonged QT intervals every time returned to control level at 6 hours after the administration, suggesting that cumulative effects do not exert on QT intervals as shown in Figure 3. No other ECG changes were observed at all.

Pharmacokinetic parameters at the final dosing were very close to those which obtained at single dose study as shown in Table 1.

Slight elevations of GOT and GPT in biochemical tests occurred in one subjects, but they returned to normal level within 1 week after the final administration. No other adverse effects were observed throughout the study.

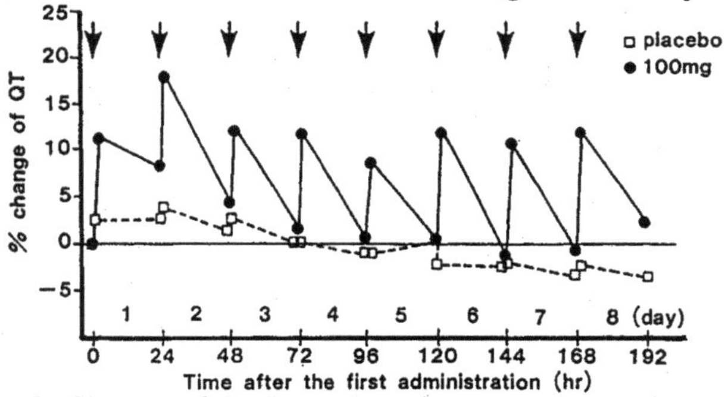

Figure 2. Changes of QT Interval During Repeated Administration

Table 3. Pharmacokinetic Parameters of Unchanged Form of MS-551 in Single Administration (100mg During Fasting) and Day 8 in Repeated Administration (22nd Administration)

	Single	Repeated
$AUC_{0-\infty}$(ng·hr/ml)	665±202	609±164
$T_{1/2}$(hr)	1.37±0.20	1.40±0.14
Cl/F(l/hr)	187±55	191±50

4. Discussion

MS-551 only prolonged QT interval of ECG without affecting on other ECG parameters in healthy volunteers, indicating that this newly synthesized compound may exert pure class III antiarrhythmic action by single and/or repetitive oral administration also in man. From results of the present phase I clinical study, MS-551 is thought to be safe and well tolerated in man, when it was administered orally. And the compound was considered to be fairly stable from the pharmacokinetic and pharmacodynamic points of view.

Since the result of CAST study indicated that class I antiarrhythmic drugs may exert severe proarrhythmic actions in patients with ventricular arrhythmias after myocardial infarction[2], reconsideration of the antiarrhythmic drug therapy is now necessary. Further clinical examinations about class III antiarrhythmic drugs including this drug are expected.

5. References

1. J. Kamiya, M. Ishii and T. Katakami, *Jap. J. Pharmacol.* **58**(1992)107.
2. The CAST Investigators, *N. Engl. J. Med.* **321**(1989)406.

EARLY ACCELERATED IDIOVENTRICULAR RHYTHM: A MARKER FOR CORONARY REPERFUSION

Armando L. Bordalo-Sá, Maria José Correia, A. Nunes Diogo, Armando Longo, Dorinda Silva, Cristina Reis, J. Lopo Tuna and Carlos Ribeiro

UTIC Arsénio Cordeiro, Hospital de Santa Maria
Av. Prof. Egas Moniz, 1699 Lisboa Codex, Portugal

ABSTRACT

With the aim of characterizing the meaning of ventricular arrhythmias occurring in patients (P) with acute myocardial infarction undergoing fibrinolytic therapy (FT), 24-hour Holter ECG was performed in 53P. FT starting time was named hour 0. The reperfusion assessment after FT was based on clinical, electrocardiographic and enzymatic criteria. Reperfusion was considered to have existed only if all 3 criteria were present. The following Holter ECG parameters were analyzed: mean PVC/h, presence and time of occurrence of accelerated idioventricular rhythm (AIVR) (≥ 3 PVC in a row; HR ≤ 120/min), ventricular tachycardia (VT) (≥ 3 PVC in a row; HR > 120/min), significant bradyarrhythmias (HR < 50/min, requiring therapy). P were divided into two groups: with reperfusion-35P; without reperfusion-18P.

AIVR appeared in 29 patients with reperfusion (83%) and in 14 patients without reperfusion (78%) (NS). AIVR within 200 min occurred in 17 patients with reperfusion (49%) and in 0 patients without reperfusion (p=0.001). The differences between the two groups concerning the other studied parameters - PVC/h, VT, VT within 200 min, bradyarrhythmias, and bradyarrhythmias within 200 min - were not significant.

We conclude that the occurrence of AIVR within 200 min after FT was highly significant as a discriminating criterion of reperfusion (p=0.001) with a 100% specificity, and consequently it can be considered as a marker for coronary reperfusion in these patients.

The widespread use of intravenous thrombolytic drugs in the treatment of acute myocardial infarction (AMI) determines an increasing interest regarding the noncoronariographic markers of coronary reperfusion. Either reperfusion took place or not, it may be possible to establish a prompt therapeutic decision after fibrinolytic therapy (FT) based on noncoronariographic criteria of reperfusion, sparing the sistematic aid of coronary angiography.

Among the noninvasive markers of reperfusion are the ventricular arrhythmias [1-4]. However, because they are extremely frequent, being nearly always present during the evolution of AMI [5-7], it is important to differentiate reperfusion arrhythmias from infarction arrhythmias. Some controversy still subsides about meaning, frequency and timing of several kinds of ventricular arrhythmias which occur in patients undergoing FT.

Methods

Patients

The study group consisted of 53 patients, admitted to a coronary care unit with a diagnosis of AMI and submitted to FT within 6 hours after the onset of symptoms. In 31 patients an intravenous infusion of 1 500 000 UI of streptokinase was administrated over 60 minutes, and the other 22 patients received an intravenous injection of 30 UI of anistreplase over 5 minutes.

An intravenous perfusion of lidocaine was prophylactically given to nearly half of the patients according to the preference of the attending physician.

Holter Electrocardiography and Arrhythmia Analysis

We started a 24-hour Holter ECG recording in all patients at the same time FT began. The time the therapy was initiated was considered hour 0. Avionics model 445 two-channel recorders were used and the tapes were analyzed in the Avionics model 660-B scanner. The quantification and the characterization of ventricular arrhythmias were performed in the compressed print of the complete recording in the Electrocardiovalidator model 9300. The count of premature ventricular complexes (PVC) was mannually performed in the compressed print at 60 seconds per line. Everytime that a succession of 3 or more PVC occurred, a paper print at 25 mm/sec was obtained to enable the study of the arrhythmia rate.

The analysis of arrhythmias was performed without knowing the FT results, and the following definitions were used:

a) *Hourly frequency of PVC* - total number of PVC counted in 24 hour recording divided by 24.

b) *Accelerated idioventricular rhythm (AIVR)* - three or more consecutive PVC with a rate ≤ 120/min.

c) *Ventricular tachycardia (VT)* - three or more consecutive PVC with a rate >120/min.

d) *Significant bradyarrhythmias* - heart rate < 50/min, requiring therapy.

Coronary Reperfusion Assessment

For the coronary reperfusion assessment the following noncoronariographic reperfusion criteria were used:

a) *Clinical* - disappearance of pain during or immediately after drug administration.

b) *Electrocardiographic* - fifty percent regression of the sum of ST segment elevation occurring within 2 hours after the start of therapy on hourly performed ECG.

c) *Enzymatic* - peak serum creatine kinase occurring until 18 hours after the beginning of pain, in blood samples being obtained every 4 hours after the time FT was started.

Using these noncoronariographic criteria, it is assumed that the simultaneous presence of all three has a virtually 100% positive predictive value that reperfusion took place [8-9]. That happened in 35 patients (66%) and we considered them the group with reperfusion. The absence of all three criteria predicts unsuccessful FT, whereas if only one or two criteria are present, reperfusion is considered doubtful. In this study we did not distinguish patients with 0 criterion, from patients with only one or two criteria; therefore the 18 patients (34%) who did not fulfill simultaneously the 3 criteria were included in the same group: group without reperfusion .

Statistical Methods

The difference between the two studied groups regarding the incidence of ventricular arrhythmias (percentage of patients with arrhythmias) and their frequency per hour were compared by the unpaired Student's t test or chi square test with Yates' correction for continuity as appropriate. Values were expressed as mean ± 1 standard deviation and range between parenthesis. p values < 0.05 were considered statistically significant.

Results

Hourly Frequency of PVC

Mean PVC/h was 30.7 ± 37.4 (range 0.1 - 218) in patients with reperfusion and 26.9 ± 33.2 (0-140) in patients without reperfusion (NS).

Arrhythmias Occurrence During 24 Hours

Considering the occurrence of ventricular arrhythmias in the total 24 hour period after FT, we found that AIVR appeared in 29 patients with reperfusion (83%) and in 14 patients without reperfusion (78%) (X^2=0.006;NS); VT in 21 patients with reperfusion (60%) and in 10 patients without reperfusion (56%) (X^2=0.00; NS); and bradyarrhythmias in 9 patients with reperfusion (26%) and in 3 patients without reperfusion (17%) (X^2=0.16;NS).

Arrhythmias Occurrence Within 200 Minutes

If the analysis was restricted to the first 200 min after FT started as is referred in another paper in this monography*, we found that AIVR occurred in 17 patients with reperfusion (49%), while did not show up in any patient without reperfusion (0%) (X^2=10.7; p=0.001); the earliest case of AIVR appeared at 9 min after therapy; of 17 patients with AIVR within 200 min, only in 9 patients the arrhythmia was detected by conventional monitoring performed by the nurse staff at the coronary care unit. VT appeared in 5 patients with reperfusion (14%) against 2 patients without reperfusion (11%) (X^2=0.11; NS); and, finally, bradyarrhythmias in 8 patients with reperfusion (23%) and in 2 patients without reperfusion (11%) (X^2=0.44; NS).

Discussion

Holter electrocardiography is the best method to characterize and quantify arrhythmias accurately. Some controversy about the significance of arrhythmias as a reperfusion criterion after FT has been related to the fact that some studies did not use this methodology and have based the characterization of arrhythmias exclusively in the surveillance of conventional monitoring performed by nurses and cardiopulmonary technicians [10-11]. Since a long time ago it is known that both coronary occlusion and reperfusion are followed by ventricular arrhythmias [12]. Simple PVC, paired PVC, VT, AIVR, and also bradyarrhythmias, have been related to reperfusion [13-14]. Otherwise, ventricular fibrillation occurs uncommonly, some authors considering it independent of reperfusion [3].

We did not find a higher occurrence of PVC, VT or bradyarrhythmias in patients with reperfusion in comparison with patients without reperfusion. Also the occurrence of AIVR during 24 hours after FT was similar in patients with reperfusion (83%) and in patients without reperfusion (78%). Our work confirms the nonspecificity of this arrhythmia as a criterion of reperfusion. However, in an early phase after FT, namely within 200 min after starting the thrombolytic drug perfusion, AIVR only showed up in patients with clinical reperfusion, and in about half of them (49%). On the contrary, VT and bradyarrhythmias did not show significant differences in their occurrence even within 200 min after FT in patients with and without reperfusion.

---

* *Bordalo-Sá et al.* How late can early accelerated idioventricular rhythm occur to be considered a marker for coronary reperfusion.

So, as a conclusion of our study, we admit that the occurrence of AIVR within 200 min after FT, in view of its high specificity, should be considered a new noninvasive marker for coronary reperfusion, its value to be confirmed in the near future with a greater number of patients.

Acknowledgment

We wish to thank Ms. Honorina Correia for the preparation of the manuscript.

References

1. W. Ganz, K. Ninomiya, J. Hashida et al., *Am. Heart. J.* **102** (1981) 1145.
2. S. Goldberg, A.J. Greenspan, P.L. Urban et al., *Am. Heart J.* **105** (1983) 26.
3. F.C. Miller, M. W. Krucoff, L. F. Satler et al., *Am. Heart J.* **112** (1986) 928.
4. B. Cercek, M. Horvat, *Eur. Heart J.* **6** (1985) 109.
5. J. T. Bigger Jr., R. J. Dresdale, R. H. Heissenbuttel et al., *Prog. Cardiovasc. Dis.* **19** (1977) 255.
6. R. S. Myerburg, C.A. Conde, R.J. Sung et al., *Sudden Death* (The Hague: Martius Nijhoff 1980) p. 219.
7. S. Sclarovsky, B. Strasberg, J. Fuchs et al., *Am. J. Cardiol.* **52** (1983) 43.
8. W. Ganz, I. Geft, J. Maddahi et al., *J. Am. Coll. Cardiol.* **1** (1983) 1247.
9. S. H. Hohnloser, M. Zabel, W. Kasper et al., *J. Am. Coll. Cardiol.* **18** (1991) 44.
10. R. M. Califf, W. O'Neil, R. S. Stack et al., *Ann. Intern. Med.* **108** (1988) 658.
11. A. J. Six, J. H. Louwerenburg, J. H. Kingma et al., *Br. Heart J.* **66** (1991) 143.
12. R. Tennant, C.J. Wiggers, *Am. J. Physiol.* **112** (1935) 351.
13. B. Cercek, A.S. Lew, P. Laramee et al., *Am. J. Cardiol.* **60** (1987);214-8.
14. D. Alexopoulos, R. Collins, S. Adamopoulos et al., *Brit. Heart J.* **65** (1991) 9.

HOW LATE CAN EARLY ACCELERATED IDIOVENTRICULAR RHYTHM OCCUR TO BE CONSIDERED A MARKER FOR CORONARY REPERFUSION

Armando L. Bordalo-Sá, Maria José Correia, A. Nunes Diogo, Armando Longo, Carlos Moreira , Cristina Reis, J. Lopo Tuna and Carlos Ribeiro

UTIC Arsénio Cordeiro, Hospital de Santa Maria, Av. Prof. Egas Moniz, 1699 Lisbon Codex, Lisbon, Portugal

ABSTRACT

Early accelerated idioventricular rhythm (AIVR) is considered a marker for reperfusion (R) in acute myocardial infarction after fibrinolytic therapy (FT), however the timing of the first episode of AIVR with this meaning is still controversial. To determine the interval between FT start and AIVR occurrence which best discriminates patients (P) with R from P without R, 24-hour Holter ECG was performed in 53P. FT starting was named hour 0. R assessment after FT was based on clinical, electrocardiographic and enzymatic criteria. AIVR was defined as ≥ 3 PVC in a row, HR ≤ 120/min. P were divided into two groups: with R, 35P (66%); without R, 18P (34%). As a marker for reperfusion the occurrence of AIVR within 200 min after FT start had a sensitivity = 49% [95% confidence interval (CI), 36 to 62%], a specificity = 100%, a positive predictive value = 100%, and an accuracy = 66% (95% CI, 53 to 79%); and the occurrence of AIVR within 260 min after FT start had a sensitivity = 66% (95% CI, 53 to 79%), a specificity = 83% (95% CI, 73 to 93%), a positive predictive value = 88% (95% CI, 79 to 97%) and an accuracy = 72% (95% CI, 60 to 84%). We conclude that the occurrence of AIVR within 200 min after FT start was a 100% specific criterion of reperfusion. However, the occurrence of AIVR within 260 min allowed the correct classification of the greatest number of patients in our population.

Recently it has been suggested that accelerated idioventricular rhythm (AIVR) usually occurs in the reperfusion phase after fibrinolytic therapy (FT) for acute myocardial infarction (AMI) [1-3]. However, some authors were not able to find a relationship between AIVR and reperfusion [4,5]. This has been imputed both to the fact that Holter monitoring has not been used as a method to characterize arrhythmias [5], and to the fact that AIVR occurrence has not been related to time after FT [4].

In another chapter of these Proceedings*, we showed that when 24 hour Holter ECG was performed after FT, the occurrence of AIVR was independent of patients having clinical reperfusion or not. However, when we considered the first 200 minutes after therapy, AIVR only took place in patients with reperfusion.

* *Bordalo-Sá et al.* Early accelerated idioventricular rhythm: a marker for coronary reperfusion.

The objective of this study was to determine the interval between FT start and the occurrence of the first episode of AIVR which best discriminates patients with coronary reperfusion from patients without coronary reperfusion.

Methods

The study group consisted of 53 patients with the diagnosis of AMI and submitted to FT within 6 hours after the onset of symptoms. An intravenous perfusion of lidocaine was prophylactically given to nearly half of the patients according to the preference of the attending physician.

A 24 hour Holter ECG recording was started in all patients at the same time FT began. The time the therapy was initiated was considered hour 0. AIVR was defined as three or more consecutive premature ventricular complexes (PVC) with a rate equal or less than 120/min.

For the coronary reperfusion assessment noncoronariographic criteria were used (clinical, electrocardiographic and enzymatic). Reperfusion was considered to have existed only if all three were present. Patients were divided into two groups: group A, including 35 patients with reperfusion, and group B, including 18 patients without reperfusion.

Descriptive analysis of population showed that the sample distribution was not normal. Contingency table was used for discrete variables. The survival curves were compared by the long-rank test calculated for the selected endpoint (occurrence AIVR). The significance level for overall results was set at 0.05. Cumulative estimates of AIVR occurrence were calculated by standard techniques with one minute intervals. All P values reported are for two tailed tests.

More details on methods used in this study are given in the chapter of these Proceedings above referred.

Results

To determine the time of occurrence of the first episode of AIVR being a marker for reperfusion, we analyzed its timing in all population by means of survival curves. The results are shown in figure 1.

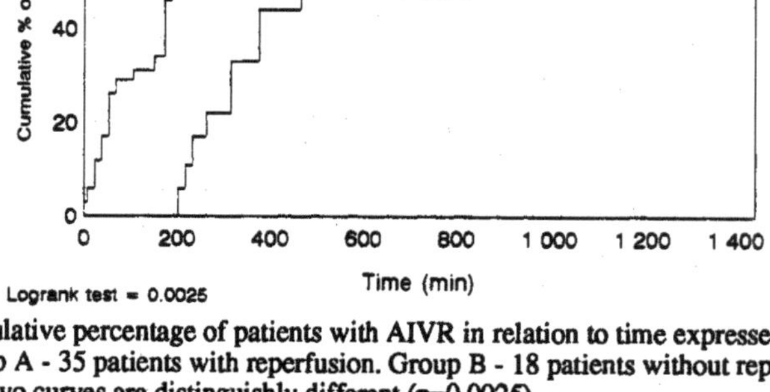

Figure 1. Cumulative percentage of patients with AIVR in relation to time expressed in minutes. Group A - 35 patients with reperfusion. Group B - 18 patients without reperfusion. The two curves are distinguishly different ($p=0.0025$).

In 6 out of the 35 patients with reperfusion (Group A), the first episode of AIVR occurred within 60 min (the earliest at 9 min), in 10 within 120 min, in 12 within 180 min, in 17 within 200 min, in 23 within 260 min, and in 29 patients AIVR occurred during the 24 hours (see Table I). In patients of group B (including 18 patients without reperfusion). None had AIVR within 200 min, three had AIVR within 260 min, and 14 had AIVR during the 24 hours.

Table I - **Sensitivity and Specificity of AIVR in the Diagnosis of Reperfusion**

	Minutes	≤60	≤120	≤180	≤200	≤220	≤240	≤260	≤300
A	Group A (35P)	6	10	12	17	19	21	23	23
I	Group B (18P)	0	0	0	0	1	2	3	4
V	Sensitivity	17%	29%	34%	49%	54%	60%	66%	66%
R	Specificity	100%	100%	100%	100%	94%	89%	83%	78%
	Accuracy	45%	53%	56%	66%	68%	70%	72%	70%

	Hours	≤6	≤7	≤8	≤9	≤12	≤24
A	Group A (35P)	24	24	27	27	28	29
I	Group B (18P)	6	9	9	10	12	14
V	Sensitivity	69%	69%	77%	77%	80%	83%
R	Specificity	67%	50%	50%	44%	33%	22%
	Accuracy	68%	62%	68%	66%	64%	62%

As the sample distribution is not normal we could not apply the discriminant analysis, but using several contingency tables we found that 260 min after FT is the the time which enables us to correctly classify the greatest number of patients of our sample. In fact, considering the timing of the first episode of AIVR as a marker of reperfusion we can see (Table I) that when it occurred within 200 min it had a sensitivity=49% [95% confidence interval (CI),36 to 62%], a specificity=100%, and an accuracy=66% (95% CI, 53 to 79%), and when it occurred within 260 min the sensitivity was 66% (95% CI, 53 to 79%), the specificity was 83% (95% CI, 73 to 93%) and the accuracy was 72% (95% CI, 60 to 84%).

Discussion

The importance of reperfusion arrhythmias as a marker for coronary reflow is still a matter of discussion. Goldberg et al. [1] initially described sinus bradycardia, in inferior infarction, and AIVR as markers of reperfusion. Gorgels et al. [3] considered AIVR highly indicative that necrosis and reperfusion have existed. Cercek et al. [6] evaluated several ventricular arrhythmias, ascribing to AIVR a sensitivity of 90% (60% in the first hour after therapy). Six et al. [7] concluded that in patients with AIVR after thrombolysis the vessel related to infarction has almost surely patency. For Hohnloser et al. [8] only AIVR, and sinus bradycardia in inferior infarctions, correlate with patency in coronary angiography. On the contrary, Gore et al. [2] confirmed the usefulness of sinus bradycardia but did not find a correlation between AIVR and coronary artery reperfusion. Also, neither Miller et al. [4], using 12-hour Holter recordings, nor Califf et al. [5], based on conventional monitoring performed by technicians and nurses, found a higher incidence of AIVR or other ventricular arrhythmias in patients with reperfusion.

To our knowledge, our study is the first one that tries to correlate the timing of the first episode of AIVR with the occurrence of coronary reperfusion. We found that the sensitivity of AIVR in the diagnosis of reperfusion rose steadily from 60 min to reach 49% at 200 min, 66% at 260 min, and 83% at 24 hours. On the other hand, AIVR had a specificity of 100% when it occurred within 200 min, to decrease to 83% at 260 min and only 22% at 24 hours. The accuracy, i.e., the capacity of AIVR to correctly classify patients with reperfusion or without reperfusion was 66% at 200 min and 72% (the highest value) at 260 min.

We conclude that the presence of AIVR within 200 min after the start of FT was a 100% specific criterion of reperfusion. However the occurrence of AIVR within 260 min after FT allowed us to correctly classify the greatest number of patients of our sample. Consequently, and knowing the obvious limitations of conventional monitoring in the diagnosis of arrhythmias which can last for 2 or 3 seconds with a heart rate similar to sinus rhythm, it will be not necessary to perform a Holter ECG longer than a 5 hour period to detect the presence of this noninvasive marker of reperfusion. The reduction of Holter recording to 5 hours, carrying natural economical advantages, allows us to obtain in a few hours time after FT administration one more clinical marker of reperfusion along with the regression of ST segment elevation (where Holter monitoring plays a role) and the resolution of symptoms, and prior to get the results of myocardial enzyme tests.

Acknowledgment

We wish to thank Ms. Honorina Correia for the preparation of the manuscript.

References

1. S. Goldberg, A. Greenspon, P. Urban et al., *Am. Heart J.* **105** (1983) 26.
2. J. M. Gore, S. P. Ball, J. M. Corrao et al., *Chest* **94** (1988) 727.
3. A. P. M. Gorgels, M. A. Vos, I. S. Letsch et al., *Am. J. Cardiol.* **61** (1988) 231.
4. F. C. Miller, M. W. Krucoff, L. F. Satler et al., *Am. Heart J.* **112** (1986) 928.
5. R. M. Califf, W. O'Neill, R. S. Stack et al., *Ann. Intern. Med.* **108** (1988) 658.
6. B. Cercek, A. S. Lew, P. Laramee et al., *Am. J. Cardiol.* **60** (1987) 214.
7. A. J. Six, J. H. Louwerenburg, J. H. Kingma et al., *Br. Heart J.* **66** (1991) 143.
8. S. H. Hohnloser, M. Zabel, W. Kasper et al., *J. Am. Coll. Cardiol.* **18** (1991) 44.

VENTRICULAR ARRHYTHMIAS AFTER MYOCARDIAL INFARCTION-IS AUTONOMIC DYSFUNCTION RESPONSIBLE ?

Stefan Trzos, Włodzimierz J.Musiał, Jerzy W.Kozłowski, Piotr Rozentryt

Medical University, Łódź, Poland
90-123 Łódź, Kopcińskiego 22

ABSTRACT

The aim of this study was to identify patients (pts) at the risk of late postinfarction ventricular arrhythmia (VA). In 56 pts after first myocardial infarction (MI) 24-hours monitoring was performed, and presence of ventricular premature complex was assessed as arrhythmia event (AE). On the basis of these results pts were divided into two groups (Gr): Gr. 1-29 pts with AE and Gr.2-27 pts without AE. In studied groups left ventricular ejection fraction (LVEF) was measured by 2-D echo technique. In 32 pts LVEF was lower than 40%. In all pts sympathetic and parasympathetic activity of the nervous system was assessed. Sympathovagal balance was measured by low (LF-0.03-0.15 Hz) and high (HF-0.15-0.35 Hz) frequency components of heart rate variability (HRV) by autoregressive power spectral analysis. Majority of pts with severe arrhythmia had LVEF<40%. In this group significant lower HF values were recorded with the increase of LF/HF ratio. Conclusion: impaired cardiac parasympathetic activity in pts with LV dysfunction may be useful to identify pts at the risk of VA.

Controversies for prognostic value of life-threatening VA in pts after MI are still the mater of many clinical investigations[1,2]. Complex VA was considered as the main factor of high risk group. It was also confirmed that impairment of LVEF (<40%)[3] determined poor prognosis for coronary pts. Decreased HRV was known as being the predicting factor for cardiac deterioration[4,5]. New methods gave quantitative assessement of autonomic nervous system (ANS) on cardiac function. In the on-going study we were estimating the influence of ANS on the VA group of pts.

MATERIAL AND METHODS

Investigations were made in 56 pts (38 male, 18 female) aged 25-72 years (mean age 48.3 y) 1-2 years after first MI. All pts were checked clinically. Standard 12-lead Ecg and 24-hour Holter monitoring was performed. 29 pts with complex VA were clasiffied as AE - Gr. 1. Gr. 2 consisted of 27 pts without AE. LVEF using 2-D Doppler echocardiography was measured. 32 pts have LVEF value lower than 40%. HRV analysis for both supine and standing position during spontaneous breathing was made using autoregressive modeling method. Estimation of spectral density for low (LF-0.03-0.15 Hz) frequency range (sympathetic) and high (HF-0.015-0.035 Hz) frequency range (parasympathetic) was determined. LF/HF ratio was calculated.

RESULTS

Tabl. 1. shows correlation between LVEF values, AE, and sympatho-vagal balance. The AE group has significantly lower LVEF (p<0.01) and decreased LF/HF ratio indicating impaired parasympathetic activity.

Table 1.

		Gr. 1		Gr. 2	
		supine	standing	supine	standing
LVEF <40%	LF	9,1	15,2	10,8	16,2
	HF	2,3	2,0	4,6	3,5
	LF/HF	3,8	6,6	2,8	4,1
LVEF >40%	LF	8,6	13,1	10,6	14,9
	HF	5,3	3,9	5,6	3,3
	LF/HF	2,1	3,8	2,2	3,7

Fig. 1,2 - reveals HRV analysis of the pt with LVEF < 40% and AE in comparison to the case without AE and LVEF > 40 %.

DISCUSSION

The mechanisms of sudden cardiac death (SCD) after MI remain still unsolved. Holter Ecg registration is commonly used for detecting spontaneous VA, which are crucial in triggering SCD. Some investigators[1-3] however are of opinion that spontaneous VA recorded with Holter do not coincide with the onset of complex

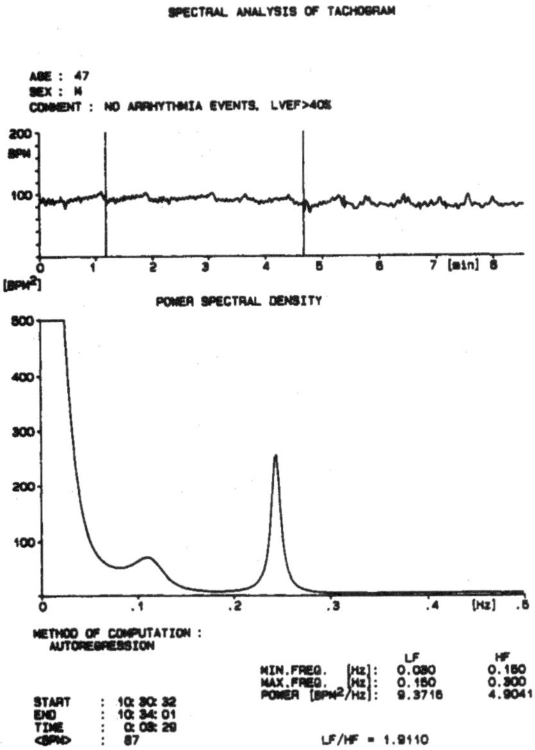

Fig. 1.
Original registration of HRV in a patient from Gr 1 without arrhythmia event. Upper tracing: spectral analysis of tachogram. Lower tracing: power spectral densities of HRV.

VA during follow-up. They do not significantly correlate with SCD cases. Prophylactic antiarrhythmic treatment is therefore under the question. Coronary impairment and ischaemia are leading to AE. HRV spectral analysis indicates relationship between decreased vagal tone and ischaemic attacks[6]. Kleiger[7] suggested that decreased HRV does not predict SCD after MI and is not related to LVEF, heart rate, and AE. However spontaneous VA can iniciate VT in certain electrophysiological conditions depending upon sympathovagal balance of the heart[8]. Parasympathetic dysfunction was significantly higher in the group with impaired LV function (LVEF<40%) corresponding to VA. Decreased HRV could lead to reentry mechanism which might be responsible for SCD in pts after MI with severely affected myocardium[9]. A field of extreme relevance in which more information is needed on its neural mechanism, concerns acute cardiovascular events and in particular the prevention of SCD. The inclusion of spectral analysis of cardiovascular variability in research protocols is promising.

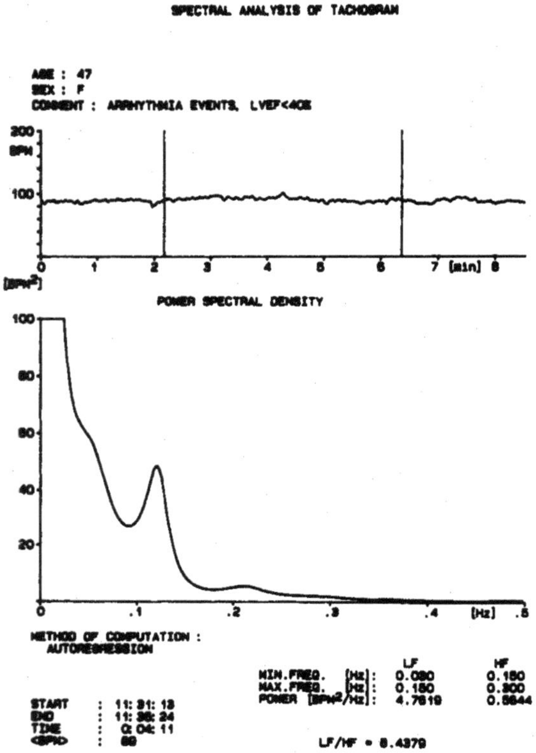

Fig. 2.
Registration of HRV in a patient from Gr 2 with arrhythmia event. Upper tracing: spectral analysis of tachogram. Lower tracing: power spectral densities of HRV.

REFERENCES

1. J.P. Zbilut, L. Lawson, *Crit.Care Med.* **16** (1988) 64
2. L.E. Hinkle, H.T. Thaler, *Circulation* **65** (1982) 457
3. A. Shiina, A.J. Tajik, H.C. Smith, M. Lengyel, *Mayo Clinic Proc.* **61** (1986) 254
4. M.Malik, T. Farrell, T. Cripps, A. Camm, *Eur.Heart.J.* **10** (1989) 1060
5. J.T. Bigger, R.E. Kleiger, K. Fleiss, *Am.J.Cardiol.* **61** (1988) 208.
6. M.V. Kenneth, D.N. Ghista, E.L. Fallen, D. Fitchett, D.Miller *Heart Vessels* **3** (1987) 33
7. R.E. Kleiger, J.P. Miller, J.T. Bigger, A.J. Moss, *Am. J. Cardiol.* **23** (1989) 245
8. G. Myers, C. Martin, N. Magin, *IEEE Trans.Biomed Eng.* **BME-33** (1986) 1149
9. T. Cripps, E. Bennett, A. Camm, D. Ward, *Br.Heart J.* **60** (1988) 181

IDENTIFICATION OF RISK OF VENTRICULAR TACHYCARDIA IN PATIENTS WITH HYPERTROPHIC CARDIOMYOPATHY

Stefan Trzos, Włodzimierz J. Musiał, Jerzy W. Kozłowski, Małgorzata Kurpesa

Medical University, Łódź, Poland
90-123 Łódź, Kopcińskiego 22

ABSTRACT

The aim of the study was to assess the main factors influencing the risk of malignant ventricular arrhythmia in patients (pts) with hypertrophic cardiomyopathy (HCM). In 55 pts 48-hour ecg monitoring was performed twice a year and presence of nonsustained ventricular tachycardia (nVT) was classified as arrhythmia event (AE). Pts were divided into two groups (Gr)- Gr.1 - 30 pts with AE and Gr.2 - 25 pts without AE. The type of left ventricular hypertrophy (LVH) and presence of systolic anterior motion (SAM) were diagnosed by 2-D echo. In all pts signal averaged ECG and assessment of autonomic regulation were carried out. Ventricular late potentials (VLP) were analysed using 40-Hz filter frequences and sympatho-vagal balance (SVB) was assessed by low (LF-0.03-0.15 Hz) and high (HF-0.15-0.35 Hz) frequency bands. Comparison of groups was made and differences in clinical features (syncope) and other symptoms such as SAM, progression of LVH, VLP and SVB were analysed. There was a significant positive relation ($p<0.02$) only between lower HF values and higher LF/HF ratio and presence of malignant arrhythmias. Conclusion: the presence of severe AE in pts with HC may be associated with impaired parasympathetic activity.

Hypertrophic cardiomyopathy (HCM) has the yearly mortality rate of approx. 4% - with over 80% sudden death events (SDE)[1]. Many investigations are made to reveal the SDE mechanism and to establish prognostic factors determining high risk group of pts. Some authors are indicating the appearance of nVT recorded in 24-hour Holter monitoring as the predicting factor for sudden death hazard[2,3]. The aim of the study was to estimate the risk factors influencing onset of ventricular arrhythmia in pts with HCM by noninvasive method.

MATERIAL AND METHODS

55 pts were investigated (34 male, 21 female) aged 18-75 y (mean age 41.2 y) with clinically diagnosed HCM confirmed by 2-D echocardiography with Doppler evaluation. Classification was made according to the type of hypertrophy and its progression, evidence of SAM, onsets of syncopal attacs. All pts underwent 48-hour Holter monitoring. The appearance of nVT was classified as arrhythmia event (AE). According to these findings two groups were analysed: Gr. 1 - 30 pts with AE and Gr. 2 - 25 pts without AE, with high gain Ecg investigation. Spectral analysis of QRS complex (final 40 ms.) was made using Fast Fourier Transform (512 points, Blackman-Harris window). VLP were estimated according to Simson-Denes criteria[2]. In all pts spectral parameters of heart rate variability (HRV) were calculated using autoregressive multivariate modelling. Total value of spectral density in low frequency range (LF - 0.03-0.15 Hz) representing sympathetic activity, high frequency (HF - 0.15-0.35 Hz) for parasympathetic function, so as LF/HF ratio were measured. Investigations were performed in supine and standing positions with spontaneous respiration.

RESULTS

Tabl. 1 presents comparison of parameters evaluated in both groups of pts. Syncopal attacs, evidence of SAM, progression of LVH were common for both groups. LP were registered commonly in Gr. 1 (no statistically significant). Statistically significant was only the relationship between the low HF values and high LF/HF ratio to nVT onsets ($p<0.02$).

Table 1.

	Gr. 1 No.	Gr. 2 No.
syncope	10	9
SAM	11	10
progression of LVH	15	13
sympatho-vagal balance		
LF (BPM^2/Hz)	7,2	7,8
HF (BPM^2/Hz)	2,5	5,1
LF/HF	2,8	1,2

Typical examples of HRV spectral analysis in patients with and without ventricular arrhythmias are presented in fig. 1, 2.

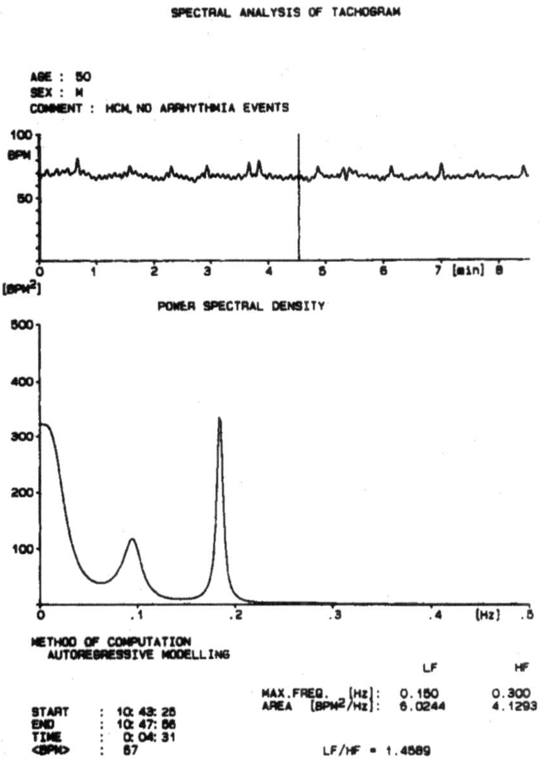

Fig. 2. Original registration of HRV in a patient from gr. 1 without nVT. Upper tracing: spectral analysis of tachogram. Lower tracing: power spectral densities of HRV.

DISCUSSION

HCM is often asymptomatic[5]. Frank[6] suggested correlation between syncopal attacs and complex ventricular arrhythmias. According to Nienaber[7] the risk of sudden death in young pts below 30 year of age with complex AE was related to syncope. However Needleman[8] is of opinion that nVT observed in 25% pts with HCM have little influence on the prognosis. Romeo[9] indicates that the LV function is of importance for estimation of the arrhythmia risk. Spectral analysis of HRV, the noninvasive method for evaluation of the function of autonomic nervous system, seems to be useful for investigation of pts with HCM especially for the arrhythmia group. Our investigations showed low HF values and increased LF/HF ratio thus indicating possibility of parasympathetic dysfunction for susceptibility of fatal ventricular arrhythmias.

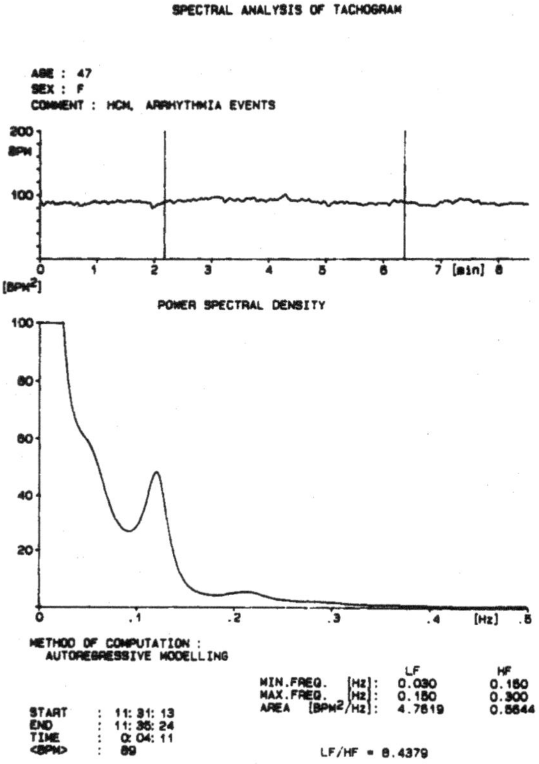

Fig. 3.
Registration of HRV in a patient from group 2 with nVT. Upper tracing: spectral analysis of tachogram. Lower tracing: power spectral densities of HRV.

REFERENCES

1. W.J. Mc Kenna, M. Davies, *Med.Clin of North Am.* **68** (1984) 983
2. B.J. Maron, A. Tajik, B. Ruttenberg, W.C. Roberts, S.E. Epstein, *Circulation* **65** (1982) 388
3. D. Savage, S. Seides, B.J. Maron, Circulation **59** (1979) 666
4. M.B. Simson, *Circulation* **64** (1981) 235
5. R.O. Brandenburg, *JACC* **15** (1990) 962
6. M.J. Frank, Z. Watkins, M. Prisant, *Am. J. Cardiol.* **53** (1984) 1608
7. Ch. Nienaber, S. Hiller, R. Spielman, M. Geiger, *JACC* **15** 948
8. C. Needleman, G. Gardiner, D. Lewin, *Cardiol.* **150** (1988) 1219
9. F. Romeo, F. Pellicio,R. Cristofani, A. Peale, *Eur. Heart J.* **11** (1990) 233

AUTONOMIC DYSFUNCTION IN PATIENTS WITH SICK SINUS SYNDROME

Włodzimierz J. Musiał, Stefan Trzos, Jerzy W.Kozłowski, Małgorzata Kurpesa, Piotr Rozentryt

I Medical Clinic, Medical Academy Łódź, Poland
93-113 Łódź, Milionowa 14

ABSTRACT

In 41 patients with symptomatic sick sinus syndrome (SSS) the activity of the autonomic nervous system was evaluated. Fast Fourier analysis of heart rate variability (HRV) was performed. Spectral density of HRV in 2 frequency domains: low frequency (LF) mostly sympathetic activity and high frequency (HF) pure parasympathetic activity were calculated. Separate samples were obtained for horizontal and vertical position before and after administration of atropine. The parasympathetic activity allowed to divide the studied pts into 4 groups. In 11-27% of pts-gr. 1 the parasympathetic activity was within the normal range. In the remaining cases this activity was disturbed. 9 pts - 22%, gr. 2 showed very low HF values accompanied by the low sympathetic activity. This finding suggested in our opinion the organic lesion of the sinus node. In 51% of studied pts (gr. 3 - 5 cases and gr. 4 - 16 cases) the parasympathetic activity was high and extremely high. There were no significant changes in HF values in 16 pts with very high parasympathetic activity after atropine.

Sick sinus syndrome (SSS) still envokes great interest, because majority of patients (pts) need implantation of a pacemaker. Despite the progress the precise mechanism of sinus node dysfunction is still unknown. In the late 70's the ecg changes were correlated with the disfunction of autonomic nervous system[1].Extrinsic and intrinsic forms of the disease were postulated[2]. Spectral analysis of heart rate variability (HRV) is a reliable noninvasive method for evaluation of the function of autonomic nervous system. The purpose of present work was to evaluate the activity of autonomic system in pts with SSS.

MATERIAL AND METHODS

41 pts (30 females and 11 males, age 21-67 years, mean age 42) with symptomatic SSS confirmed by clinical course, Holter monitoring and electrophysiologic tests were studied. Fast Fourier analysis of HRV was performed using a autoregressive modelling method. Spectral densities of HRV in 2 frequency domains : low frequency (LF) - 0,05-0,15 Hz mostly sympathetic activity and high frequency (HF) - 0,15-0,35 Hz pure parasympathetic activity were measured. Separate samples for horizontal and vertical position were obtained with spontaneous respiration and the HF/LF ratios were calculated before and after administration of atropine (i.v. 0,04 mg/kg body weight).

RESULTS

The parasympathetic activity allowed to devide studied pts into 4 groups (gr) - fig. 1.

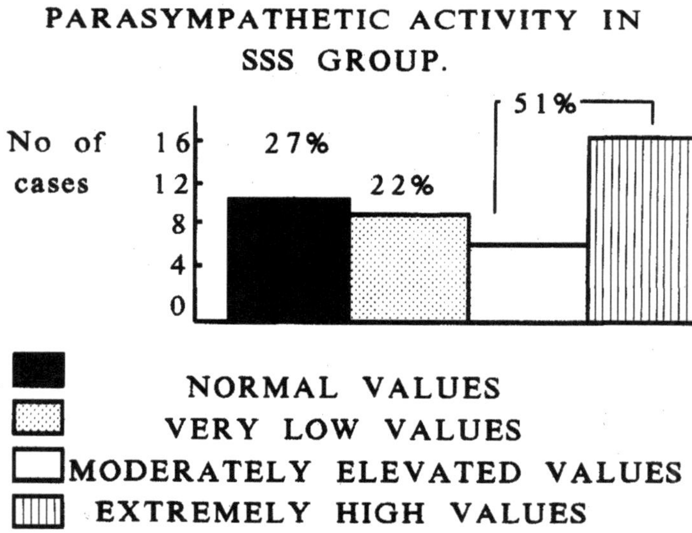

Fig. 1.
Parasympathetic activity in 41 SSS pts. Details in the text.

In the first gr (11 cases- 27%) the parasympathetic activity was within the normal range comparable to the values obtained in our laboratory in 55 control cases (LF_1 3,5 BPM^2/Hz, HF_1 3,0 BPM^2/Hz in supine position, LF_2 8,5 BPM^2/Hz, HF_2 1,5 BPM^2/Hz in standing position; $LF_2 + LF_2 + HF_1 + HF_2 > 7{,}5$ BPM^2/Hz). In the second gr (9 cases - 21%) the HF values vere very low and were accompanied by low sympathetic activity. In 51% of pts gr 3 (5 cases - 12%)

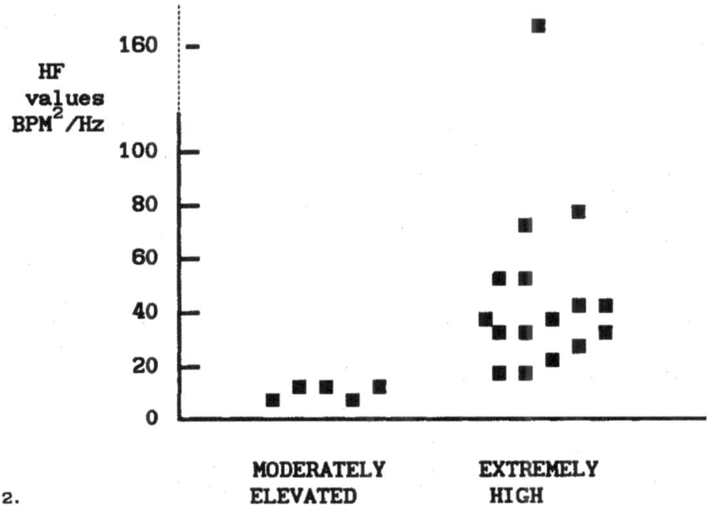

Fig. 2.
Parasympathetic activity in pts with moderately elevated (gr 3) and extremely high (gr 4) HF values in the control conditions before atropine.

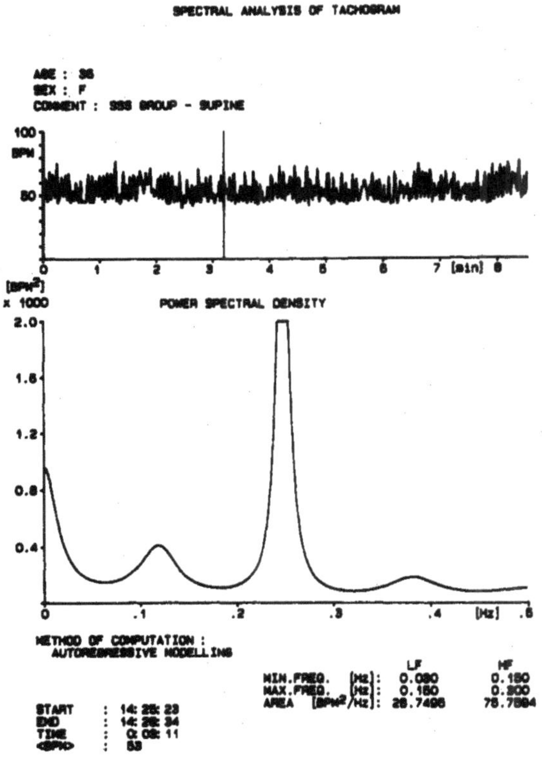

Fig. 3.
Original registration of HRF in a patient with a very high parasympathetic activity. Upper tracing: spectral analysis of tachogram. Lower tracing: power spectral densities of HRV showed very high HF values (75,7 BPM^2/HZ). Registration made in supine position before atropine.

and gr 4 (16 cases - 39%) the parasympathetic activity was high or extremely high, about 10 times greater than in control group - fig. 2, 3. In gr. 3 with elevated parasympathetic activity atropine caused normalization of the values. However there were no significant changes in HF values after atropine in cases with very high parasympathetic activity - gr. 4.

DISCUSSION

Spectral analysis of heart rate variability is a new non-invasive method for assessment of activity of autonomic system. Till now evaluation of autonomic regulation of the circulatory system was based mainly on reflexes. Estimation of sympatho--vagal balance using HRV was recently performed in some clinical conditions, but not in SSS. It was used for prediction of serious ventricular arrhythmias or sudden cardiac death in acute phase of myocardial infarction or in pts after infarction[3,4]. It also appeared as a useful parameter for assessment of transplant rejection in heart transplant pts[5].

The results of our study indicated that in great number of SSS cases the autonomic nervous function was abnormal. Nearly half of them showed high or very high parasympathetic activity. In the group with extremely high HF values they can't be significantly changed by artropine.

Enhanced parasympathetic activity in SSS pts was also shown during electrophysiologic studies with pharmacological denervation. Basing on this findings intrinsic and extrinsic forms of the disease were postulated[2]. These two different types of changes had also clinical implications. Pacemaker had to be implanted more frequently in pts with intrinsic sinus node dysfunction because of accompanying disease. In extrinsic form of SSS syncope is more frequently observed[2]. Low sympathetic and parasympathetic activity diagnosed with spectral analysis in 22% of cases represent in our opinion the intrinsic form of sinus node dysfunction. However further studies are necessary to correlate the clinical picture, electrophysiologic data and spectral analysis of HRV in a greater group of patients.

REFERENCES

1. J.L. Jordan, I. Yamaguchi, W.J. Mandel, *Circulation* **57** (1978) 217
2. Z. Ciemniewski, L. Zając, E. Świderska et all. *Kard. Pol.* **35** (1991) 3
3. D. Mc Areavey, J. Neilson, D. Ewing, D. Russel, *Brit. Heart J.* **62** (1989) 165
4. F. Lombardi, G. Sandrone, S. Pernpruner et all. *Am.J.Cardiol.* **60** (1987) 1239
5. K. Sands, M. Appel, L. Lilly et all. *Circulation* **79** (1989) 76

ADENOSIN TRIPHOSPHATE: MECHANISMS OF REVERSION OF THE PAROXYSMAL SUPRAVENTRICULAR TACHYCARDIA

Cabrera Sole, R.[*]; Lucas Imbernón, F.J.; Peñalver Pardines, C.; Jiménez Hernández, P.A.; García García, C.; Galán Traba, M.A.; Paya Berbegal, J..

Departments of Cardiology[*] and Emergency from the Albacete General Hospital. Albacete. Spain.

ABSTRACT

To evalue the different electrocardiografhic characteristics of the paroxismal supraventricular tachycardia (PST), during reversion to sinus rhythm (SR) with adenosine triphosphate (ATP), we have prospectively studied 50 spontaneus episodes of PST in 41 patients, who were treated with 0,3 mg/Kg/dose of ATP given intravenously. We found the following results:

Group I: 19 episodes of PST reverted to SR by A-V block (AVB),
Group II: 9 episodes of PST reverted by VPC+AVB,
Group III: 9 episodes of PST reverted by AVB + Ventricular Premature Complexes (VPC),
Group IV: 8 PST converted by VPC, and
Group V; 5 PST reverted to SR by non sustained ventricular tachy - cardia (ns VT).

The average time of conversion was 27.8+8.9 seconds. We found a lengthening of R-R intervals in 42 cases of PST and 20 of the had electrical alternancy, both previous to conversion to SR.
We can conclude that there are five predominant ways to reversion of PST treated with ATP, being AVB significantlymore frecuent with respect to another forms. We did not observe any dangerous arrhythmias when PST were converted to SR with ATP

Keys words: Paroxysmal Supraventricular Tachycardia. Adenosine Triphosphate.

INTRODUCTION

The efficacy of ATP in the conversion of paroxysmal supraventricular tachycardia (PST) to sinus rhytm (SR) has been demostrated in several studies, being at this time one of first ejection drug in the treatment of PST[1,2]. Conversion porcentage are between 90 to 100 % of cases depending of the different studies[3,4], however, litle has been writen about the mechanisms of reversion of this PST evaluating a standard electrocardiogram. We know that one of the principal effects of ATP is the auriculo-ventricular node block (AVB), but, until now, nobody have demostrated any effect neither ventricular[5] or Hissien conduction systems[6]. Herein, we pretend to make a description of different electrocardiographic morphologies which are possible to find analysing a standard electrocardiogram of this PSV, when they are converted to SR with ATP.

MATERIAL AND METHODS

We have prospectively studied 50 episodes of PST in 41 patients, who were admitted at the emergency room of our hospital. Our exclusion criteria were previus bronchospasm history, a known allergy to ATP or cardiac failure at the moment of admission. After this, all patients submited to a physical examination, we measured heart rate, blood presure and we made a carotid sinus massage. If this latest was negative we administered intravenously in bolo 0.3 mg/kg/dose of ATP. During this time a continuous electrocardiogram strip in V1 or II leadswas recorded, in order to obtain the transicion of PST to SR.

After, we evaluated the different forms in which the PST were converted to SR, time to start the ATP effect, duration of transition time and the different electrocardiografic alterations inmediatly before and after the conversion of PST.

Statistical Analysis

All data were expresed as media with standard desviation. We compared the different parameters using Student T for parametric data and Chi square test for non parametric data. We considered significant p value equal or less than 0.05.

TABLE I: DIFERENT PARAMETERS EVALUATED IN THE CONVERSION OF PST TO SINUS RHYTHM

PARAMETERS	AVB	VPC+AVB	AVB+VPC	VPC	nsVT
Number of cases	*19 (38 %)	9 (18 %)	9 (18 %)	8 (16 %)	5 (10 %)
Heart rate of PST	179,8±27,6	185,8±21,5	189,4±15,1	193,4±22,0	205,0±20,5
Heart rate of SR	101,6±12,1	86,6±14,9	100,0±12,2	86,2± 6,9	100,0±18,7
On set time to start effect of ATP (sec.)	24,5±10,5	27,6± 6,1	27,5±10,6	33,8± 6,2	27,9± 5,4
Time of reversion to SR (sec.)	*0,8± 0,3	3,2± 0,9	1,8±1,4	4,9± 2,1	3,7± 2,5
Electrical alternance	4 (21,1%)	3 (33,3%)	3 (33,3%)	7 (87,5%)	3 (60%)

AVB: Auricle Ventricular Block. VPC: Ventricular Premature Complexe.
nsVT: Non Sustained Ventricular Tachycardia
* $p < 0{,}05$.

RESULTS

There were not statitical differences with respect to age and sex of the groups, being the average of age of 47,6 + 14,2 years. We detected five different groups considering the mechanisms of reversion of the PST: Group I with 19 episodes of PST converted to - SR by AV block, bein the communest way of reversion: Group II with 9 PST which were finished by premature ventricuar beats followed by AV block: Group III with 9 PST converted to SR by EV block followed by premature ventricular beats: Group IV with 8 episodes reverted by isolated premature ventricular beats and finally group V with 5 PST - converted to SR by non sustained polimorphic ventricular tachycardia. The mean heart rate during the PST was of 187.3±24.3 beat per minute (bpm) and during SR was of 96.3± 14.3 bpm without differences between groups. Mean time of conversion was 27.8±8.9 seconds from the time in which the drug was administered. Electrical alternacy inmediatly before of conversion we have found in 20 cases of PST (40%), without differences - between groups.

DISCUSSION

ATP depress the sinus and auriculo-ventricular nodes conduction[5]. These effects do to this drug a very useful tool in the treatment of PST in the acute phase and translated these effect in the convertional electrocardiogram we find a AV block when we use ATP.
Auriculo ventricular block is the most frecuent way which ATP convert PST to SR, being possible to find it in 80% of cases in which ATP is used[3]. We found this study in 56% of our cases. Other investigators have found third degree AV block in 70% and second degree AV block in 30% of their patients treated with ATP[1].However it is possible to find another forms of conversion, different of AV block such as ventricular premature beats which represent in our study 18% of all conversion forms and 20% in the serie of Belhassen and coworker[3]. AV block followed by ventricular premature complexes we found in 18% of our cases but we did not find any previous references on this way of conversion in the literature. Non sustained ventricular trachycardia is an unfrecuent way if conversion of PST which we found in 10% of cases, while other authors[3] found in 5% of their patients.
Electrical alternancy, seconds before conversion of PST, frecuently seen with verapamilo, we found in 40% of this serie. This is a phenomena which is difficult to explain, suggesting an effect of the tachycardia on the conduction system and not of the ATP properly speaking[7].
Other studies have shown several arrhythmias using ATP, like as auricular fibrilation or flutter[8], supraventricular premature beats[9],which show that ATP has different ways of termination of PST although there are predominants patterns.

CONCLUSIONS

ATP must be considered a drug of first election in the treatment of PST in acute phase, because is very effective, does not have any dangerous effects on the patients, and despite its different ways to convert the PST to SR we did not find any threatening arrhythmias when we used it.

REFERENCES

1-S. Favale; M. Di Biase; U. Rizzo et al: effect of adenosine triphosphate and adenosine Triphosphate and Adenosine on Atrioventricular conduction in patients. J. An Coll Cardiol 5 (1985) 1212.

2-JP. Di Marco; T.D. Sellers; RM. Berne et al: Adenosine: Electrophysiologic effects and Therapeutic Use for Teminating Supraventricular Tachycardias. Circulation 63 (1983) 1254.

3-B. Belhassen; A.Glick; S. Laniado et al: Comparative. Clinical and Electrophysiologic effects of Adenosine Triphosphate and Verapamil on Paroxysmal Supraventricular Tachycardia. Circulation 77 (1988) 795.

4-R. Cabrera Sole; M. Abeytua; L. Lopez Bescos; R. Rubio: Treatment of Verapamilo.Circulation II-80 (1989) 632.

5-L. Bellardinelli; EC. Mattos; R. Berne: Evidence for Adenosine Mediation Of Atrioventricular Block in the Ischemic Canine Myocardium. J. Clin Invest 68 (1981) 195.

6-L. Bellardinelli; RA. Fenton; A. West et al: Extracellular action of Adenosine and the Antagonism by Aminophylline on the Atrioventricular conduction of Isolated Perfused Guinea Pig and Rat Hearts. Cir Res 51 (1982) 569.

7-DH. Spodick: Electrical Alternation of the Heart. Am. J. Cardiol 10 (1962) 155.

8-B. Perrot; Clozel JP.; Faivre G.: Effects of Adenosine Triphospphate on the accesory pathways. Europ Heart J. 5 (1984) 382.

9-L. Garrat; A. Antonion; M. Griffith; D. Ward; J. Gamm: Use of Intravenons adenosine in Sinus Rhythm as a Diagnostic Test for Latent Preexitation. Am. J. Card. 65 (1999) 868.

4:2 SINO-ATRIAL BLOCK DUE TO HYPERKALEMIA WITH ELECTROTONIC INFLUENCE OF A-V JUNCTIONAL IMPULSES UPON THE SINUS NODE

Gaetano Satullo, Giovanni Sergi, Giuseppe Busà, Antonino Coglitore, Lucio Cavallaro and Giuseppe Oreto *

Servizio di Cardiologia con UTIC, Ospedale Papardo, USL 41, 98122 Messina, Italy.
(*) Istituto Pluridisciplinare di Clinica Medica, Cattedra di Malattie Cardiovascolari, Università di Messina, Messina, Italy.

ABSTRACT

This presentation reflects a rather uncommon manifestation of hyperkalemia, namely the influence exterted by an A-V junctional rhythm upon the S-A node in the absence of any manifest atrial activation. A patient with Addison disease and hyperkalemia manifested with sino-atrial block; at the end of long pauses occasioned by the block, A-V junctional escape beats occured, but the A-V junctional impulses did not result in retrograde atrial activation. Calculation demonstrated a relationship between the duration of the escape intervals and the sinus cycle length; namely short escape intervals were associated with relatively short sinus cycles. This suggested an influence of the A-V junctional impulses on the sinus node. And since no manifest retrograde atrial activation occured the influence of the A-V junctional rhythm upon the sinus node was probably mediated by conduction of the impulses across the crista terminalis, with further electrotonic influence on the sinus pacemaker cells. Laboratory research has demonstrated that A-V junctional impulses may indeed affect the sinus node without the occurrence of any manifest atrial depolaritation. This is the opposite of the so-called sino-ventricular conduction, namely the direct trasmission of the sinus impulse to the ventricles without depolaritation of the entire atrial mass.

Hyperkalemia is frequently associated with S-A block, and even with disappearance of P waves due to inexcitability of atrial fibers. In the latter condition, however, sinus impulses may at times reach the A-V node throughth the atrial conduction pathways despite lack of depolarization of the entire atrial chamber. This has been termed "sinoventricular conduction".[1]

This presentation reflects a somewhat opposite phenomenon with respect to sinoventricular conduction: namely, the influence exerted on the sinus node by an A-V junctional pacemaker in the absence of manifest retrograde atrial activation by the A-V junctional impulses.

CASE REPORT

The electrocardiograms were recorded from a 67-year-old female affected by Addison disease. At the time of the observation the serum Potassium was 7.3 mEq. Figure 1 show a Type II S-A block with 4:2 conduction ratio. It is evident that sinus P waves occur in pairs, and the pairs are separated from each other from pauses whose duration is approximately 3 times the basic sinus cycle length. The first P wave in each pair always closely follows an A-V junctional escape beat, and is often superimposed upon the preceding T wave. The sinus origin of such an "early" P wave is proved by its configuration,that is identical to that of the ensuing "late" P wave.

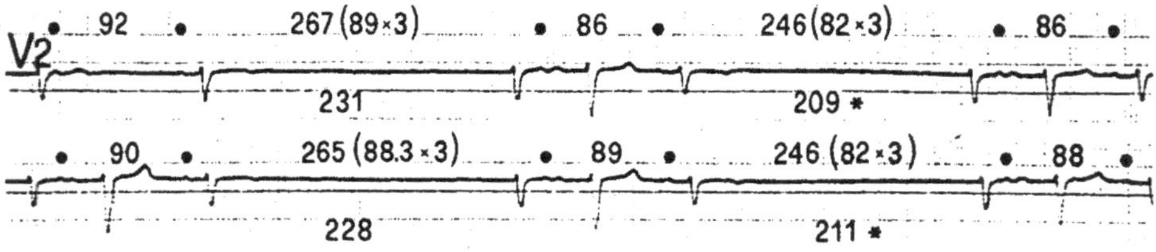

FIGURE 1

"Early" P waves occur with coupling intervals ranging from 0.08 to 0.36 sec; very early sinus impulses are blocked in the A-V node, whereas impulses with relatively long coupling intervals are conducted to the ventricles with P-R intervals whose duration is directly related to the prematurity. Several conducted impulses, in addition, are associated with aberrant ventricular conduction, as reflected by an increased S wave voltage, with respect to the S waves of normally conducted beats.

The diagnosis of 4:2 S-A block is strongly suggested by pauses whose duration is three times the sinus cycle length. For example, the first pause in the second strip of Figure 1 measures 2.65 sec, that corresponds to 3 times the ensuing sinus cycle of 0.89 sec.

The normalization of serum potassium levels resulted in disappearance of the S-A block and restoration of normal sinus rhythm.

Several pauses are shorter than expected, namely less than 3 times the manifest sinus cycle length. For example, the pause of 2.46 sec in the 2th strip corresponds to 0.82 x 3, whereas both the preceding and the following P-P intervals are longer than 0.82 sec, and measure 0.89 sec and 0.88 sec respectively. The sligth difference beetween manifest sinus cycle (or P-P interval) and sinus cycle calculated by dividing the long pause could theoretically be casual, or related to sinus arrhythmia. Analysis of the entire recording, however, reveals that pauses shorter than expected are always associated with shortened A-V junctional escape intervals. Escape intervals ranging from 2.01 to 2.11 sec (labeled with asterisks) are always associated with pauses shorter than expected, whereas with escape intervals of 2.20 sec or more the corresponding pauses are 3 times the preceding or the ensuing P-P interval.

Definition of terms:

P1,P2 = The first and the second sinus P wave in a pair <u>preceding</u> a pause.
P3,P4 = The first and the second sinus P wave in a pair <u>following</u> a pause.
P2-P3 = The long pause containing 2 consecutive blocked sinus impulses.
The same pair of P waves may be therefore defined as P1,P2 with respect to the ensuing pause, and as P3,P4 with respect to the preceding pause.

Figure 2 represents the data deduced from a continuous 5-minute recording. The abscissa reflects the escape interval duration, and the ordinate reflects the ratio between the pause (P2-P3) and the sum of the P-P intervals that precede and follow the pause (P1-P2 + P3-P4). Since any pause contains 3 sinus cycles, in the presence of an exactly regular sinus discharge the ratio

$$\frac{P2\text{-}P3}{P1\text{-}P2 + P3\text{-}P4}$$

should be 1.5, namely 3/2. The diagram of Figure 2 shows two distinct zones: 1) A zone 1 (plateau), corresponding to escape intervals ranging from 2.22 to 2.46 sec. In this zone the ratio is about 1.5, ranging from 1.46 to 1.54. No relationship occurs between the escape interval and the ratio. This reveals that the pause length (P2-P3) is independent of the escape interval duration. 2) A zone 2, corresponding to escape intervals of 2.16 sec or less. In this zone there is a clear relationship between the escape interval and the ratio, a decrease in the escape interval duration being associated with a parallel decrease in the ratio and viceversa. The reduction of the ratio indicates that, with relatively short escape intervals, the pause (P2-P3) is reduced, and the reduction is related to the decrease of the escape interval.

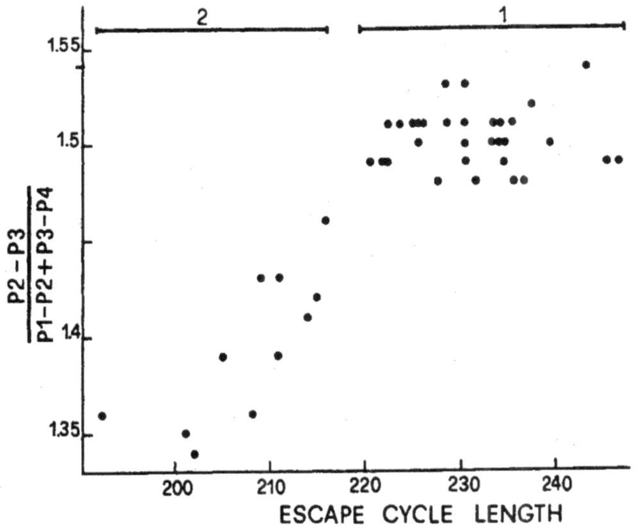

FIGURE 2

DISCUSSION

This patient had a rather uncommon form of S-A block, a 4:2 block. HyperKalemia was almost certainly responsible for the conduction disturbance. The sinus cycle is relatively constant, apart from some exceptions, in such a way that the long pauses, containing 2 blocked sinus impulses, correspond to roughly 3 times the P-P interval. This holds true as long as the A-V junctional escape interval is longer than 2.20 sec. Contrarywise, escape intervals shorter than 2.18 sec are associated with pauses that are less than 3 times the manifest sinus cycle. It is thus very likely that the A-V junctional rhythm affects in some way the sinus node automaticity. In other words, a relatively early A-V junctional escape impulse accelerates the ensuing sinus discharge, resulting in shortening of the pause. This phenomenon is, at first glance, very difficult to be explained, since the A-V junctional escape impulse does not depolarize the atria, so that the influence of the escape rhythm on the sinus node is independent of atrial activation.

It is well know that in the presence of hyperkalemia the sinus impulse may still be conducted to the A-V node through the specialized atrial conduction pathways without depolarization of the atrial working myocardium, namely without occurrence of the P wave. This is defined as sino-ventricular conduction.[1] Sanchis and Coll[2] have recently demonstrated that in hyperkalemia an A-V junctional rhythm may influence the S-A node without activation of the entire atrial mass. The influence was mediated by impulse conduction across the crista terminalis, resulting in electrotonic influence upon the sinus pacemaker cells. In the experimental work by Sanchis, the electrotonic influence exerted by the AV junctional rhythm upon the S-A node was governed by a monophasic curve: A-V junctional impulses that occured either very early or very late within the sinus cycle did not exert any effect, whereas intermediate impulses accelerated the ensuing sinus discharge.

The phenomena observed in the present case are quite similar to those described by Sanchis[2] in his laboratory research. The A-V junctional escape impulse, thus, does not result in manifest atrial depolarization, but could still be conducted across the crista terminalis and reach the S-A node. The most evident effect due to electrotonus is acceleration of the ensuing sinus discharge. This occurs only when the A-V junctional impulse is relatively early, in accordance with the experimental data. It could be inferred, in addition, that the electrotonic influence of the A-V junctional impulse facilitates the S-A conduction, allowing the sinus impulse to traverse the S-A junction.[3] This is likely, but cannot be proven in the present case.

REFERENCES

1. De Carvalho AP, Langan WB: Influence of extracellular potassium levels on atrioventricular transmission. Am J Physiol 205 (1963) 375.

2. Sanchis J, Opthof T, Wilde AAM, Janse MJ: Mutual electrotonic interaction between the rabbit sinoatrial node and atrioventricular node. J Cardiovasc Electrophysiol 1 (1990) 318.

3. Antzelevitch C: Electrotonus and reflection. In Cardiac electrophysiology: a textbook. Eds Rosen MR, Janse MJ, Wit AL (Futura Publishing Company, Inc., Mount Kisco, NY 1990)

PART IV

Cardiac Electrophysiology and Conduction

EFFECTS OF VARIATION OF LEFT VENTRICULAR CONDUCTING SYSTEM TERMINATIONS ON THE VECTORCARDIOGRAM

VAVRINEC SZATHMÁRY, IVAN RUTTKAY-NEDECKÝ, RÓBERT OSVALD
Institute of Normal and Pathological Physiology,
Slovak Academy of Sciences, Sienkiewiczova 1, Bratislava,
Czech and Slovak Federative Republic

ABSTRACT

A realistic computer model of the propagation of ventricular activation was used to study the effects of varying the position of places of initial activation in the left ventricle on resulting spatial heart vectors. The foci of initial activation were on the left ventricular endocardial surface: in the central part of septum, posteriorly about one third of the distance from apex to base and in the upper part of the anterior free wall. Variations of their positions were achieved by shifting them ± 5 mm in the vertical and lateral directions. Shifting of the basal focus led to significantly smaller changes of the vectorcardiographic loop than shifting of the more apically localized focus.

1. Introduction

The influence of interindividual differences of the localization of specific conductive system terminations on the shape of the vectorcardiogram is not sufficiently known, because of limitations of in vivo or in vitro experiments, focused on this problem. The use of a suitable computer model for this purpose may be informative.

2. Method

In our computer model of ventricular activation propagation [1] the ventricular dimensions were determined analytically in agreement with published data for human hearts[2]. The left and right ventricles as well as the interventricular septum consisted of 149017 elements, leading to a resolution of about $1mm^3$.

The position of starting points of ventricular activation corresponded to regions of earliest activation on the endocardial surfaces as published by Durer et al.[3] : 1 - on the mid-septum, between its anteroseptal and inferior segments; 2 - at the region between the middle and apical parts of the postero lateral segment; 3 - at the basal part on the boundary between the antero-septal and antero-superior segments. The activation of the left ventricle was started in three consecutive steps.

The localization of starting points was varied by shifting their position in apical-basal (meridional) and lateral (equatorial) directions. The extent of these small shifts was five arbitrary model units, which corresponded approximately to 5 mm.

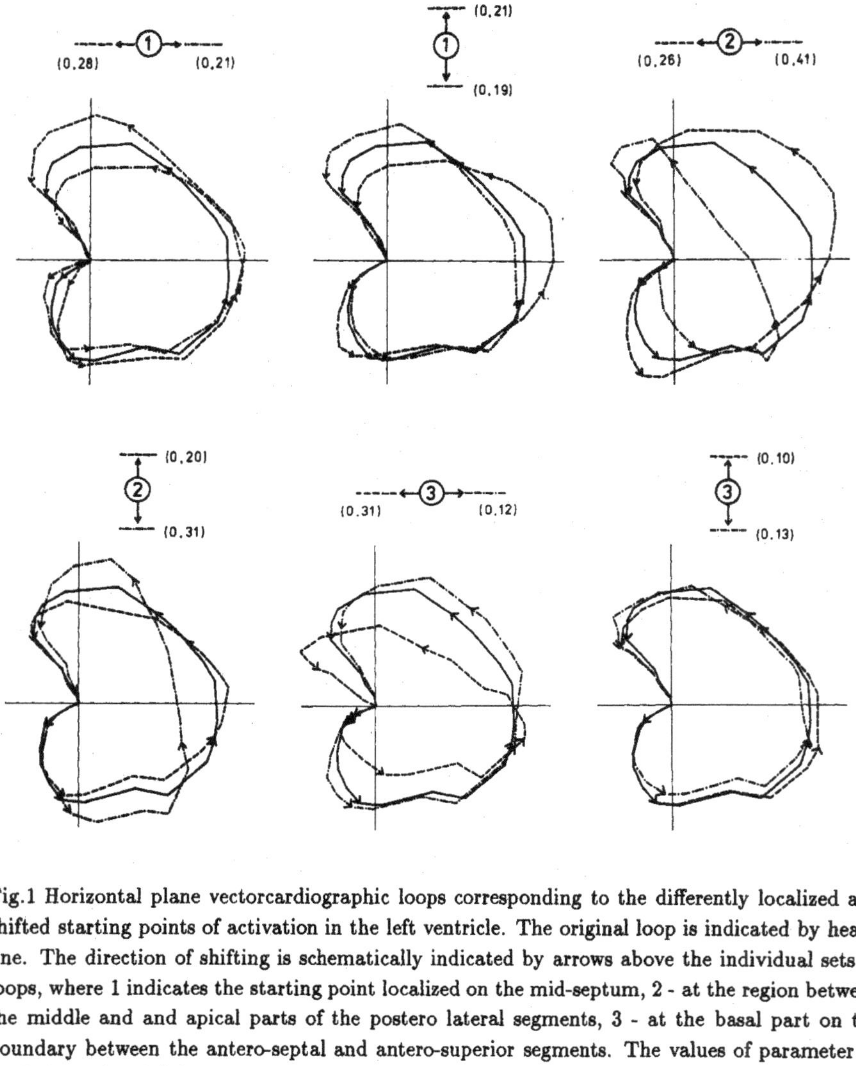

Fig.1 Horizontal plane vectorcardiographic loops corresponding to the differently localized and shifted starting points of activation in the left ventricle. The original loop is indicated by heavy line. The direction of shifting is schematically indicated by arrows above the individual sets of loops, where 1 indicates the starting point localized on the mid-septum, 2 - at the region between the middle and and apical parts of the postero lateral segments, 3 - at the basal part on the boundary between the antero-septal and antero-superior segments. The values of parameter D are indicated in brackets.

For evaluation of effects of this procedure on the resultant heart vectors a parameter D was defined as the ratio of the mean square deviation of the "shifted" vectors with respect to the original ones (MD) to the mean square value of original resultant heart vectors (MV).

$D = MD/MV$

where

$$MD = ((\sum_{t=1}^{T}(x(t) - x_o(t))^2 + \sum_{t=1}^{T}(y(t) - y_o(t))^2 + \sum_{t=1}^{T}(z(t) - z_o(t))^2) \; / \; T)^{1/2}$$
$$MV = ((\sum_{t=1}^{T} x_o(t)^2 + \sum_{t=1}^{T} y_o(t)^2 + \sum_{t=1}^{T} z_o(t)^2) \; / \; T)^{1/2}$$

$x(t), y(t), z(t)$ and $x_o(t), y_o(t), z_o(t)$ are the instantaneous values of orthogonal components of the "shifted" and original resultant heart vectors respectively. T is the duration of activation.

3. Results and Discussion

The effect of small variations of the position of starting points of activation, localized in the left ventricle, on the time course of the end points of resultant heart vector, represented by its horizontal plane projections, is shown on Fig.1.

The shifting of the mid-septal starting point in equatorial sense influenced mainly the magnitude of the terminal vectors. The anterior shift increased the posterior and rightward forces and vice versa. This kind of changes are indicative of right ventricular enlargement. The meridional shift towards the cardiac base, increased the leftward and posteriorly oriented forces, which are indicative of left ventricular hypertrophy.

Higher degree of deviation from the original loop was achieved by equatorial shifting of the starting point in the apical postero-lateral part of the left ventricle - shift towards the center of the lateral free wall led to a decrease of the magnitude of left posterior vectors and their counterclockwise rotation. These changes resemble to vectorcardiographic signs of diminishing participation of left ventricular forces in the cardiac electric field. Meridional shifts did not have characteristic effects.

The change of the position of initial activation in the basal part of left ventricle did not give significant results if they were displaced meridionally, with exception of the displacement towards the center of the lateral free wall, which diminished both the anteriorly and posteriorly oriented vectors and increased the maximum of the to the right amplitude of the loop.

Different sensitivities of vector parameters with respect to positional variations of starting points are illustrated in the graph, where vertical positions of shifted staring points are related to the parameter D (Fig.2). They are less evident if the positions of the basal starting points were changed and more pronounced if apical starting points were manipulated.

In conclusion, this model study shows that relatively small changes in localization of starting points of ventricular activation have as a consequence diagnostically

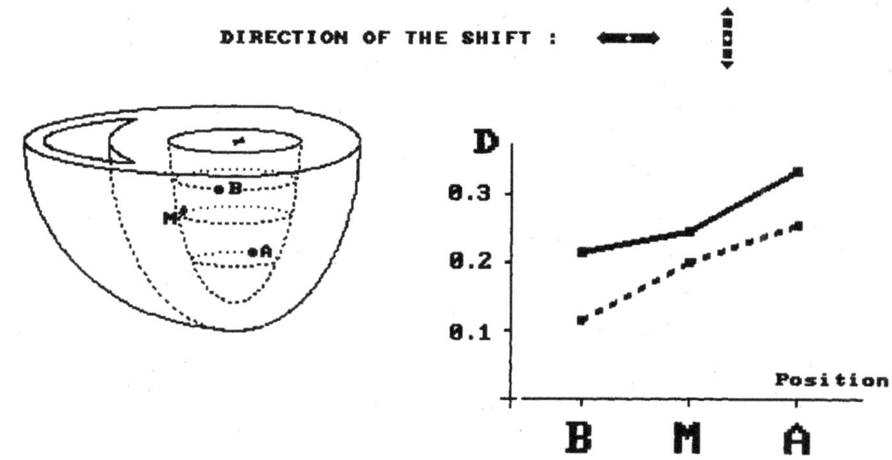

Fig.2 Graphical representation of the relation between the parameter D and vertical position of the starting points. Heavy line - mean values for shifting in apical-basal direction, broken line - mean values for shifting in lateral direction. B indicates the localization of starting point in basal, M in middle and A in apical parts of left ventricle, as it is evident from the scheme in the left part of the figure.

meaningful changes of configuration of simulated cardiac vectors and so also of the vectorcardiographic loops. It should be stressed, that such small variations in the topography of starting areas may be not only constitutional, but they may occur also as a consequence of local pathologic alterations of the myocardium.

4. References

1. I.Ruttkay-Nedecký, A. Drkošová, V. Szathmáry , in *Advances in Electrocardiology*, ed.P.d' Alché (Publications de l' Université de Caen, 1985).
2. G.M. Hutchins, B.H. Bukley, G.W. Moore, M.A. Piasion, F.V. Lohr, *Am. J. of Cardiology* **41** (1978) 646.
3. D. Durrer, R.Th. van Dam, G.E. Freud, M.J. Jause, F.L. Meijler, R.C. Azbaecher, *Circulation* **41** (1970) 899.

QUALITY OF LIFE EVALUATION IN PATIENTS WITH AUTOMATIC CARDIOVERTER DEFIBRILLATOR

Mestre J.L., Moro C., Madrid A.H., Novo L, Marín-Huerta E.
Arrhythmia Unit. Ramón y Cajal Hospital
Ctra de Colmenar Km 9,100. 28034. MADRID. SPAIN

Abstract

This article describes the psychological aspects of 54 patients with an AICD (Automatic Implantable Cardioverter Defibrillator). All they were evaluated by means of a questionnaire refered to discharges, occupationnal status, social life, sexual activity and psychological responses to device as sense of well-being, depression, optimism, dependance and security.

Fifty-seven per cent of the patients were reemployed after AICD implantation, their functional class was better than those unreemployed. Two thirds of our patients continued with their usual activities, social life and hobbies unchanged after the implant. Those with clinical discharges gave up more frequently their hobbies than those without. Sexual activity was unchanged in 48% of the patients and advanced age and poor functional class were the best predictors of the decrease in the sexual activity.

A increase in their sense of security was reported by 100% of the patients. Depression and other negative psychological responses were related with a poor functional class, more frequent discharges and inability to work.

Introduction

Automatic implantable cardioverter defibrillator is being widely used for the management of patients with malignant ventricular arrhythmias. However, psychological aspects of response to AICD implantation has been poorly studied.

We performed this study in order to asses the quality of life and the psychological profile of our patients with AICD and to identify the factors that determine it. Psychological responses to device , degree of reemployment after implantation, changes in daily activities, sexual activity, etc, and its relation with functional class and with the presence and number of discharges were specifically investigated in every patient

Material and methods

All patients who underwent implantation of the AICD in three differents medical centers were elegible for participation in this retrospective study. Fifty - four completed the specially designed questionnaire refered to number and characteristics of discharges, occupational status, social life, sexual activity, and sense of well-being, depression, optimism, dependence and security. Their mean age was 58 ± 12 years and the mean follow-up was 24 ± 18 months. Sixteen patients (30%) were in functional class III of the New York Heart Association, and no patient was in class IV.

Statistical analyses. Data are summarized as mean ± standard deviation. Qualitative group differences were evaluated using the chi-square test with Yates correction. Statistical significance was defined as $p < 0.05$.

Results

Twenty- seven patients received one or more clinic discharges during the assesment, with a mean of 14 ± 16 discharges. Ten patients (36%) received more than 10 discharges and painful discharges were experienced by 14 patients (15%).

Twenty - one patients were employed before implant, however only 12 (57%) returned to work after AICD. It wasn't significant difference of mean age between these two groups (table 1). Only 16% of the reemployed patients were in functional class III, versus 77% of patients who did not returned to work ($p < 0.05$).

TABLE 1

	Reemployed	Unemployed	p
Mean age (years)	49 + 7	50 + 10	N.S.
Functional class III	16%	77%	<0.05
Discharges	16%	55%	N.S.

About the usual activities, 63% of the patients continued with their hobbies, over 70% continued with their social life and 66% travelled as they used to.

Only 26% of the patients who continued with their hobbies received discharges versus over 90% in the group discontinuing their hobbies ($p<0.01$).

Eighty - four percent of the patients who continued with their social life were in acceptable functional class (I or II), however over 60% of the patiens who gave up their social life were in poor functional class ($p<0.01$).

Sexual activity was unchanged in 26 patients (48%), diminished in 12 (22%) and abolished in 16 patients (30%). It was a significantly more frequent presence of poor functional class and advanced age in the group who reduced their sexual activity. There was too a trend, not statistically significant, towards more frequent discharges in this group (table 2).

Concerning the psychological response, the results of the questionnaires are summarized in table 3.

Increase of their sense of security was reported by 100% of the patients and sense of well-being good or normal by 70% percent.

TABLE 2

Sexual activity	Maintained	Not maintained	p
Age (years)	46 ± 8	63 ± 10	<0.01
Functional class III	11%	46%	<0.05
Discharges	34%	64%	N.S.

TABLE 3

	Frequently	Occasionally	Never
Depression	19%	26%	55%
Dependence	64%	15%	21%
Optimism	67%	22%	11%
Security	100%	0%	0%

Functional class, presence of discharges and occupational status were related with the sense of depression (Table 4). Poor functional class presence of clinical discharges and inability to work were significantly more frequents in depressed patients.

TABLE 4

Depression		Never	Frequently/occasionally	p
F.C.	I-II	26 (86%)	12 (50%)	<0.05
	III	4 (14%)	12 (50%)	
Discharges	Yes	10 (33%)	17 (71%)	<0.05
	Not	20 (67%)	7 (69%)	
Employed	Yes	10 (33%)	2 (8%)	<0.05
	Not	20 (67%)	22 (92%)	

Discussion

Return to work after the implantation of an AICD is an important factor in evaluating the quality of life of these patients (1). In our group it was a high frequency of retirement both before and after the implant.Initially, thirty three patients were medically disabled before implantation , retired or not employed outside of the home. Due to patient limited job expectations, some patients elected early medical retirement after the implant. In addition return to work is a ongoing and gradual process, and there may yet be a group of patients returning to work after the cutoff point for the follow-up period, it is possible a late reemployment.

Surprisingly in our group it was not difference of the mean age between both groups, reemployed and unreemployed, after the implant. However, poor functional class was significantly more frequent in patients unreemployed.

In this group, over two thirds of the patients continue with their usual activities: hobbies, travels, social life with their family and friends. This is too a important factor to establish their quality of life. Patients who did not resume their usual activities were limited by urderlying cardiopathy and were in poor functional class (2).

Patients with clinical discharges gave up more frequently their hobbies after the implant and during the assesment.

Over 50% of patients maintained unchanged their sexual activity after the implant. Advanced age and poor functional class were the best predictors of the decrease in the sexual activity in these patients. In this patients with malignant ventricular arrhythmias and in their sexual partners sex becomes frequently stressful because of fear of dying or of causing a partner's death.

Sense of depression was present frequently or occasionally in 45% of the patients. This sense was significantly more frequent in patients in functional class III, in these who experienced clinical discharges and in the group not reemployed after AICD. In these cases, the severity of their heart conditions (poor functional class and, probably, more frequent discharges) prevents further job activity, leading to feelings of wothlessness, low self- esteem and depression (3,4). Changes in mood are, then, related primarily to health status, degree of functioning and ability to work (5).

Feelings of dependence were presents frequently in 64% of the patients. Overprotective and oversolicitious attitudes toward the patient are frequents from their family.

The AICD increase the sense of security in all our patients. (100%). They came to view the device as a lifesaver and symbol of psychological security.

The quality of life paremeters in this group were satisfactory in over two thirs of the patients. The aceptance of device was high and the negative psychological responses were related primarily with poor health status secondary to advanced cardiopathy.

Bibliography

1.- KR Kalbfleisch, MH Lehmann, RT Steinman,K Jackson, K Axtell, CD Schuger, PJ Tchou. **Reemployment Following Implantation of the Automatic Cardioverter Defibrillator.** Am J Cardiol 1989;64 : 199-202.

2.- C Pycha, AD Gulledge, J Hutzler,N Kadri, J Maloney. **Psychological responses to the implantable defibrillator: Preliminary observations.** Psychosomatics 1986; 27: 841-845.

3.- SC Vlay, LC Olson, GL Fricchione,R Friedman. **Anxiety and Anger in Patients with Ventricular Tachyarrhythmias.Responses after Automatic Internal Cardioveter Defibrillator Implantation.**PACE 1989; 12: 366-373

4.- DK Cooper, RM Luceri, RJ Thurer, RJ Myerburg. **The impact of the Automatic Implantable Cardioverter Defibrillator on quality of life.** Clin Prog Electrophysiol Pacing 1986; 4: 306-309.

5.- Keren R, Aarons D, Veltri EP. **Anxiety and depression in patients with life threatening ventricular arrhythmias: impact of the implantable cardioverter defibrillator.** PACE 1991; 14: 181-187.

INCREASING DOMINANCE OF CONCORDANT VENTRICULAR REPOLARIZATION SEQUENCE IN NORMAL OLDER ADULTS

Zhou S.H., Wong S., Rautaharju P.M.

EPICORE Centre, Division of Cardiology, University of Alberta, Edmonton, Alberta, T6G 2S2, Canada

ABSTRACT

Ventricular excitation time (QRS duration) has been shown to have a significant positive association with repolarization time (QT duration). QRS duration is significantly longer in males than in females. However, QT intervals in females at reproductive age are longer than in males of comparable age.

We investigated patterns of variations with age in the influence of excitation time on the QT interval in a pooled community-based population sample of 18,725 North American adults aged from 20 to 99 years with a normal resting ECG. Linear regression models were derived separately for each 10-year age group for regression of QT on QRS after forcing in the first step an optimal correction term for heart rate. QRS duration had a minimal (although still significant) influence on QT at age 20, suggesting that the reverse sequence of ventricular repolarization is most dominant in young adults. The value of QRS regression coefficient on QT increased progressively with age both in men and women, indicating that the repolarization sequence in myocardial regions excited during the second half of QRS becomes more and more concordant with the sequence of excitation.

It is concluded that the traditional concept of reverse sequence of repolarization is not uniformly valid in all myocardial regions, and that the concordant sequence tends to become increasingly prominent with increasing age.

1 Background

It has been documented that QRS duration has a significant positive association with QT interval[1]. This association suggests that the traditional concept of reverse sequence of ventricular repolarization is not uniformly valid in all myocardial regions.

The purpose of the present study was to investigate patterns of variation with age in the dominance of the influence of excitation time on the repolarization time in normal subjects.

2 Methods

2.1 *Study Population*

The source data for the study were derived from a large computer-ECG data bank of the EPICORE Centre, University of Alberta. This data file contains 18,725 normal adult subjects, including 7,408 males and 11,317 females. Excluded from this group were individuals with primary ECG abnormalities known to influence QT interval, such as ventricular conduction defects and various other abnormal Minnesota Code categories such as Q, QS waves and related items, ST-T abnormalities and ventricular hypertrophies.

2.2 *ECG Methodology*

QT and JT measurements were made by using NOVACODE software[2] after selective averaging of normally conducted complexes contained in a 10-second ECG record. Proper detection of correct QRS onset and offset (J point) and T offset was verified visually. Leads with excessive noise were rejected automatically and occasional wave detection errors with difficult waveforms were corrected by trained operators.

2.3 *Statistical Methods*

Two multiple regression models were used for each 10-year age group with the SAS statistical software to evaluate the regression of QT and JT interval on heart rate (HR) and QRS duration:

$$\mathrm{QT} = \alpha_1 \mathrm{RF} + \beta_1 \mathrm{QRS} + \gamma_1,$$
$$\mathrm{JT} = \alpha_2 \mathrm{RF} + \beta_2 \mathrm{QRS} + \gamma_2.$$

RF is the rate factor derived for optimal correction of QT and JT for HR[1], with $\mathrm{RF} = 1/(1 + 0.01\mathrm{HR})$.

3 Results

There were no significant sex differences in the absolute QT values in adults. The HR values in males are significantly lower than those of females following puberty and remain significantly lower until about the age of 45 years. Consequently, the rate-corrected QT values are significantly lower in females than in males throughout the reproductive years although there are no significant age trends in uncorrected or rate-corrected QT values in adult females.

Regression coefficients for QT regression on QRS duration after rate correction in males (Fig.1) demonstrates that QRS duration makes a relatively small contribution on QT interval in the two younger age groups, but a sudden increase occurs at age group 30 to 40 years and remains approximately constant in the older age groups.

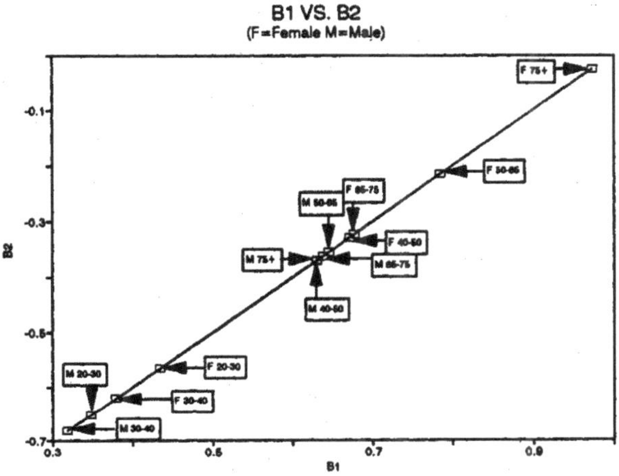

Figure 1: Regression coefficients for QRS regression on QT (β_1) and JT (β_2) intervals in various age groups of males and females demonstrating an increase of QRS contribution on QT by age and a parallel decrease in the inverse association between QRS and JT interval with age.

Regression coefficients for QT regression on QRS duration after rate correction in females (Fig.1) shows that QRS duration makes a progressively increasing contribution to QT interval with advancing age. Value of the QRS regression coefficient for QT increases from about 0.40 in the two youngest age groups to 0.91 in the age group 75 years and older.

Coefficients of QRS regression on QT (β_1) and JT (β_2) from multiple linear regression models containing heart rate correction term (Fig.1) demonstrate a progressively increasing contribution of QRS duration on QT (β_1) with advancing age and a parallel decrease in the inverse (negative) association between QRS duration and JT interval with age in such a way that for all age groups $\beta_2 = \beta_1 - 1$. This relationship is due to the linear regression models used for QT and JT prediction whereby JT = QT − QRS.

4 Discussion

Experimental evidence and empirical observations support the concept that repolarization sequence is reverse in the free left ventricular wall[3]. In contrast, the significant association between excitation time and the QT interval implies that the concept of reverse sequence of repolarization is not universally valid in all myocardial regions and that mainly concordant sequence prevails in myocardial regions excited during the terminal portions of QRS or perhaps during the major portions of the second half of QRS.

QRS duration has a minimal influence on the QT interval at the age of 20 years, suggesting that reverse sequence of repolarization is most dominant in young adults. The increasing values of QRS regression coefficient on QT (β_1) reflect the fact that the repolarization sequence during the second half of repolarization becomes more and more concordant particularly in adults over 40 years old.

Differential age trends in QT interval between males and females have revealed longer QT interval in females in reproductive age than in males. However, these differences were shown to be due to a shortening of the QT interval in males following puberty, with no significant age trends in females during reproductive age or following menopause[4].

5 Conclusions

QRS duration has a significant influence on the QT interval. Excitation time has minimal influence on QT interval in young adults and the contribution of QRS to QT increases progressively with age. These observations indicate that the reverse sequence of repolarization is not universally valid in all myocardial regions. Reverse sequence is most dominant in young adults and concordant sequence of repolarization becomes increasingly dominant with increasing age in myocardial regions excited during the second half of QRS.

6 References

1. P. M. Rautaharju, J. W. Warren and H. P. Calhoun, *J. Electrocardiol.* **23** (1991) 111-117.

2. P. M. Rautaharju, H. P. Calhoun, B. R. Chaitman, *J. Electrocardiol.* **24** (1992) 179-187.

3. S. H. Zhou, S. Wong, P. M. Rautaharju, N. Karnik, H. P. Calhoun. *J. Electrocardiol.* (1992) in press.

4. P. M. Rautaharju, S. H. Zhou, S. Wong, H. P. Calhoun, G. S. Berenson, R. J. Prineas and A. Davignon, *Can. J. Cardiol.* (1992) in press.

PROLONGATION OF REPOLARIZATION TIME IN VENTRICULAR CONDUCTION DEFECTS

Wong S., Zhou S.H., Karnik N.S., Calhoun H.P., Rautaharju P.M.

EPICORE Centre, Division of Cardiology, University of Alberta, Edmonton, Alberta, T6G 2S2, Canada

ABSTRACT

It is well established that the conventional QT prediction formulas are not valid for detection of QT prolongation in ventricular conduction defects (VCD). We investigated the influence of QRS duration on QT interval in an ECG data bank derived from community-based population samples classified for the presence of various types of VCD according to the Minnesota Code (MC). R-square values were determined to estimate the contribution of QRS to QT. The results indicate a strong influence of duration of excitation on QT in complete bundle branch blocks, with a 15% increase in R-square value by the inclusion of QRS in the regression model. In contrast, the JT interval was essentially uninfluenced by QRS duration in all VCD categories. It is also noted that the values of regression coefficients differ substantially between various VCD categories, reflecting differing degrees of concordance vs. discordance of repolarization with respect to the excitation sequence. It is concluded that it is essential to include QRS duration in QT prediction formulas to achieve reliable estimation of QT prolongation in VCD, otherwise, it is preferable to use JT as the dependent variable in rate correction formulas.

It is well known that the conventional formulas for detection of QT prolongation are not valid in ventricular conduction defects and that QRS duration has a highly significant influence on the QT interval in normal subjects with ventricular conduction[1]. Das[2] recently observed in a small groups of patients with VCD that QT prolonged in direct proportion to QRS prolongation. We investigated the association between excitation time and QT interval in a large sample of VCDs with the objective to derive new formulas for QT prediction in the presence of VCD.

1 Methods

Our study population was a subset of 2865 persons with VCD and 20,687 normal adult subjects with normal ventricular conduction derived from large community-based population samples. The group with various categories of ventricular conduction defects was stratified into subgroups of complete and incomplete bundle branch block (BBB), using the Minnesota criteria, including 231 LBBB (MC7.1), 673 RBBB (MC7.2), 616 IVCD, complete block of unspecified type (MC7.4), 607 incomplete LBBB (MC7.3) and 738 in incomplete RBBB (MC7.3). QT and JT measurements were made by the NOVACODE computer programs[3,4], from simultaneously sampled 8 independent components of the standard 12-leads ECG.

Stepwise multiple regression was used to derive coefficient estimates for QT and JT regression on QRS duration after adjustment for heart rate in the first step using the following statistical models:

$$\mathrm{QT} = \alpha_1 \mathrm{RF} + \beta_1 \mathrm{QRS} + \gamma_1,$$
$$\mathrm{JT} = \alpha_2 \mathrm{RF} + \beta_2 \mathrm{QRS} + \gamma_2,$$

where the rate factor $\mathrm{RF} = 1/(1+0.01\mathrm{HR})$ is a recently established optimal heart rate correction factor for QT. R-square values were determined after each step in order to estimate the individual contribution of QRS duration to the overall variance of QT. Coefficient β_1 and β_2 indicate to what extent excitation sequence and QRS duration will influence QT and JT intervals.

2 Results

Incremental R^2 values in Table 1 indicate that QRS duration explains about 15% of QT variation in all complete BBB categories. The values of regression coefficients for QRS (β_1) are very high in these conditions, ranging from 0.77 in RBBB to near unity (0.99) in IVCD. QRS duration makes a significant although from a practical point of view, a modest contribution to QT in normal conduction ($\beta_1 = 0.55$) and in incomplete RBBB ($\beta_1 = 0.56$). However QRS duration is not significantly associated with QT in incomplete LBBB (Table 1).

In contrast to QT regression on QRS, JT interval was not significantly associated with QRS duration in any of the complete BBB categories or in incomplete LBBB. In normal conduction QRS duration explained 7% of the total JT variance and 3% in incomplete RBBB (Table 2).

It is noted that as the values of QRS regression coefficients for QT progressively increased from 0.29 for incomplete LBBB to near unity for IVCD, the values of

Table 1: Coefficient estimates for regression of QRS on QT.

ECG Category	α_1	β_1	γ_1	R^2	ΔR^2
Normal	596	0.55	-7	0.62	0.03
LBBB	577	0.87	-20	0.60	0.16
RBBB	503	0.77	20	0.54	0.16
IVCD	563	0.99	-38	0.54	0.15
Incomplete RBBB	591	0.56	-7	0.66	0.04
Incomplete LBBB	523	0.29	65	0.50	0.00

Table 2: Coefficient estimates for regression of QRS on JT.

ECG Category	α_2	β_2	γ_2	R^2	ΔR^2
Normal	596	-0.45	-7	0.62	0.07
LBBB	577	-0.13	-20	0.50	0.00
RBBB	503	-0.23	20	0.43	0.01
IVCD	563	-0.01	-38	0.48	0.00
Incomplete RBBB	591	-0.44	-7	0.62	0.03
Incomplete LBBB	523	-0.71	65	0.50	0.01

QRS regression coefficient for JT increased from -0.71 for incomplete LBBB to near zero for IVCD in such a fashion that for all categories $\beta_2 = \beta_1 - 1$.

3 Discussion

The fact that QRS duration has a significant (although in practical terms a relatively modest) influence on QT interval in normal conduction implies that the traditional concept of reverse sequence of repolarization is not uniformly valid. Reverse sequence of repolarization is more pronounced in incomplete LBBB (low value of QRS regression coefficients β_1 on QT). High values of QRS regression coefficients on QT (β_1) in complete BBB suggest that in these conditions the repolarization process is largely concordant with the sequence of excitation.

4 Conclusion

It is concluded that the relative degree of discordance vs. concordance of repolarization with respect to the sequence of excitation varies a great deal depending on the type of ventricular conduction on ventricular excitation patterns.

It is essential to include QRS duration in QT prediction formulas to achieve reliable estimation of QT prolongation in VCD, otherwise, it is preferable to use JT as the dependent variable in rate correction formulas.

5 References

1. P. M. Rautaharju, J. W. Warren and H. P. Calhoun, *J. Electrocardiol.* **23** (1991) 111

2. G. Das, *J. Electrocardiol.* **23** (1990) 49

3. P. M. Rautaharju, P. J. MacInnis, W. J. Warren, H. K. Wolf, P. M. Rykers and H. P. Calhoun, *Meth. Infor. in Med.* **29** (1990) 362

4. P. M. Rautaharju, H. P. Calhoun and B. R. Chaitman *J. Electrocardiol.*, **24** (1992) 179

POLICARDIOGRAPHY IN PACEMAKER PATIENTS

Balbi M., Bertero G., Meng J., Caponnetto S.

Cardiology Chair, University of Genoa, Italy.

INTRODUCTION

Since the first pacemaker implantation in nineteen-fiftyeight, cardiac pacing has continued to grow. For example, presently more than 500.000 patients have pacemakers in the United States. But the most meaningful progresses in this field were obtained in the mode of pacing. The evolution from ventricular (VVI) to dual chamber (DDD) pacing mode allow to achieve normal or near normal hemodinamics at rest and exercise, by restoring syncronized atrial systole. In fact about 30% of entire cardiac output is due to a normal timing between atrial and ventricular contraction (1).

Several invasive and noninvasive approaches have been advanced in these years to evaluate the role of atrial contraction on the left ventricular function: hemodinamic studies (2), ECHO-doppler evaluation (3) and policardiographyc methods (4).

Policardiography is an easy, low cost and feasible test that describes with accuracy left ventricular function by means of the so-called sistolic time intervals (STI):

QS2 : from the onset of QRS complex in the ECG to the beginning of 2° sound in the phonocardiogram.

LVET (left ventricular ejection time) : from the upstroke of the carotid pulse to the incisural notch.

PEP (pre-expulsive period) : from the onset of QRS to the beginning of left ventricular ejection.

PEP/LVET ratio : the best index of left ventricular performance.

With this study we want to demonstrate the usefulness of STI to evaluate the role of atrial contraction on left ventricular function, and in second istance to recognize the atrio-ventricular (A-V) intervals that yeld the best ventricular performance.

PATIENTS AND METHODS

The study population consists in fourthy patients with VVI pacemaker. We devided them in group A (20 patients with 3° degree A-V block without retroconduction) and group B (20 patients with atrial fibrillation and slow ventricular response). the clinical characteristics of patients were similar in the two groups.
During scheduled controls we performed in those patients a prolonged recording of ECG, PCG and carotid pulse with a Siemens Elema Mingodoc Polyanalyzer. Then we calculated the STI related to random A-V couplings.

RESULTS

Our results show that the best performances of left ventricular function, expressed by prolongation of LVET and shortening of PEP, with a lower PEP/LVET ratio, were obtained within the 110 and 300 msec. A-V interval. There is statistical significance between the values of this group and the values of goup B (atrial fibrillation): p<0,0 (T Student test for nonpaired data).

Table 1

	Q-S2	LVET	PEP	PEP/LVET
n.v.(msec.)	360-400	220-340	80-110	0,31-0,38
af	435	268	167	0,62
PR 0	433	252	180	0,72
PR 10-50 msec	439	276	163	0,59
PR 60-100 "	455	292	163	0,55
PR 110-150 "	449	295	154	0,52
PR 160-200 "	441	296	148	0,50
PR 210-250 "	446	295	152	0,51
PR 260-300 "	437	292	145	0,49
PR 310-350 "	451	292	159	0,54
PR 360-400 "	435	275	160	0,58
PR 410-450 "	443	271	172	0,63

When A-V interval fall to zero (P wave inside the QRS complex) STI are worst than those of group B. We can explaine this fact with atrial contraction against closed A-V valves, as we can see in the so-called pacemaker syndrome.

CONCLUSIONS

Poligraphic assessment is a useful test able to identify the role of syncronized atrial systole on the left ventricular performance. Such test allows: to identify

the patients who need a dual-chamber pacemaker (i.e. among patients that undergo pacemaker substitution for end of life); to select the best interval for improving the left ventricular function.
In our experience the best indexes of left ventricular function were obtained at A-V intervals within the 160-300msec.

REFERENCES

1) Samet P., Bernstein W., Levine S.: Significance of atrial contribution to ventricular filling. Am J Cardiol, 1965; 15: 195-202.
2) Ogawa S., Dreifus L., Shenoy P. et al.: Hemodinamic consequen-ces of atrioventricular and ventriculoatrial pacing. PACE, 1978; 1.
3) Mehta D., Gilmour S., Ward D. et al.: Optimal AV delay at rest and during exercise in patients with dual chamber pacemaker: a noninvasive assessment by continuous wave Doppler. Br Heart J, 1989; 61: 161-172.
4) Weissler A.M., Peller R., Roehllw H.: Relationship between left ventricular ejection time, stroke volume and heart rate in normal individuals and patients with cardiovascular disea-se. Am Heart J, 1961; 62:367-378.

EPICARDIAL ELECTRIC SHOCK ABLATION OF ACCESSORY PATHWAYS IN PREEXCITATION SYNDROME

KAZIMIERZ SUWALSKI
Department of Cardiovascular Surgery National Institute of Cardiology, Spartanska 1, Warsaw, Poland.
MARIUSZ PYTKOWSKI, DARIUSZ WOJCIECHOWSKI, PIOTR ZELAZNY,
WACLAW SITKOWSKI, ZYGMUNT SADOWSKI.
National Institute of Cardiology, Spartanska 1, Warsaw, Poland.

Abstract

Twenty two years have elapsed since the first successful division of an accessory pathway (Kent bundle) was performed by Cobb and Sealy .Recently, many authors described preexcitation syndrome. Progress in this field is based, for the most part, on improvement of existing techniques of Kent bundle ablation and on the newly developed methods. The authors present simple method of surgical treatment of preexcitation syndrome, based on the application of current through the myocardium, called "epicardial electric shock ablation", focusing on the use of this techniques to ablate accessory pathways (EESA of AP). We have used the EESA of AP in 28 patients (ranging from 6 to 66 years of age) presenting with disabling supraventricular tachycardias who were resistant to antiarrhythmic drug therapy. Results: We have obtained a success rate of 100 percent in the first group. This was documented by postoperative epicardial mapping of atria and ventricules.

In patients with life threatening and drug-resistant tachyarrhytmias, in course of WPW syndrome only non pharmacological treatment can cure the patient. Recently, the closed-chest electrical ablation methods have been rapidly developed and become more popular. However in many cases surgery is the only effective treatment. At the beginning destruction of the accessory pathways (AP) was performed by dissection of appropriate anatomical spaces. Later a cryoablation and some other methods were introduced(2,3). One of them was an epicardial electric shock ablation (EESA) which was introduced by Bockeria et al (1). We would like to present our experience and results which we have obtained with this method.

Patients

Twenty eight consecutive patients who presented at our department between 1989 and 1991 were included in this study. There were 4 females and 24 males with age of 6 to 66 years. 18 patients had manifested preexcitation on the surface electrocardiogram (Wolff–Parkinson–White syndrome), and 10 were found to have a concealed AP. Fifteen had no evidence of organic heart disease; 9 patients had coronary artery disease, 4 congenital heart diseases. All patients were referred to our department because of symptomatic spontaneous tachyarrhythmias related to AP. Symptoms included disabling palpitations,nausea, dizziness and presyncope. One patient had an antitachycardia pacemaker implanted at a different hospital that failed to control recurrent supraventricular tachycardia. The duration of symptom ranged from 12 months to almost 20 years. The underlying type of arrhythmia was atrioventricular reentrant tachycardia in 26 patients, atrial fibrillation with a rapid ventricular response in 18 patients. Before therapy, all patients had undergone drug trials with a median of 3 antiarrhythmic agents (range one to seven) that neither failed to control the arrhythmia nor caused intolerable side effects.

Preoperative studies

Each patient underwent a diagnostic electrophysiologic study. Three 6F quadripolar catheters (üSCI) with 1–cm interelectrode spacing were inserted into a femoral vein and positioned in the following positions: high right atrium, His bundle, and right ventricle. In patients with left–sided or concealed AP, a 7F quadripolar catheter (üSCI) was positioned in the coronary sinus via the right subclavian vein. Programmable pacing was carried out with a Biotronik VSN 30 stimulator. The goals of the diagnostic portion of the electrophysiological test were to confirm the presence of an accessory AV connection, to determine the baseline electrophysiological properties of the AV node and accessory AV connection, and to localize the accessory AV connection to a general region of the heart. 24 patients had one left lateral AP, 4 patients had both left lateral and right lateral or septal AP.

Intraoperative studies

We did an epicardial intraoperative mapping using three electrodes. A ventricular timing reference signal is provided by electrode sewn directly to the right ventricle near the apex. An atrial reference signal is provided from a modified clip electrode , which has been attached to the right atrial appendage. For the mapping of peri a–v groove area we used a hand–held mapping probe. All electrodes are fabricated locally.

Operative procedures

The principle of EESA is to deliver a series of two to five ECG synchronized shocks of 50 to 150 joules by a cardiac electrode along the ventricular margin of the AV groove fat pad. The cardiac electrode in connected to the negative output of a DC defibrillator (Hellige). The back paddle of the DC defibrillator is the anode and is placed under the patients left scapula.
The damage induced by this method is based on coagulation of the myocardium, ionic gradient disturbances, disruption of the capillary network and haematoma formation at the site where the electric shock is delivered. This contributes to the dehiscence of cell membranes, cell structure damage, and myocitenecrosis. In order to perform EESA of AP in a posterior location, we lifted the heart with a special hook, the handle of which was covered with isolating material. In patients with second AP localized either in septum or in right lateral area we used Sealy's method.

Results

The first group consisted of 18 patients with the preexcitation syndrome. In four patients EESA of AP was performed without cardiopulmonary bypass, in the others EESA of AP was performed under normothermic cardiopulmonary bypass. Total duratation of cardiopulmonary bypass didn't exceed 20 minutes (average duration was 4 – 14 min.). The second group consisted of 10 patients with either the second AP or other cardiac pathology. AP localized in the left lateral area was eliminated by EESA at the first stage of the operation. The second stage involved: ablation of second accessory pathway (in 3 cases), ablation of second AP and closure of ASD (1 pt.), closure of VSD (1 pt.) and a coronary by–pass (4 pt.). The second stage was performed under cardiopulmonary by–pass with moderate hypothermia and pharmacological cardioplegia with cooled potassium solution. The postoperative electrophysiological studies didn't reveal neither delta waves nor conduction through AP and possibility of tachycardia induction.

Discussion

The method of surgical dissection of AP introduced by Sealy

involves an administration of cooled cardioplegia under cardiopulmonary by-pass and can be followed by damage of valves and coronary vessels (3,4). The usage of EESA in patients with left lateral AP eliminates these problems. In cases with two AP a combination of both Sealy's method and EESA allows to avoid damage of interatrial septum. The EESA in comparision with epicardial cryoablation reduces the risk of damaging coronary arteries and veins (3,5). The usage of EESA allows to reduce markedly the overall time of the operation. Hence, considering anatomical relationships in between various important structures and vessels localized in the right lateral and septal area we prefered EESA only in left lateral localization.

References

1. L.A.Bokeria, S.I.Mikhailin, A.S.Revishvili, L.J.Baturkin, A.G.Rybalov, *Epicardial electric shock ablation of accessory pathways in preexcitation syndrome. in Ablation in Cardiac Arrhythmias*, edited by G.Fontaine, M.M.Scheinman,(Futura Publishing, Mount Kisco,New York 1987).
2. T.B Ferguson, J.L.Cox, *Surgical therapy for patients with supraventricular tachycardia.* Cardiology Clinics 1990;8:535-555.
3. J.J.Gallagher, J.G.Selle, R.H.Svenson, J.M.Fedor, S.H.Zimmern, W.C.Sealy, F.R.Robicsek, *Nonpharmacologic treatment of supraventricular tachycardia.*
4. G.M.Lawrie A.Pacificio, *The role of surgery in the treatment of tachyarrhythmias.* J.Cardiol.1989;25:155-158.
5. E.N.Prystowsky,D.Packer, *Nonpharmacologic treatment of supraventricular tachycardia.* Am.J.Cardiol 1988;62:74L-77L.

PROGRAMMED ELECTRICAL STIMULATION IN PATIENTS WITH VENTRICULAR TACHYCARDIA AND NO STRUCTURAL HEART DISEASE

Anna–Maria WNUK–WOJNAR,
Leszek GIEC, Janusz DRZEWIECKI

1st Cardiologic Clinic
Silesian Medical Academy, Silesian Heart Center
Katowice, Poland

ABSTRACT

Clinical and electrophysiological data were analyzed in 34 patients with apparently normal heart and serious ventricular arrhythmia: 17 of them with VT/VF (Group A) and 17 with palpitations only (Group B), who underwent a baseline drug free electrophysiologic study with programmed electrical stimulation (PES) using 1–3 decremental stimuli delivered from 2 right ventricular (RV) sites during sinus rhythm as well as 100, 120, 140 bpm and burst stimulation. VT was induced in 36% of group A pts and in 6% of group B, $p<0.05$. No one from our group died in follow–up period (up to 3 years), in one patient automatic defibrilator was implanted..

In conclusion: In patients with spontaneous VT, but with apparently normal heart VT is often noninducible. Prognostic value of this fact, however, is still controversial.

Programmed electrical stimulation (PES) allows reproducibility of clinical ventricular tachycardia in approximately 90% of patients after myocardial infarction[1], but the value of the results of PES in the evaluation of patients with ventricular arrhythmia and apparently normal heart is still uncertain. The aim of this study was to establish the rate of inducibility of ventricular tachycardia (VT) as well as the character and prognostic value of evoked VT in patients with normal heart and ventricular arrhythmia.

1. Methods

The study comprised 34 patients, 19 males and 15 females at mean age of 40 ± 11 years, with apparently normal hearts, suffered from serious ventricular arrhythmia. Myocardial or valvular heart disease as well as coronary artery disease were excluded using both noninvasive and invasive methods including coronarography and myocardial biopsy. Group A consisted of 17 patients with ventricular tachycardia (VT) documented in ECG (in 9 patients) or suspected (in 8 patients) because of syncopal episodes in history and ventricular arrhythmia in 24 hrs Holter ECG monitorings. Group B consisted of 17 patients with palpitations due to ventricular arrhythmia (Lown's grade 4 in 5 patients and grade 1 or 2 in 12 patients).

All antiarrhythmic drugs were discontinued for at least five half–lives. After written, informed consent was obtained, multipolar electrode catheters were positioned in right ventricular (RV) apex and outflow tract (RVOT). Stimuli were 2 ms rectangular pulses delivered at twice diastolic threshold. The standard protocol included one or two decremental extrastimuli from the RV apex at sinus rhythm and ventricular pacing 100,120 and 140 bpm. If it failed to induce sustained monomorphic VT (lasting more than 30 seconds or requiring termination in less time because of hemodynamic collapse) the extensive protocol was used with up to 3 extrastimuli during sinus rhythm and burst stimulation from RV apex and after that the whole protocol repeated from RVOT.

The incidence of VT inducibility during PES was related to the type of protocol needed to evoke VT and to the QT interval in standard ECG. The QT was measured from 3 R–R cycles in each standard 12 ECG leads and expressed as QTc using Bazett formula[2]. The dispersion of QT (dQTc) on surface ECG was estimated as the difference between the maximal and minimal QTc calculations in all 12 ECG leads (dQTc = QTc max – QTc min). Basic comparative statistics were calculated with chi square test, analysis of variance, or Student's t test.

2. Results

2.1. Induced arrhythmias

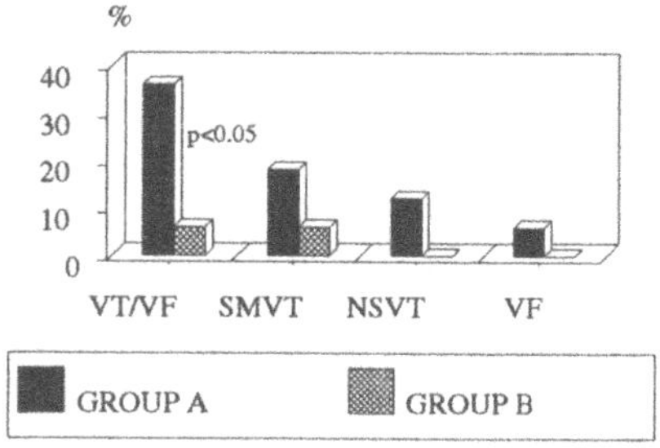

Fig. 1. Ventricular arrhythmia evoked during programmed electrical stimulation. See text for abbreviations

Ventricular tachycardia or fibrillation (VT/VF) was induced in 36% of patients from group A and only 6% of patients from group B, $p<0.05$ (Fig 1.) In 18% of group A patients it was sustained VT (SMVT), non–sustained (NSVT) in 12% and in 6% it was ventricular fibrillation (VF). In group B induced VT was sustained one. In group A VT was inducible during standard protocol of PES in 12% of patients: in 6% it was SMVT and in 6% NSVT, in further 24% extensive protocol provoked VT/VF: in 12% the provoked arrhythmia was SMVT, in 6% NSVT, and in 6% it was VF. In group B VT was inducible only during extensive protocol of PES. The evoked VT had LBBB morphology and normal or right axis in both groups of patients with mean cycle length 260 ± 38 ms.

2.2. Relation to QTc

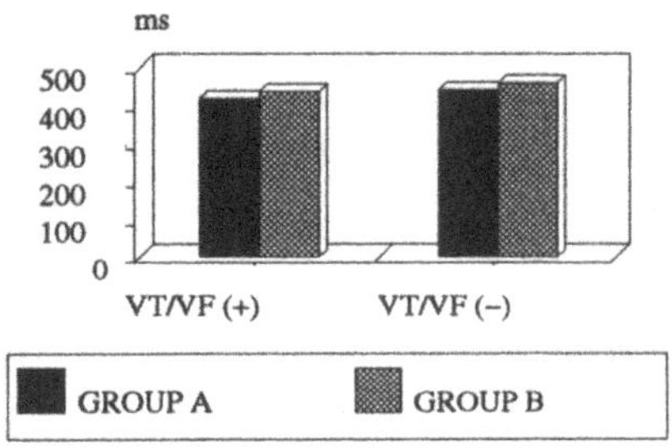

Fig. 2. Inducibility of VT in relation to the QTc interval. See text for abbreviations

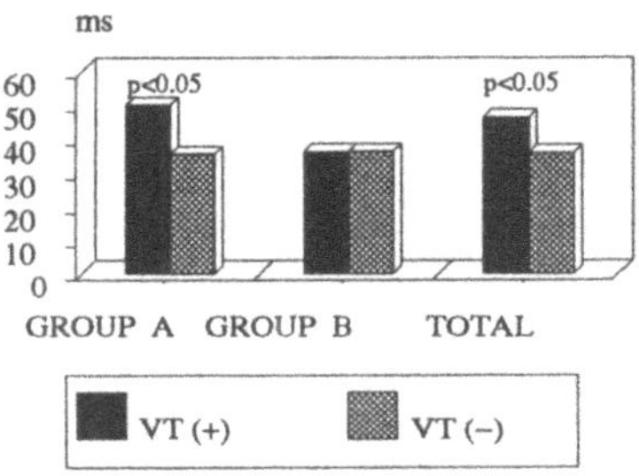

Fig. 3. Inducibility of VT in relation to dispersion of QTc interval. See text for abbreviations

In group A patients QTc interval was slightly shorter (432 ± 37 ms) than in group B (458 ± 46 ms). The shorter QTc interval (Fig.3) was observed in patients with inducible VT (422 ± 33 ms: in Group A 419 ± 18 ms and in group B 436 ± 32 ms) than in patients without VT during PES (452 ± 45 ms: in group A 442 ± 32 ms and in group B 458 ± 45 ms), NS. However, signifficant difference was found in the dispersion of QTc (Fig. 4). In patients with inducible VT the dQTc was greater: 46 ± 11 ms vs 36 ± 9 ms, $p<0.05$ (in Group A: 50 ± 24 ms vs 35 ± 15 ms, $p<0.05$ and in group B: 36 ± 27 ms vs 36 ± 18 ms, NS)..

Nobody died in up to 3 years follow–up period. No one from group B patients had clinical VT during follow–up. In one patient from group A, a woman with VF in history, who was noninducible to VT during PES, automatic implantable defibrillator (AICD) was implanted because of VT recurrences.

3. Discussion

Ventricular tachycardia was evoked by PES in a small rate of patients with apparently normal heart. In standard protocol it was provoked only in patients with VT in history (Group A). It confirms the observations of Swerdlow et al.[3] that prior spontaneous SMVT is and independent predictor of induced SMVT. The incidence of induced VT/VF does not depend on the time from spontaneous incident to electrophysiologic study. The relative low incidence of induced sustained arrhythmias is caused probably by the fact, that VT is inducible in patients with documented spontaneous VT, but is not inducible in patients with only unexplained syncopal episodes[4]. In patients with no structural heart disease VT/VF may be precipitated by possible transient arrhythmogenic condition such as metabolic abnormalities, or changes in the autonomic nervous system, which may have resolved too rapidly to be detected in electrophysiologic study. Our observation, that the inducibility of VT is more often observed in patients with bigger dispertion of QTc may support this hypothesis.

The prognostic value of the VT/VF inducibility during PES is still open question. In Leclerq et al.[5] 10 years observation of patients with inducible VT, but no structural heart disease no cardiac death was observed, while in the similar group of patients with coronary artery disease the mortality rate was 53%. In our study, however, one patient who aborted sudden death because of VF, has had recurrent VT/VF episodes after negative PES, what is in concordance with Hwang et al.[6] observations that VT is noninducible in almost 40% of patients after cardiac arrest, but the prognosis in those patients is not better.

4. Conclusions

1. In patients with apparently normal heart VT is often noninducible despite of the presence of spontaneous VT in history.
2. The prognostic value of noninducibility of VT during programmed electrical stimulation in this group of patients is still uncertain.

5. References

1. P. Brugada, R. Lemery, M. Talajic, P. Della Bella, H.J.J. Wellens, *Treatment of patients with ventricular tachycardia or ventricular fibrillation: First lessons from the "parallel study"*. In : *Cardiac Arrhythmias: Where to go from here ?*, eds. P.Brugada, H.J.J. Wellens (Futura Publishing Company , New York, 1987)
2. H.C. Bazett, *An analysis of the time relation of electrocardiograms*. Heart **7** (1920) 353.
3. C.D. Swerdlow, G.H. Bardy, J. McAnulty, J. Kron, J.T. Lee, E. Graham, J. Peterson, L. Greene, *Determinants of induced sustained arrhythmias in survivors of out–of–hospital ventricular fibrillation*, Circulation, **76** (1987) 1053.
4. B. Krol, F. Morady, G.C. Flaker, L.A. DiCarlo Jr., J.M. Baerman, J. Hewett, M. deBuitleir, *Electrophysiologic testing in patients with unexplain syncope: Clinical and noninvasive predicttors of outcome*. J. Am. Coll. Cardiol. **10** (1987) 358 .
5. J.–F. Leclerq, P. Coumel, I. Denjoy, P. Maisonblanche, B. Cauchemez., F. Chouty, A. Leenhardt, R. Slama, *Long–term follow–up after sustained monomorphic ventricular tachycardia: Causes, pump failure, and empiric antiarrhythmic therapy that modify survival.* Am. Heart J. **121** (1991) 1685
6. S.Hwang, W.G. Stevenson, I. Wiener, *Hearts too good to die: Ventricular fibrillation due to small infarctions or ischemia*, Am. Heart J. **121** (1991) 938.

THE ROLE OF QTc DISPERSION IN VENTRICULAR TACHYCARDIA

Anna–Maria WNUK–WOJNAR,
Cezary CZERWINSKI, Janusz DRZEWIECKI, Leszek GIEC

1st Cardiologic Clinic
Silesian Medical Academy, Silesian Heart Center
Katowice, Poland

ABSTRACT

The dispersion of QTc interval in standard 12–leads ECG (dQTc) and the adptation of QT to the heart rate (HR) during cardiac pacing 100, 120 and 140 bpm were evaluated in 70 patients with serious ventricular arrhythmia: 37 with coronary heart disease (group A) and 33 with no manifest heart disease (Group B). There was no significant difference in dQTc between patients with and without clinical VT (43±22 ms vs 40 ± 20 ms). The dQTc was significantly higher in group A patients in whom VT was inducible during programmed electrical stimulation: 50 ± 21 ms vs 36 ± 19ms ($p<0.05$) in patients noninducible to VT. No significant difference was observed between patients with HR–dependent QT interval and those with QT unchanged during cardiac pacing in the incidence of clinical VT: 14% vs 20% as well as VT inducibility: 57% vs 50%,

We conclude, that the dispertion of QTc in normal ECG rather than HR–adaptive variability of QT may be related to the higher rate of VT inducibility, mainly in patients with coronary heart disease.

The QT interval on surface electrocardiogram is an indirect measure of myocardial depolarization and repolarization. Abnormalities of the QT interval, which indicate abnormal repolarization and thus myocardial refractoriness, have been linked with the development of ventricular arrhythmias. The aim of this study was to determine the role of QT variability and of the dispersion of QTc in arrhythmogenesis in patients with spontaneous and inducible serious ventricular arrhythmia.

1. Methods

1.1. Patients

Seventy patients, 41 males and 29 females at mean age 55 ± 7 years, suffered from serious ventricular arrhythmia, were included in the study. Group A consisted of 37 patients with coronary heart disease (CHD): 13 of them without myocardial infarction (MI) in history (group A_1) and 24 patients after MI (group A_2). Group B consisted of 33 patients with no structural heart disease diagnosed both by means of noninvasive and invasive methods.

In every patient all antiarrhythmic drugs were discontinued for at least five half-lives. To provoke ventricular tachycardia (VT) all patients underwent programmed electrical stimulation (PES) with 1–3 decremental extrastimuli during sinus rhythm and 3 drives of ventricular pacing: 100, 120 and 140 bpm.

1.2. QT measurements

In all patients QT interval was measured in all 12 standard surface ECG leads (paper speed 100 mm/s) from 3 R–R cycles and expressed as QT corrected to heart rate (QTc) using Bazett[1] formula. The dispersion of QTc (dQTc) was calculated as the difference between maximal and minimal Qtc measurements (dQTc = QTmax – QTmin). In addition, QT interval was measured from 5 R–R cycles during ventricular pacing 100, 120 and in some patients 140 bpm to determine the QT adaptation to HR.

Basic statistics was calculated with chi–square test, analysis of variance or Student's *t* test.

2. Results

Spontaneous incidents of VT were observed in 18 patients from group A and 9 patients from group B. VT has been evoked during PES in 66% of group A patients and in 21% of group B.

There were no signifficant difference between groups in QTc interval: 438 ± 21 ms in group A and 432 ± 18 ms in group B, as well as in the dQT : 42 ± 21 and 38 ± 16, respectively. No difference in dQTc was also observed between patients with or without spontaneous VT regardless to underlying disease: 43 ± 22 ms vs 39 ± 20 ms. However, dQTc was significantly bigger in patients with VT inducible during PES: 47 ± 21 ms vs 36 ± 19 ms in noninducible group , $p<0.05$.

The analysis of QT adaptation to heart rate during ventricular pacing showed the strong relationship between QT interval and HR in group A_2 ($p<0.02$) and group B patients ($p<0.005$). No difference was seen between the patients with spontaneous VT (Fig.1) or VT inducible during PES (Fig.2) in any group of patients. There was also no significant difference in the rate of spontaneous and inducible VT incidence between

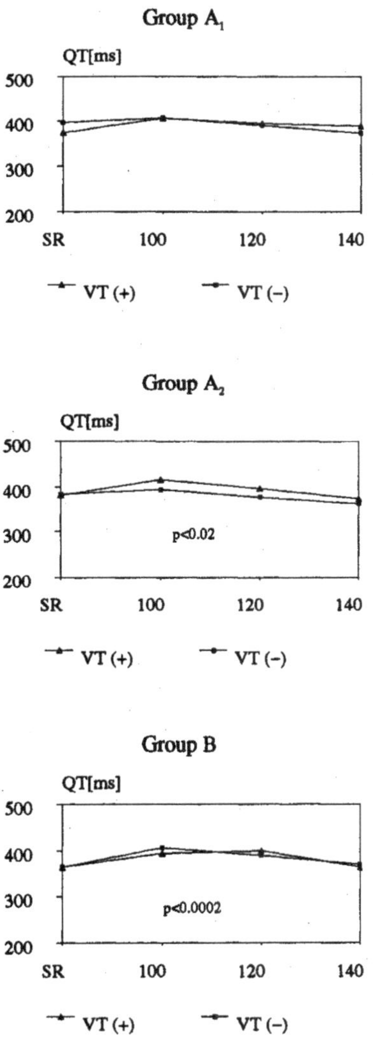

Fig. 1. Adaptation of QT to heart rate in relation to the presence of spontaneous ventricular tachycardia. SR – sinus rhythm; 100, 120, 140 – ventricular pacing 100, 120 and 140 bpm

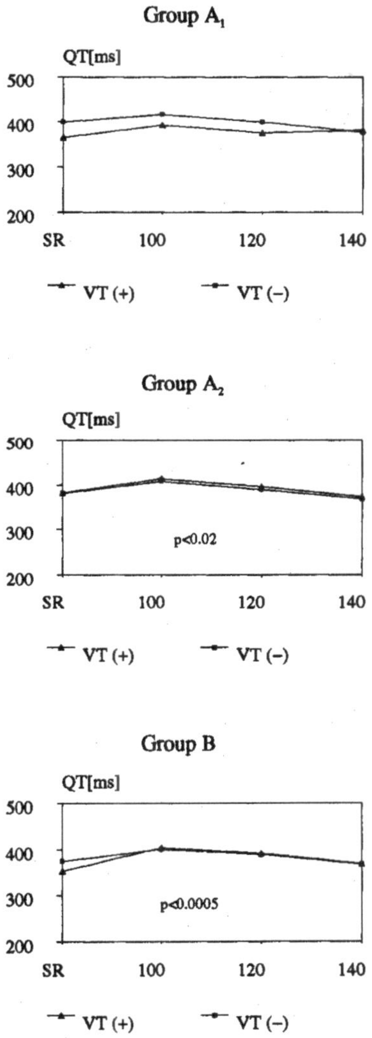

Fig. 2. Adaptation of QT to heart rate in relation to the presence of ventricular tachycardia inducible during PES. SR – sinus rhythm; 100, 120, 140 – ventricular pacing 100, 120 and 140 bpm

patients in whom QTc was or was not related to HR: 14% vs 20% for spontaneous VT and 57% vs 50% for VT inducible during PES.

3. Discussion

The QT interval is essentially a reflection of the overall ventricular refractory period. Conventionally, the ECG repolarization duration is quantified by measuring QT interval or the heart rate – corrected form (QTc), both of which are used clinically to assess the propensity to VT in certain subsets of patients[2]. In concordance to previously published reports[3] our data confirmed that the dispersion of refractory periods predisposed to malignant arrhythmias.

Recently, there has been considerable interest in the dynamic nature of the QT interval, both normal and pathological[4]. The mechanism of the effects of sudden changes in heart rate on ventricular refractory periods are not well understood. The rapidity with which the QT intervals adapt to a new cardiac cycle length may have clinical implications. Santinelli and Chiariello[5] reported woman who developed VT associated with an increase in heart rate without the expected QT interval shortening. These authors suggested that this might be a variant of the long QT syndrome. Our data did not confirm the relationship between the ability to HR–QT adaptation and propensity to serious ventricular arrhythmias, peharps because permament pacing might be efficiacious in decreasing the dispersion of refractoriness[6].

4. Conclusions

The dispersion of QTc as an indirect measure of abnormal repolarization may be the cause of the higher rate of VT inducibility in patients with coronary heart disease.

5. References

1. H.C. Bazett, *An analysis of the time relation of electrocardiograms.* Heart **7** (1920) 353.
2. D. Sadeh, D.C. Shannon, S. Abboud, P. Saul, S. Akselrod, R.J. Cohen, *Altered cardiac repolarization in some victims of sudden infants death syndrome* N. Engl. J. Med. **317** (1987) 1501
3. R.E. Haynes, A.P. Hallsrom, L.A. Cobb, *Repolarization abnormalities in survivors of out–of–hospital ventricular fibrillation* . Circulation **57** (1978) 654.
4. R.S. Bexton, H.O. Vallin, A.J. Camm. *Diurnal variations of the QT interval – influencece of the autonomic nervous system.* Br. Heart J. **55** (1986) 253.
5. V. Santinelli, M. Chiariello, *Heart rate acceleration without changes in the QT interval and severe ventricular arrhythmias: a variant of long QT Syndrome?* Int. J. Cardiol. **4** (1983) 69.
6. J. Han, D. Millet, B. Chizzonitti, G.K. Moe, *Temporal dispersion of recovery of excitability in atrium and ventricle as a function of heart rate.* Am. Heart J. **71** (1966) 481.

ATRIO-VENTRICULAR CONDUCTION DISTURBANCES AFTER OPEN HEART SURGERY IN CHILDHOOD. DYNAMIC 24 HOURS - ELECTROCARDIOGRAPHIC STUDY

Fernández-Pineda L., López-Zea M., Quero-Jiménez M., Rico-Gomez F., Casanova-Gómez M., Cazaniga M., López-Checa S. y Maitre-Azcárate MJ.

Servicio de Cardiología Pediátrica
Hospital Ramón y Cajal, MADRID

ABSTRACT

The incidence of atrioventricular (AV) conduction disturbances is studied by means of 24 hours electrocardiography in 60 children submitted to cardio-pulmonary bypass surgery (BS) for congenital heart disease from August 1.990 to December 1.991. Patients (pts) with preoperative first degree A-V block (most of the times related to digitalis effect) and those with AV septal defects have been excluded from this study. Complete A-V block has been encountered in 9 (15%) pts: 2 after Mustard, 2 after atrio-pulmonary anastomosis and 5 of other origines (Table). A second degree A-V block was present in 4 (6,6%) pts: 2 after corrective surgery for Tetralogy of Fallot (TOF), 1 after correction of double outlet right ventricle (DORV) and another one of surgery of atrial septal defect and ductus. This apparent high incidence of 21% should be compared with the general incidences of 7% (17 pts) encountered in 243 cases studied with 24 hours ECG during the same period of time: 6 of them which were complete were unrelated to cardiac surgery (5 congenital and 1 following an ablation procedure for incessant atrial tachycardia) and among the 8 with a second degree A-V block, only one had an structural heart disease with a palliative surgical procedure.

INTRODUCTION

Diverse conduction disturbances have been observed in the follow-up of cardiac surgery patients, most of the times transitory in nature [1,2]. Complete atrioventricular block (CAVB) is sometimes related to cardiac surgery at the atrial and/or ventricular level, which is also responsible of a high percentage of second degree AVB. Attempts have been made to establish a relationship between the conduction abnormalities and the kind of surgical technique utilized [1,3]. The present study has been realized aiming at getting information on A-V conduction derangements after different types of cardiopulmonary bypass surgery (CPBS).

MATERIAL AND METHODS

From August 1.990 to December 1.991 225 CPBS procedures have been performed in our Medico-Surgical Unit of Pediatric Cardiology ; cases with A-V septal defects (both complete and incomplete) and those with first degree A-V block related to digitalis efect have been excluded. During the same period of time, 60 pts have been studied with a Holter electrocardiogram (Holter-ECG) due to different types of disrryhthmias and degrees of A-V block, ages ranging from 9 months to 14 years (mean 8.9 years) and time of registration from inmediate postoperative period to several years thereafter.

All studies were interpreted by means of a compatible IBM-PC properly programmed and provided with the adequate software to detect premature beats, maximal and minimal heart rate, slow and rapid disrrhythmias and ST level alterations. In all pts this analysis followed a general routine heart exammination (physical examination, chest XR, basal surface ECG with a long lead II recording and intregral echo-Doppler investigations).

RESULTS (Table)

The incidence of CAVB among the 60 infants and children studied was of 15% (9 cases, Table). It is worthwhile to point out on 4 pts in whom CAVB appeared in the inmediate postoperative period after a Mustard procedure in 2 and following an atriopulmonary anastomosis in other 2; in 4 pts a second degree AVB appeared after CPBS: : 2 with Tetralogy of Fallot (TOF), 1 with double outlet right ventricle (DORV) and 1 with atrial septal defect (ASD) plus patent ductus arteriosus (PDA).
Because of this, and as a complementary analysis, 243 24 hours ECG (Holter) studies of either operated or non operated pts performed during the same period of time were reviwed. Age varied from 13 days to 21 years (mean 9.5 yrs.). A Holter diagnosis of CAVB was reached in 17 (7%) pts: 9 after CPBS (just quoted in this paper), 7 of congenital origin (CCAVB) and 1 appearing after fulguration for incessant supraventricular tachycardia. A second degree AVB was encountered in 8 pts: 4 after a CPBS, 3 of congenital origin and 1 after a pulmonary artery banding in a case of univentricular heart (UVH).

DISCUSSION

Disturbances of the AV conduction constitute an important item in the field of Pediatric Cardiology. For diagnosis documentation and treatment, obviously a basal surface ECG is not enough. A 24 hours ECG recording continuously the electrical activity during the normal life a complete day is necessary. Recording cassettes are of a reduced appropriate size to be used in babies. Recordings may be now easyly analyzed and adequately displayed by means of the specific software; a graphic display of heart rate (HR) changes, frequency of premature ventricular contractions (PVC) and repolarization alterations is now possible [4,5].

It seems that the incidence of disrrhythmias is progressively increasing as survival of postcorrective-surgical congenital heart pts is augmenting as well and the physcian ability for detection improves [6].

Advanced degree AVB relative to cardiac surgery represents a substancial proportion among the different etiological features in AVB in infants and children. According to the published series, its relative incidence depends on the experience and expertise of the team, surgical technique and underlying pathology.

Our series is in agreement with the previously reported ones, although the incidence in our experience may be in part byssed by the fact of applying 24 hours ECG only to pts with clinical suspicion of advanced AVB and to those with very low heart rates, in the borderline concerning a pacemaker implantation.

To the already well known incidence of advanced AVB after surgery involving either the ventricular (TOF, DORV, etc..) [3,7] or atrial (ASD, single atrium physiological TGA correction, etc.. [8,9,10] septa, we have to add that occurring after the atriopulmonary anasastomosis, a widely applied procedure for many types of complex

TABLE: A-V CONDUCTION DISTURBANCES

(Incidence according to the underlying pathology and surgical procedure)

Postsurgical CAVB 9

FOLLOWING:

(.) Atriopulmonary anastomosis 2

1 patient with UVH and PS

1 patient with UVH and PA

(.) A Mustard procedure 2

(.) A resection in a subaortic stenosis... 1

In 1 patient with UVH+narrowing of the bulbo-ventricular foramen).

(.) Correction of TAPVD 1

(.) VSD closure 1

(.) DORV corrective surgery 1

(.) ASD + PS corrective surgery 1

Postsurgical partial AVB 4

FOLLOWING:

(.) TOF corrective surgery 2

(.) DORV corrective surgery 1

(.) ASD + PDA 1

<u>Abbreviations:</u> PS. Pulmonary stenosis; PA: Pulmonary atresia. TAPVD: Total anomalous pulmonary venous drainage.

congenital heart disease [11,12], and the one occurring after invasive management of disrrhythmias.

This paper support once more the view that 24 hours ECG remains as a most useful technique for early detection and management of disrrhythmias, which in turn will be responsible for a better control of morbidity and mortality after surgical treatment of congenital heart disease.

REFERENCES

1.- P. Silva Orrego, M. Urina Triana, H. Mora Montenegro, X. Escudero Canedo, G. Fernández de la Reguera. Trastornos de la Conducción en el Post-operatorio de la Cirugía Cardíaca con Circulación Extracorpórea. Arch Inst Cardiol Mex 58 (6) 1988, p 569.

2.- A. Garson, in Pediatric Arrhythmias: Electrophysiology and Pacing, ed. W.B. Saunders (1990).

3.- A.M. Basagoitia, P. Iturralde, O. Galvan, J. Rosado, C. Vazquez, L. Colin, L. Romero, J. González Hermosillo. Trastornos del Ritmo y de la Conducción en Pacientes Operados de Corrección Total de Tetralogía de Fallot. Arch Inst Cardiol Mex 61 (1) 1991, p 27.

4.- H.B. Wiles, D.S. Buckles, V.L. Zeigler, in Pediatric Arrhythmias: Electrophysiology and Pacing, ed. W.B. Saunders (1.990).

5.- C.J. Porter, P.C. Gillette, D.G. McNamara. 24-Hour Ambulatory ECGs in the Detection and Management of Cardiac Dysrhytmias in infants and Childrens. Pediatr Cardiol 1, 1980, p. 203.

6.- J. Deanfield, W. McKenna, H.S. Yen. Congenital Heart Disease: Postoperative Follow up and Dysrhytmias. Am J Cardiol 49, 1982, p. 998.

7.-L. Houyel, G. Vaksmann, A. Fournier, A. Davignon. Ventricular Arrhytmias after Correction of Ventricular Septal Defects: Importance of Surgical Approach. J Am Coll Cardiol 16 (5) 1990, p. 1224.

8.- L. Houyel, J. Petit, J. Langlois, R. Nottin, C. Planche, J.P. Binet. Surgery for incomplete atrioventricular Canal. Mid-Term follow-up Apropos of 128 Patients. Arch Mal Coeur 81 (4) 1988, p. 501.

9.- V.L. Vetter, C.S. Tanner, L.N. Horowitz. Electrophysiologic Consequences of the Musta Repair of D-Transposition of the Great Arteries. J Am Coll Cardiol 10, 1987, p. 1265.

10.- C. Hayes, W.M. Gersony. Arrhytmias after the Mustard Operation for Transposition of the Great Arteries: A Long-Term Study. J Am Coll Cardiol 7, 1986, p. 133.

11.- K.E. Ward, J.P. Moak, A. Garson. Appearance and Disappearance of Arrhytmias after the Fontan Operation. J Am Coll Cardiol 5, 1985, p. 427.

12.- C.C. Kurer, C.S. Tanner, W.I. Norwood, V.L. Vetter. Perioperative Arrhytmias after Fontan Repair. Circulation 82 (5 Suppl) 1990, p. IV190.

SINUS NODE FUNCTION AND HEMODYNAMICS

Naoyuki Takahashi
Department of Cardiology, Surugadai Nihon University Hospital,
1-8-13 Kanda-Surugadai, Chiyoda-ku, Tokyo 101, Japan

and

Hiroshi Yagi, Hideo Suzuki, Keiichi Sugino, Takayoshi Watanabe,
Kenji Sugimoto, Mikio Sasaki, Kagari Wada, Ryuitsu Kang, Satoshi Uenishi,
Makiko Matsuyama, Jirou Tokita, Sumito Ohguchi, Kazutaka Yamaguchi,
Kagari Matsudaura, Shinobu Imai, Katsuo Kanmatsuse,Nagao Kajiwara,
Department of Cardiology, Surugadai Nihon University Hospital,
1-8-13 Kanda-Surugadai, Chiyoda-ku, Tokyo 101, Japan

ABSTRACT

This study was aimed to investigate whether systolic blood pressure (SBP) and/or right atrial pressure (RAP) during right atrial overdrive pacing influence on the sinus node function in thirteen normal subjects .

All patients had 30 seconds of atrial pacing at a 1 to 1 A-V conduction, with continuous arterial and right atrial pressure monitoring.

There was no significant correlation between the atrial pacing rate and the corrected sinus node recovery time (CSRT). The atrial pacing rate correlated significantly with the change in the RAP($r=0.40$) and SBP ($r=-0.68$), and CSRT correlated significantly with the change in the RAP($r=-0.26$) and SBP ($r=0.33$) before and the first 10 seconds of pacing. No significant correlation was observed among the RAP and SBP during pacing and sino-atrial conduction time (SACT).

These results suggest that either elevation of RAP which produces a stretch effect on the sinus node, or a decrease in SBP which activates the sympathetic nervous system during right atrial pacing may contribute to the enhanced sinus node automaticity in normal subjects.

Methods

Subjects

Thirteen subjects with normal sinus node function with a mean age of 55.3±20.2 years (6 men and 7 women) were hospitalized for examination of arrhythmias. Informed consent were obtained before this procedure.

Pacing protocol and Hemodynamic measurements

For all patients, a 5F quadripolar catheter (1 cm interelectrode distances Vygon Corp.) was looped in the superior vena cava and the recording poles were placed at the right atrial-superior vena caval junction. High amplification (100 to 200 μV/cm) was used with filter settings of 0.1 to 50 Hz. A 6F multipolar electrode catheters (USCI Corp., Elecath Corp., and Mansfield Corp.) were positioned in the high right atrium, His bundle, and in the right ventricular apex. One 7F tipped-manometer catheter (Miller Corp.) was positioned in the mid-right atrium to obtain RAP recordings. SBP was measured with intra-arterial catheters. Pacing was performed with a custom-built stimulator (SEC-3102 Nihonkouden Corp.) using 2-msec rectangular pulses at twice late diastolic threshold. Surface leads were displayed on a multichannel oscilloscope (Model RMC-1100 Nihonkouden Corp.) simultaneously with sinus node, high right atrial, his bundle and ventricular electrograms, RAP and SBP. All parameters were recorded at a paper speed of 50 or 100 mm/sec. The right atrial pacing rate was increased every 10 beats for 30 seconds from 10 beats above the basic sinus beat to development of second degree A-V block. CSRT was defined as the difference between sinus node recovery time measured by the direct method and basic cycle length. SACT was measured by the direct method at the first recovery period after the cessation of rapid atrial pacing.

SBP and RAP(A wave) were monitored continuously throughout the pacing period by a intra-arterial catheter and a tipped manometer, respectively.

SBP in the pre-pacing period (SBPpre) and RAP in the pre-pacing period (RAPpre) were defined as an average of SBP and RAP of 5 beats before pacing. SBPi and RAPi were defined as an average of SBP and RAP of the first 10 seconds of pacing. ΔSBP was calculated from the difference of SBPpre and SBPi. ΔRAP was calculated from the difference of RAPpre and RAPi(Table 1).

Statistical Analysis

Statistical significance was defined as p values of less than 0.05.

Results

Fig1. shows a correlation between the pacing rate and CSRT at 1 to 1 A-V conduction. There was a no significant correlation between the atrial pacing rate and CSRT. Fig2. shows a correlation between the pacing rate and ΔSBP at 1 to 1 A-V conduction. The atrial pacing rate correlated significantly with ΔSBP. Fig3. shows a correlation between the atrial pacing rate and ΔRAP at 1 to 1 A-V conduction. The atrial pacing rate correlated significantly with ΔRAP. Fig4. shows a correlation between ΔSBP and CSRT. CSRT correlated significantly with ΔSBP for the first 10 seconds during rapid atrial pacing. Fig5. shows a correlation between ΔRAP and CSRT. CSRT correlated significantly with ΔRAP for the first 10 seconds

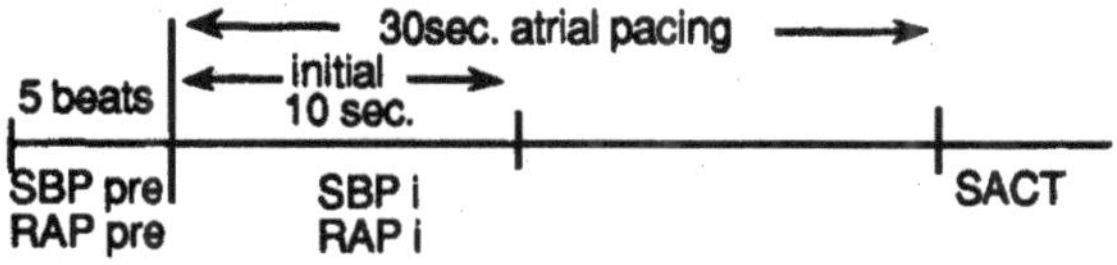

Table 1 Pacing protocol and Hemodynamic measurement

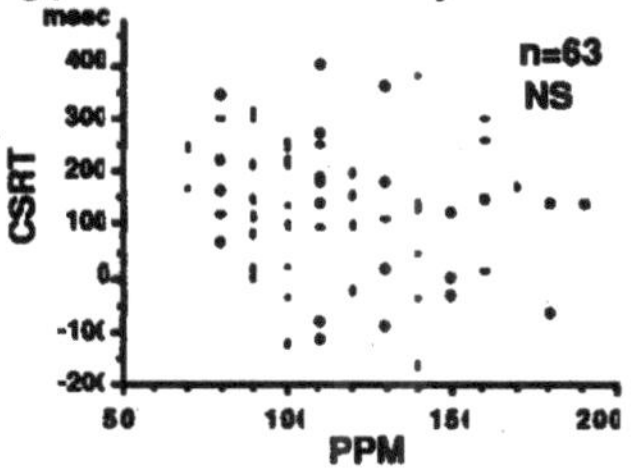

Fig 1 Correlations between pacing rate and CSRT at 1 t0 1 A-V conduction
n= periods of measuring CSRT ppm= pacing per minute

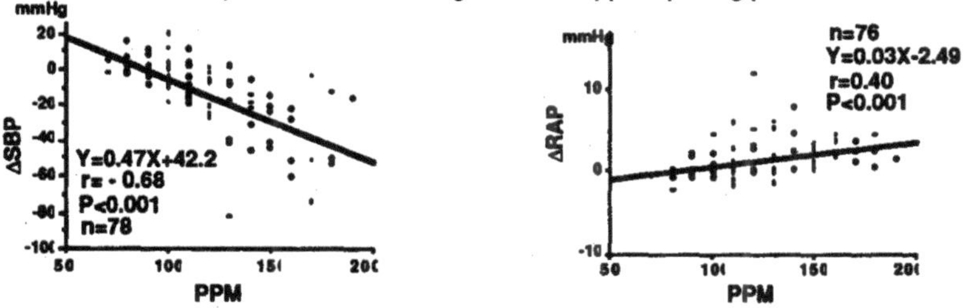

Fig 2,3 Correlations between Pacing rate and ΔSBP, ΔRAP at 1 to 1 A-V conduction

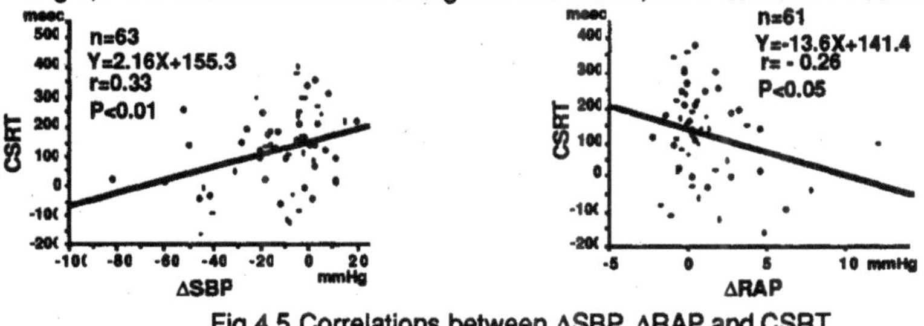

Fig 4,5 Correlations between ΔSBP, ΔRAP and CSRT

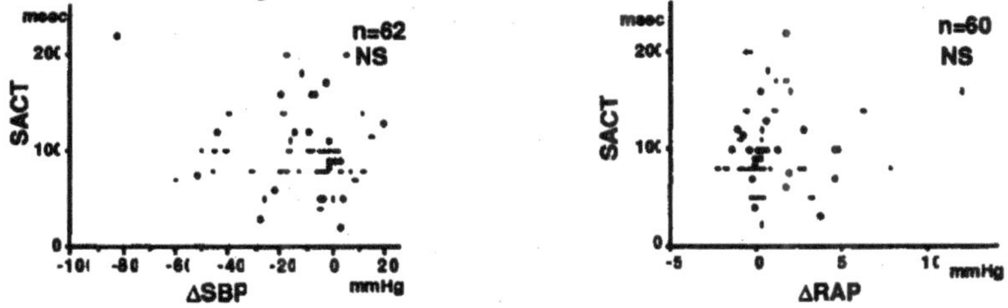

Fig 6,7 Correlations between ΔSBP, ΔRAP and SACT

during rapid atrial pacing. Fig6. shows a correlation between ΔSBP and SACT. No significant correlation was observed between ΔSBP and SACT.Fig7. shows a correlation between ΔRAP and SACT. No significant correlation was observed between ΔRAP and SACT.

Discussion

We have previously reported that the CSRT, measured indirectly by an atrial electrogram (indirect method), was affected by changes in SBP at 1 to 1 A-V conduction during rapid atrial pacing before pharmacological denervation in patients without sinus node dysfunction[1]. However the CSRT estimated by the indirect method derived from the two components which consisted of sinus node automaticity and sino-atrial conductivity. Furthermore a rapid atrial pacing sometimes induced a dominant sinus node pacemaker shift[2,3], sino atrial entrance and/or exit block[4]. Therefore, in the present study, for overcoming the limitations of indirect methods, both CSRT and SACT were evaluated by a direct sinus node electrogram (direct method).

This study was performed to re-investigate the influence of hemodynamic changes on the sinus node function by direct method at 1 to 1 A-V conduction during rapid atrial pacing in thirteen normal subjects.

These results suggest that either elevation of RAP which produces a stretch effect on the sinus node, or a decrease in SBP which activates the sympathetic nervous system during right atrial pacing may contribute to the enhanced sinus node automaticity in normal subjects.

References

1. M Sasaki, H Yagi, and N Kajiwara, *The influence of the systolic blood pressure and right atrial pressure on the sino-atrial conduction time.* **Vol.10 No.1**, Japanese Journal of Electrocardiology, 1990, 89-101
2. JAC Gomes, RI Hariman, and IA Chowdry, *New application of direct sinus node recordings in man: Assessment of sinus node recovery time.* **Vol.70**, Circulation 1984, 663
3. HH Lu, G Lange, and CMC Brooks, *Factors controlling pacemaker action in cells of the sino-atrial node.* **Vol.17**, Circ Res 1965,460
4. P Assemann, B Berzin, D Desry, P Durand, C Delmonte, EH Sarkis, J Lekieffre, C Thery, *Persistent sinus nodal electrograms during abnormally prolonged post pacing atrial pauses in sick sinus syndrome in Humans: sino-atrial block vs overdrive suppression.* **Vol.68** Circulation 33,1983

AN ATTEMPT TO LOCALISE THE ACCESSORY PATHWAY IN WPW SYNDROME USING ELECTROCARDIOGRAPHIC METHODS

MIHAI STEFANESCU,CONSTANTIN GEORGESCU
University of Medicine and Pharmacy,Clinic of Cardiology,
Tirgu Mures,Romania

ABSTRACT

In 5o patients with WPW syndrome,the standard ECG,vectorcardiogram(VCG) and precordial map(PM) were used together in order to better localize the pre- excitation.Correlated with the electrophysiologic(EP)study,theese three noninvasive methods revealed a rather good sensitivity and specificity(92) to establish the site of bypass tracts.

The advent of surgical techniques to interrupt accessory pathways as a treatment modality of medically resistant arrhythmias has made more apparent the necessity to localize pre- operatively the site of pre-excitation [6,8,18].The ECG in standard lead system cannot be used alone to reliably predict the site of anatomic bypass tract with the precision needed for operative interventions.Therefore,together with the standard ECG lead system,we have used vectorcardiography and body surface isopotential mapping of delta wave,and correlated the data with the localize of accessory pathways by electrophysiologic study [1,10,13].

Patients and Method

The investigations were carried out in 5o patients, 39 males and 11 females,ranging in age from 9 to 6o years,selected usind ECG criteria for WPW syndrome.

In all patients,in supine position,the following examinations were done:

- standard 12 lead ECG;

- orthogonal X,Y,Z electrocardiogram in Frank system,with the corresponding deduced loops [12];
- precordial mapping,recorded from 36 anterior thorax sites provided to a FORTRAN program performed on a FELIX-256 computer(determining the amplitude,duration and surface of the delta wave)[1,4,11].

The recordings were made using a six channel 6 NEK 4 RFT electrocardiograph,on standard ECG paper running at a speed of 5o mm/sec,with a standardization of 1 cm/1 mV.All the recordings and the measurements were done by the same observer(S.M.).

The criteria used to localize the site of pre-excitation were:
- For ECG:the Gallagher lo types of classification[8].
- The 4 VCG types described by Medvedowsky,[10].
- The 6 types of PM proposed by Ambroggi,[1].
- EP study: - right atrial and ventricular pacing for the right-sided accessory pathways
  - coronary sinus or esophageal left atrium pacing for the left-sided accessory pathways.

Results

The localization of pre-excitation in our 5o patients taking into account the ECG,VCG and PM criteria is shown in Table I.

Table I.
The site of accessory pathway in WPW syndrome
(nr. of patients)

	LEFT LATERAL	RIGHT LATERAL	PARA-SEPT. LEFT POST.	PARA-SEPT. RIGHT POST.	TOTAL	UNCERTAIN LOCATION
ECG, VCG, PM	15	18*	8	5	46	4
EP study	16	19	8	6	49	1
CORRELATION INDEX	94%	95%	100%	83,3%	92%	

* 2 cases possible paraseptal right anterior(ECG and PM)

It is obvious that,using together these three methods,a rather precise localization of pre-excitation was obtained in all patients,except 4.

Table II
The lack of correlation between ECG,VCG and PM (4 patients)

Patients	ECG Type	VCG Type	PM Type	EP Study
Nr.7	6 (paraseptal left posterior)	I (left lateral)	e (left posterior)	James-Mahaim
Nr. 22	1 (paraseptal left anterior)	I (left lateral)	d (left anterior)	? possible left an terior ventricular wall
Nr. 29	3 (right lateral)	IV (paraseptal right posterior)	d (right anterior)	James-Mahaim
Nr. 49	10 (left anterior)	III (paraseptal left posterior)	f (right)	right lateral ventricular wall & left paranodal accesssory pathways

In patients Nr.22 and 49 from Table II,the lack of concordance of theese methods could be explained only during an intracavitary examination,as multiple abberant pathways,and in patients Nr.7 and 29 we found combination of James and Mahaim fibers [5].

Discussion and Conclusion

Noninvasive and easy to be performed without special equipment,used together,the ECG,VCG and PM confer upon a rather precise location of the accessory pathways in the WPW syndrome.[1,4,6,8,10,13]. The simpleway of ECG,VCG and PM performing,classification and interpretation used in this study are almost as effective as the invasive procedures in the determination of preexcitation.For the rapide,preoperative orientation in a patient with WPW syndrome,the computer techniques are not quite neccessary,the delta wave vector orientation beeing easily detected by electrocardiographic pattern.The lack of concordance of the three methods and the impossibility of localizing the pre-excitation suggest multiple aberrant pathways and the patient should be studiated separately by intracavitary examination.For operative reasons,ECG,VCG and PM should be considered only as preliminary steps to more refined electrophysiologic study.Theese three methods utilised in our study have not been correlated with surgical or pathological findings,so that we cannot draw definitive conclusions as their advantage in a very precise localization of the preexcitation.[6,11].

References

1. L.Ambroggi,F.D.Taccardi,E.Macchi,*Circulation*,54(1976)251.
2. S.Bellet,*Clinical disorders of the heart beat*,ed.Lea & Febiger(Philadelphia,1971).
3. J.P.Boineau,E.N.Moore,J.F.Spear,W.C.Sealy,*Circulation*,32 (1973)32.
4. G.Bonneau,G.Tremblay,P.Sarvad et al,*IEEE Trans Biomed Eng*,34(1987)415.
5. G.E.Burch,*Am.Heart J.*,9o(1975)307.
6. J.L.Cox,J.J.Gallagher,M.E.Cain,*J.Thorac.Cardiovasc.Surg*.90 (1985)49o.
7. R.Frank,G,Fontaine,G.Quiraudon,C.Cabriol,Y.Grosgoceat, I.Facquet,*Arch. Mal.Coeur*,7o(1977)441.
8. J.J.Gallagher,W.C.Sealy,A.G.Wallace,J.Kassel, in *The conduction system of the heart*,ed.H.J.J.Wellens, K.I.Lie, H.J.Janse (Senfert-Kroese,Leiden,1976).
9. J.Machecourt,B.Denis,P.Martin-Noel,*Ann.Cardiol.Angeiol*, 27(1978)1.
lo. J.L.Medvedowsky,P,Nicolai,C.Barnay,J.Delaage,J.C.Agelou, *Arch.Mal.Coeur*, 9 (1978) looo
11. H.J.Vidaillet,J.E.Lowe,L.D.Germanet al,*Am.J.Cardiol*, 58(1986)94o.
12. C.A.Witham.in *A system of vectorcardiographic interpretation* (Year Book Medical Publishers,Chicago,1975).
13. K.Yamada,K Toyama,J.Wada et al,*Am.Heart J*.90 (1975)721.

PACEMAKER CELLS OF ATRIOVENTRICULAR NODE AND ATRIOVENTRICULAR VALVES FORM A SINGLE PACEMAKER?

PROSHEVA V.
Institute of Physiology, Syktyvkar, 167610, Russia

ABSTRACT

The dimension of pacemaker in the atrioventricular area of the avian (pigeon, chicken) and mammal (rabbit) heart were estimated by the method of microelectrode mapping of action potentials. Electrophysiological properties of pacemaker cells in atrioventricular node (AVN) and atrioventricular valve (AVV) were compared. Our findings suggest that the pacemaker of the atrioventricular area is more extended than is generally accepted, that is it includes both the pacemaker area of compact AVN and pacemaker zones of AVV.

1. Introduction

It is known that in the atrioventricular area of the heart not only cellular elements of atrioventricular node but those of atrioventricular valves possess pacemaker properties[1-4]. In the present study we compare the electrophysiological properties and functional organization of pacemaker cells in atrioventricular node and atrioventricular valves of the mammal and avian heart. We put forward a new conception about the structural-functional organization of the atrioventricular area of the heart. In our opinion this area includes both the pacemaker area of the atrioventricular node and the pacemaker zones of the atrioventricular valves.

2. Material and Methods

The objects of our investigation were adult rabbits (29), chickens (16) and pigeons (31). The experiments were conducted on the isolated preparations of the atrioventricular area, including atrioventricular node, right atrioventricular valve and adjacent parts of free walls of the right atrium and right ventricle and interventricular septum, on the isolated right atrioventricular valves and on the isolated atrioventricular nodes. In the right atrioventricular opening of the heart in adult mammals there is a multicuspid valve, but in bird's heart there is another type of the valve, namely: muscle and unicuspid.
Action potentials were registered with glass microelectrodes on the automatized electrophysiological set-up. The period of discretization is 0.5 ms. We applied the method of microelectrode mapping of action potentials because only this method allows to perform an accurate differentiation of the cells in the

transitional areas of the heart. Microelectrode mapping of pacemaker area was performed with a various "step" beginning from 10 μm.

3. Electrophysiological organization of pacemaker cells in the atrioventricular node and right atrioventricular valve

Both the isolated preparations of atrioventricular node and atrioventricular valve possess stable regular spontaneous activity during several hours in the rabbit, chicken and pigeon hearts. The ratio between spontaneous rate of pacemaker cells of atrioventricular node and sinoatrial node is similar to that between spontaneous rate of cells of atrioventricular valve and sinoatrial node. Fig. 1 shows the results of the typical experiment on the mapping of action potentials in the atrioventricular area of the rabbit heart. The microelectrode was moved from the area of the atrioventricular node to the leaflets of the tricuspid valve. The distance in which pacemaker cells action potentials were registered in given case was 32 mm. Then we cut this preparations into its two parts, which can be named the area of the atrioventricular node and the area of the valve. Both preparations showed spontaneous activity during eight hours. In the given experiment the area of the atrioventricular node contracted 1.8 times more frequently than the area of the valve.

It should be noted that the microelectrode mapping of the pacemaker area of the atrioventricular node in the direction from the atrium to interventricular

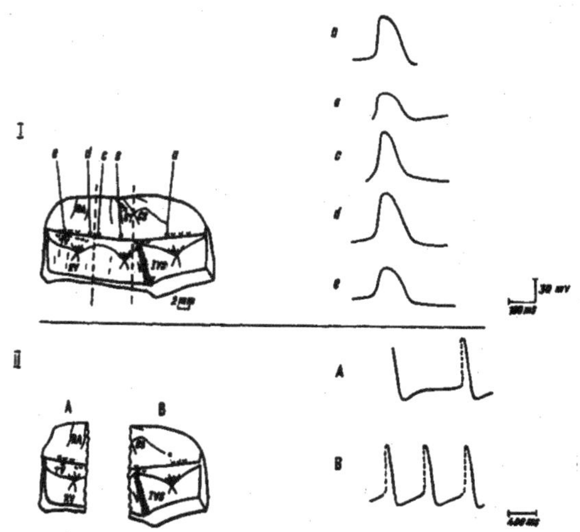

Fig.1. Microelectrode mapping of the pacemaker in atrioventricular area of the rabbit heart. *I* - scheme of the preparation and action potentials of pacemaker cells, registered from the atrioventricular node (*a*) and right atrioventricular valve (*b-e*). The plotted points are the places of registration of these action potentials. The dotted lines point out the places of the subsequent cut of the preparation; *II* - scheme of the preparations after the cut and action potentials recorded from the area of the right atrioventricular valve (*A*) and atrioventricular node(*B*). The plotted points are the places of registration of these action potentials. *RV* - right ventricle, *TV* - right atrioventricular valve, *RA* - right atrium, *CT* - crista terminalis, *CS* - coronary sinus, *IVS* - interventricular septum.

septum showed that the width of the pacemaker in this region is 2.8 mm. According to our data[3] the width of the pacemaker area in the leaflets of the rabbit tricuspid valves is 2-3 mm. In pigeons and chickens the length of the pacemaker area is coincided with the length of the valve of the investigated individual and is equal from 13 to 20 mm. The width of the pacemaker zone is about 2 mm.

Low maximal diastolic potential, slow rate of depolarization and low amplitude of action potentials of pacemaker cells in atrioventricular valve are similar to the characteristics of transmembrane action potentials of pacemaker cells in atrioventricular node.

Electrophysiological heterogeneity of the cells in the atrioventricular node is generally-known fact. Variability of the configurations of the registered pacemaker cells action potentials in rabbit[3], chicken and pigeon[2,4] atrioventricular valves points out at the electrophysiological heterogeneity of the cells forming this area of the heart. In the transition area atrial myocardium - pacemaker of atrioventricular node and also atrial myocardium - pacemaker of atrioventricular valve, pacemaker cells action potentials with the prepotential on the upstroke are registered. The duration of the plateau of pacemaker cells action potentials in atrioventricular node and atrioventricular valve increases in the antegrade direction.

Pacemaker cells in atrioventricular valve like the cells in atrioventricular node are sensitive to agents blocking the slow channel, to the manganese, cobalt ions, verapamil and pluronics[1,5].

4. Conclusion

Thus the pacemaker area of the atrioventricular valves in the bird and mammal heart is organized like that of the atrioventricular node.

The obtained findings give the possibility suggest that the pacemaker of the atrioventricular area has a larger extent than it is generally accepted. Namely in our opinion it includes both the pacemaker zone of the compact atrioventricular node and the pacemaker zone of the atrioventricular valves. The original scheme of the topography of the pacemaker and conducting system in the bird heart is shown on the Fig.2. In our opinion the structural formation of great extent having pacemaker properties should be named a pacemaker of the atrioventricular area, but not an atrioventricular node or atrioventricular ring of specialized fibers.

At present in monographs and handbooks usually one can meet the scheme where the location of pacemaker in the atrioventricular area of mammal heart is shown as a compact atrioventricular node.

Our findings show a considerable extent of the pacemaker zone in the atrioventricular area in the mammal heart also. That is we dare to suggest a modified scheme of the topography of pacemaker in the mammalian heart (Fig.3). We believe that the information concerning large extent of pacemaker

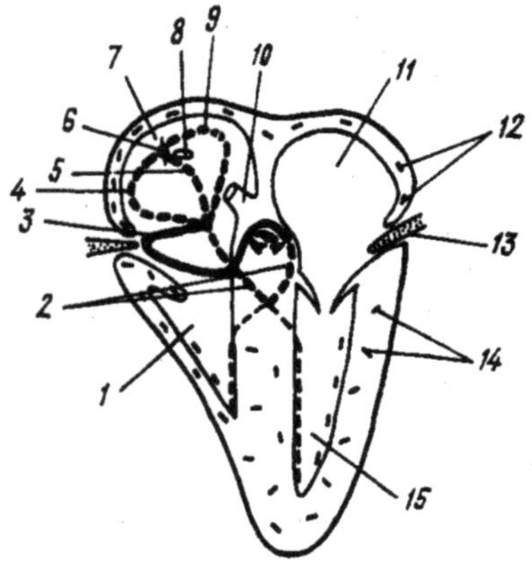

Fig.2. The scheme of topography of the pacemaker and conducting system in the bird heart. *1* - right ventricle, *2* - atrioventricular bundle, *3* - pacemaker of the atrioventricular area, *4* - right atrial bundle, *5* - middle atrial bundle, *6* - pacemaker of sinoatrial area, *7* - right atrium, *8* - right cranial vena cava, *9* - left atrial bundle, *10* - aorta, *11* - left atrium, *12* - Purkinje fibers in atria, *13* - fibrous tissue, *14* - Purkinje fibers in ventricles, *15* - left ventricle.

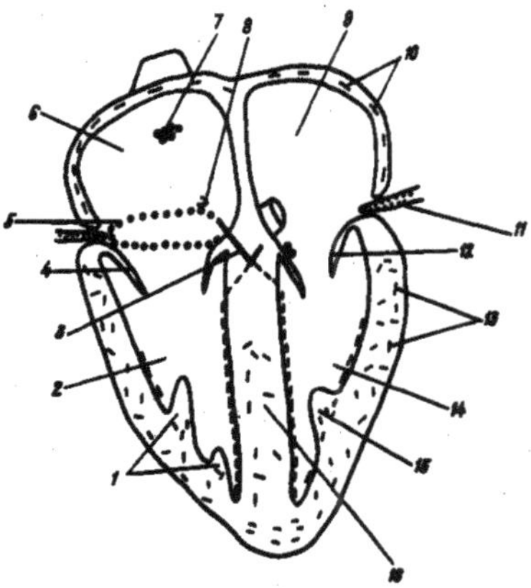

Fig.3. The scheme of topography of the pacemaker and conducting system in the mammal heart. *1* - papillary muscles, *2* - right ventricle, *3* - atrioventricular bundle, *4* - right atrioventricular valve, *5* - pacemaker of atrioventricular area, *6* - right atrium, *7* - pacemaker of sinoatrial area, *8* - coronary sinus, *9* - left atrium, *10* - Purkinje fibers in atria, *11* - fibrous tissue, *12* - left atrioventricular valve, *13* - Purkinje fibers in ventricles, *14* - left ventricle, *15* - papillary muscles, *16* - interventricular septum.

zones in the atrioventricular area is absolutely necessary to take into consideration at surgical interference in the given area of the heart. Probably we are approaching some new understanding of structural organization and functioning of the pacemaker in the atrioventricular area of the heart.

5. References

1. G.J.Rozansky, *Amer.J.Physiol.* **253**(1987)H720-H727.
2. V.Prosheva and I.Rapota, in *Electrocardiology 87*, ed. E.Shubert (Academie-Verlag, Berlin, 1988) p. 127-130.
3. V.Prosheva, in *Advances in electrocardiology*, ed. Z.Antaloczy et al (Excerpta Medica, Amsterdam, 1990) p.83-86.
4. V.Prosheva, *Successes of Physiological Sciences*, **21**(1991) p.83-93 (in Russian).
5. V.Prosheva, in *Abstracts of the 19th Intern.Cong.on Electrocardiol.* (Lisbon, 1992) p.173.

DO TYPES OF THE QRS_{V1} CORRESPOND TO INTERRUPTED SITES IN THE RIGHT BUNDLE BRANCH?

RYOZO OKADA, M.D.

Research Laboratory for Cardiovascular Pathology, Juntendo University School of Medicine, Tokyo 113, Japan

ABSTRACT

Sixty three autopsied hearts with a right bundle branch block, were histopathologically studied to determine interrupted sites in the atrioventricular conduction system. The AV node, bundle of His and bilateral bundle branches (R-and L-BB) were cut serially and each one from 10 or 20 serial thin sections, was examined under a light microscope. The R_{V1} type corresponded with a proximal RBB interruption in 6 out of 7 cases associated with a normal QRS axis, with an interruption of the distal bundle of His in 8 out of 10 associated with a QRS left axis deviation (LAD) and also with the former or latter interruption in 4 or 2 out of 6, respectively, with a QRS right axis deviation (RAD). The rsR'_{V1} type corresponded with a middle RBB interruption in 21 out of 36, in which 9 with LAD were combined with a lesion in the anterior radiation of LBB and 6 with RAD were combined with either a lesion in the posterior and anterior radiations of LBB or the ventricular septum. The qR_{V1} type showed an interruption in the same manner as the rsR' and an association of a ventricular septum lesion in all 7 cases. The rSr'_{V1} type corresponded with a distal RBB interruption in 3 cases. It is worth mentioning that an RBB interruption proximal or distal to the first anterior fascicle of the RBB determined either an R or rsR' type at the V_1 lead.

The aim of this paper is to compare variations of the QRS_{V1} morphologies and histologically proven interrupted sites in the right bundle branch (RBB) using human autopsied hearts.

Materials and Methods

A total of 69 autopsied hearts with an electrocardiographically proven right bundle branch block (RBBB) was examined histologically. The patients' age was distributed from 12 to 91 years with an average of 67.3 years, and the sex distribution was 45 males and 24 females. Their basic diseases consisted of 20 cases of ischemic heart disease, 14 of hypertensive heart disease, 7 of myocarditis and sequelae, 4 of specific heart muscle disease, 3 of isolated conduction system disease, 2 each of idiopathic cardiomyopathy, congenital heart disease and valvular heart disease, 7 of malignant neoplasms, 6 of respiratory disease, 4 of cerebrovascular disease, 4 of diabetes mellitus and 3 of miscellaneous diseases.

The AV conduction system was cut from the AV node to the periphery of the bundle branches, according to Lev's method[1]. Each one from 10 or 20 serial thin sections was stained by hematoxylin-eosin, azan and elastica-van Gieson's methods, respectively. Pathological lesions, such as necrosis, degeneration, adiposis or lipomatosis, fibrosis and calcification of the conducting cells, were carefully checked under a light microscope, and the grade of cell loss was estimated as +, ++ and +++, corresponding to 25%, 50% and more than 75% reduction, respectively.

Results

Diagnosis of an interrupted site in the conduction system was made by determining the site of the most proximal lesion of maximal conducting cell loss. The grade of cell reduction at the interrupted site, exceeded a 75% loss in 97% of the studied cases and was close to a 50% loss in only 3% of the cases.

Fig. 1 shows a 70-year-old male case, having an R type QRS_{V1} and a normal QRS axis (NA). The RBB has a fibrotic interruption starting from its proximal to upper middle portion. The conducting cells of the RBB are completely lost there, but a small number of myocytes in the first anterior fascicle of the RBB, still persists. Fig. 2 shows an 83-year-old female case, having an R_{V1} and a QRS left axis deviation (LAD). The distal bundle of His has been replaced completely by a calcified mass, which interrupted 100% of the conduction system. Fig. 3 shows a 73-year-old male case with an rsR'_{V1} and NA. More than 75% of the conducting cells have been replaced by fibro-adiposis at the middle RBB. Fig. 4 shows 12 year-old male case with an rSr'_{V1}.

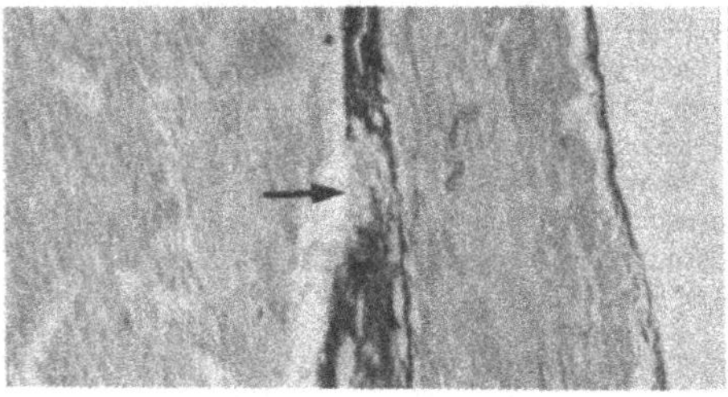

Fig.1 Photomicrograph of the RBB of a case with R_{V1} and NA. Elastica-van Gieson's stain. x40. Arrow mark shows a remnant of the first anterior fascicle of the RBB.

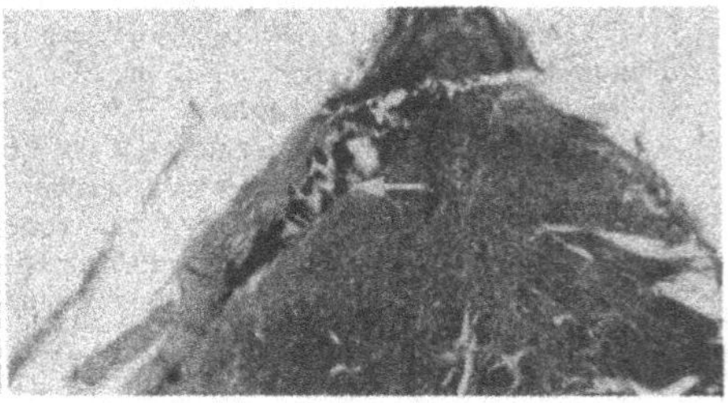

Fig.2 Photomicrograph of the His' bundle of a case with R_{V1} and LAD. H-E stain. x13. Arrow mark shows calcified distal end of the His' bundle.

The corresponding pathology is a focal necrosis and bleeding in the peripheral RBB.

Results of the study are shown in the table. In R_{V1} cases, 6 out of 7 cases with NA, showed a proximal RBBB, 8 of 10 associated with LAD showed a block at the distal bundle of His, including the anterior radiation of the LBB, and 4 or 2 out of 6 associated with RAD showed either a block at the proximal RBB or the distal His' bundle, respectively, combined with a lesion in both the posterior and anterior radiations of the LBB or in the ventricular septum. Twenty one of 36 cases with rsR'_{V1}, corresponded with a middle RBBB. Among these, all 9 cases with LAD were associated with a block in the anterior radiation of the LBB, and 6 with RAD were associated with a lesion in

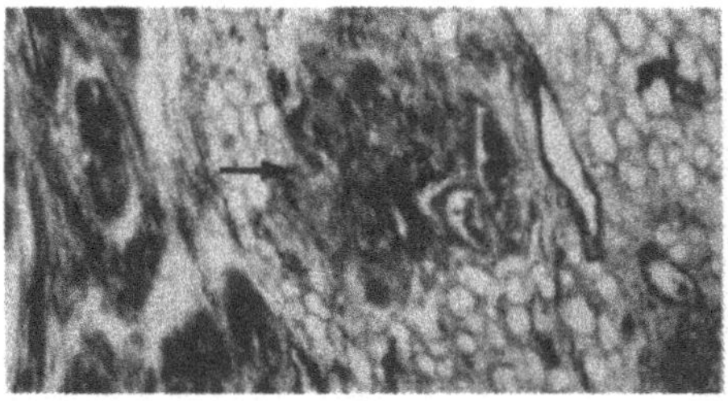

Fig.3 Photomicrograph of the RBB of a case with rsR'$_{V1}$. Azan stain, x40. Arrow mark shows a fibro-adiposis at the middle RBB.

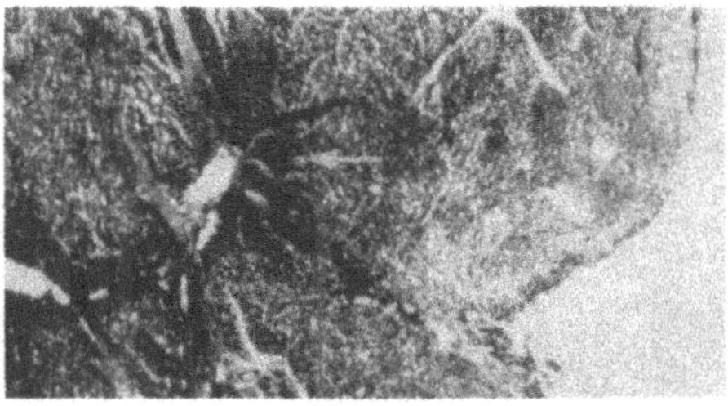

Fig.4 Photomicrograph of the RBB of a case with rSr'$_{V1}$. Azan stain x40. Arrow mark shows a necrosis and bleeding at the peripheral RBB.

Table. Relationship between QRS$_{V1}$ morphology and site of RBBB.

QRS$_{V1}$ morphology	R			rsR'			qR			rSr'
Interrupt.site/QRSaxis	NA	LAD	RAD	NA	LAD	RAD	NA	LAD	RAD	NA
Distal His' bundle		8	2	3	1		1			
Proximal RBB	6	1	4	1	1		1			
Middle RBB	1	1		15	5	6		4	1	
Distal RBB				2	2					3
Post.radiation of LBB*		2	4	1	2	4	1			
Ant. radiation of LBB*		9	4	1	9	4	1	4		
Ventricular septum*		1	1	3	2	2	2	4	1	1
No. of cases	7	10	6	21	9	6	2	4	1	3

NA: Normal QRS axis. LAD: Left axis. RAD: Right or north-west axis.
*LBB and ventricular septum lesions are doubly counted to RBB lesions.

both the posterior and anterior radiations of the LBB or in the ventricular septum. All 7 cases with qR$_{V1}$, showed a similar RBBB as the rsR'$_{V1}$ group, but were also accompanied by a massive ventricular septum lesion. All 3 cases with rSr'$_{V1}$ corresponded with peripheral RBBB.

Comment

An RBBB proximal or distal to the first anterior fascicle, corresponds either to an R$_{V1}$ or rsR'$_{V1}$ type[2]. An end of the His' bundle block corresponds with an R$_{V1}$ and LAD[3], because both the RBB and the anterior radiation of the LBB interrupt at a point lesion of their bifurcating portion. A peripheral RBB lesion forms a similar pattern to an incomplete RBBB. Lesions in the ventricular septum including the LBB, modifies the rule through a loss of the initial r or an association of RAD.

References

1. M. Lev, J. Widran and E.E. Erickson, AMA Arch. Path. 52 (1951) 73.
2. K. Fukuda, Y. Nakata, R. Okada and T. Takagi, Jpn Heart J 20 (1979) 831.
3. M. Sugiura, R. Okada, K. Hiraoka and S. Ohkawa, Jpn Heart J 10 (1969) 121.

Permanent Pacemakers in the Paediatric Age Group

Dulce Brito
Med. 4 Department, Sta Maria Hospital
Lisboa/Portugal

and

Margarida Telo
Paediatric Cardiology Department
Sta Maria Hospital
Lisboa/Portugal

ABSTRACT

Pacemaker (PM) implantation is seldom required in the paediatric age group. We present our 11 years (y) experience. From Nov. 80 to Sept. 91, 15 patients (pts), 8 boys and 7 girls, aged 4 days to 14 y ($\bar{5}$ y) had permanent PM implantation. The indications were congenital complete A-V block (CAVB) in 8 pts, cquired CAVB in 6 and bradycardia-tachycardia syndrome in 1. Seven of the 8 pts, with congenital CAVB had heart failure or syncope; the other had assymptomatic severe bradycardia. The age at initial PM implantation was lower in 4 pts with associated congenital heart disease than in those with isolated congenital CAVB: 3 to 10 months ($\bar{6}$ m) vs 4 days to 8.9 y ($\overline{4.2}$ y) - $p < 0.05$. Acquired CAVB was postoperative in 5 pts (following VSD closure in 3 and ressection of sub-aortic membrane in 2) and secondary to diphtheritic myocarditis in 1 pt.

Pacemaker leads were epicardial in 13 pts (VVIM) and endocardial in 2 pts (1 VVIM, 1 DDDM). Generator case was abdominal in 13, pectoral in 1 and intrathoracic in 1. During a follow-up period of 3 m to 11.8 y ($\bar{4}$ y), 7 pts underwent a total of 13 reoperations due to battery replacement in 7 and lead failure in 6. Two pts developed infection at the PM case. One pt died due to the associated heart defect. The 14 survivors are well with regard to PM function and cardiac rhythm.

In this series congenital CAVB was the most common indication for PM implantation. Morbidity requiring reoperation was significant but the incidence of true complications was low and the long term outlook is good.

Introduction

Pacemaker (PM) implantation in children is seldom required. Nevertheless, when this procedure becomes necessary it can be performed safely and with short and long term good results. We analysed the clinical features and outcome of our paediatric population submitted to permanent PM implantation during the last 11 years.

Material and Methods

Between November 1980 and September 1991, 5 pts-8 boys and 7 girls-aged 4 days to 14 y (mean 5 y), underwent permanent PM implantation. The reasons were complete atrioventricular block (CAVB) in 14 cases and bradycardia-tachycardia syndrome in one. CAVB was congenital in 8 pts and acquired in 6. Regarding congenital CAVB, 7 out of 8 pts had threatening symptoms (cardiac failure or syncope). In the other child, PM was implanted prophylactically because severe bradycardia (during sleep) was detected by Holter monitoring. Four of these pts had associated heart defects-complex cardiophaties or isolated ventricular septal defects (VSD)-and they needed PM implantation at a younger age than those with isolated congenital CAVB: 3 to 10 m (mean 6 m) vs 4 days to 8 y 9 m (mean 4 y 2 m). In 3 out of 4 pts with isolated congenital CAVB, diagnosis was made "in utero" (by fetal echocardiography) and anti SS-A (RO) antibodies were detected in 2 pts (both in children and their mothers).
Acquired CAVB was the reason for 6 permanent PM implants in a population ranging from 2 to 14 y (mean 7 y 5 m): 5 were postsurgical (following VSD closure in 3 pts and ressection of sub-aortic membrane in 2) and in 1 pt (a 5 y old girl) CAVB appeared during the course of diphtheritic myocarditis.
Pacing was initially epicardial in 13 pts (VVIM units) and endocardial in 2 (1 VVIM, 1 DDDM), being positioned by thoracotomy in 14 pts and by transvenous approach in 1. Generator site was abdominal in 13, pectoral in 1 and intrathoracic in another child.

Results

During a follow-up period of 3 m to 11 y 8 m (mean 4 y 2 m) 7 pts underwent a total of 13 reinterventions, due to battery replacement in 7 and lead failure in 6 (fibrosis with exit block or breakage of the wire). Two pts developed infection at the PM case, successfully treated. Two pts with epicardial leads changed later to endocardial pacing. One pt died, due to her associated heart defect. The 14 survivors are well with regard to PM function and cardiac rhytm.

Discussion

Indications for PM implantation in children are nowadays well defined [1]. In our series, as in others[2,3] congenital CAVB prevailed being acquired CAVB (surgically induced) the second main reason for implantation.

Congenital CAVB was associated in 4 pts with structural heart disease: 2 were compex cardiophaties (including single ventricle and L-transposition of the great arteries) and 2 were simple large VSD, abnormalities frequently found in association with congenital CAVB. Isolated congenital CAVB has a strong association with autoimmune abnormalities [4] and in 2 of 4 pts, the presence of anti-RO antibodies was documented. Symptoms were most severe in pts with congenital CAVB and associated heart disease, demanding permanent PM sooner than pts with isolated CAVB, as others also reported[5]. In a child with congenital CAVB, PM was implanted prophylactically because 9 seconds pauses were detected, during sleep, by Holter. Althought previously asymptomatic, once the permanent PM was implanted the child felt much better.

Surgical correction of congenital heart disease is often the cause for PM implantation in children[3,5,6]. The risk of development of heart block following surgery appears to be decreasing[7]. However, in our series, it was the second most frequent reason for PM implantation. The CAVB appearing during the course of diphtheritic myocarditis persisted beyond the cure, with marked bradycardia, therefore justifying permanent PM implantation.

In 9 out of 13 pts submitted initially to epicardial implant, this approach seemed the most suitable [6]: 5 were in their first year of life; in 4, the indication for PM developed immediatly after cardiopulmonary bypass. Nowadays there is a strong trend towards endocardial leads[5,6] because transvenous pacing is less traumatic and carries less morbidity. Children who require pacing often benefit from the most sophisticated dual chamber stimulation mode but their size may preclude the use of such a system. We used initially a small programmable ventricular synchronous pacing (VVIM) in almost all pts. Today we are increasingly using dual chamber PM, when the child has a sufficient growth to permit it.

During follow-up period, reintervention was frequently necessary (13 in 7 pts). However, 7 of them were for battery replacement and only 6 because of lead failure. There was only one death and unrelated to the PM system. The 14 survivors are growing and developing normally.

Conclusions

In this series congenital CAVB was the most common indication for PM implantation but surgically induced CAVB remained also an important one. Morbidity requiring reintervention was significant but the incidence of true complications was low.

Permanent pacing in children is now an acceptable treatment with low risk and good longterm outlook.

Acknowledgements

The authors wishes to thank Mrs. Ana Maria Madeira for assistance in preparing this manuscript.

Bibliography

1. L.S. Dreifus, C. Fisch, J.C. Griffin, P.C. Gillette, J.W. Mason, V. Parsonnet, *Circulation* 84 (1991) p. 455
2. C.A. Walsh, H.F. McAlister, C.A. Andrews, C.N. Steeg, R. Eisenberg, C. Furman, *Pace* 11 (1988) p. 1940
3. M. Jimenez, A. Fournier, E. Hery, M. Montigny, C. Kratz, C. Chartrand, P. Stanley, A. Davignon. *Arch. Mal. Coeur* 81 (1988) p. 665
4. B. A. Ross, *Pediatric Clinics of North America* (W.B. Saunders Company, Philadelphia) 37 (1990) p. 69
5. B. Dodinot, F. Marccon, B. Mouna, F. Ribeiro-Lages, J.P. Godemir, C. Pernot. *Arch. Mal. Coeur* 81 (1988) p. 673
6. R. Sutton, I. Bourgeois, *The Foundations of cardiac pacing* (Futura Publishing Inc. Mount Kisco, New York, 1991) p. 223
7. L.B. McGrath, L.L. Gonzalez, D.P. Morse, J.M. Levett, *Pace* 11 (1988) p. 1182.

PART V

Holter Monitoring, Heart Rate Variability and Signal Averaged ECG

THE EXPANSION OF ELECTROCARDIOLOGICAL INFORMATION BY FREQUENCY ANALYSIS OF SINUSARRHYTHMIA

ERNST SCHUBERT, ANDREAS PATZAK, WOLFGANG LAUBE
Institute of Physiology, Humboldt-University of Berlin
Hessische Straße 3/4, O-1040 Berlin, FRG

ABSTRACT

Sinusarrhythmia and heart rate deliver information about efferent chronotropic control pathways. Fast Fourier Transformation allows to separate components of sinusarrhythmia. In respiration experiments and exercise tests connections of the components with different input mechanisms are investigated. Central origins are detected for respiratory frequency and the control command in exercise besides baro-, chemo- and metaboreceptive peripheral afferents.

1. Rhythm analysis of sinusarrhythmia vs. heart rate informs about the efferent chronotropic control pathways

Sinusarrhythmia (SA) frequently has been utilized as evaluation of the heart rate variability. SA describes the rhythmical oscillations of heart rate (HR) measured by the mean differences of consecutive heart period durations. The reactions of SA on physical load [1], its resetting after fatiguing exercise [2], its diurnal changes [3] and the influences of age [4], training conditions and diseases [5] accentuate diverse regulatory mechanisms for SA in contrast to HR. Pharmacological blockades of cardiac vagus or sympathicus verify increasing SA as caused by growing vagal activity and increasing HR as determined by rising sympathetic activity coupled to diminishing of vagal tone up to HR values of about 120 beats/min [5]. These facts allow to consider this rhythm analysis as the noninvasive electrocardiological approach to the evaluation of the efferent pathways of cardiac control.

Slow traced records of HR and the spectral analysis of heart rate variability demonstrate the existence of several frequency components included in SA [6]. These observations stimulate to an expansion of the interpretation of such data in order to receive direct diagnostic information about afferent pathways of the cardiac control by analyzing the single components of heart rate variability. This study serves for finding direct connections between parameters of respiration and such of the "respiratory" peak in the frequency spectrum as well as between reactions of the spectral components and conditions of physical load in different intensity.

2. The spectral components of heart rate variability show characteristic dependencies on respiratory frequency and physical load

2.1. Methods and experimental procedures

Experiments were made in two groups of young healthy volunteers. The first group (n = 22, aged: 23,5 + 3,3 yrs.) performed resting respiration at 11 voluntarily controlled frequencies between 0,07 and 0,5 Hz following an acustical signal with freely chosen tidal volumes or at a constant volume of 15 % of vital capacity. The second group (n = 16, aged: 25,4 + 5,8 yrs.) underwent an bicyle ergometer test of 6 load steps from 0,5 to 3,0 W/kg body weight for 5 min each step followed by 5 min for recovery. From each partizipant the ECG lead NEHB-A was picked up and stored continuously for the evaluation of the heart period time series out of the RR-distances. In respiratory experiments the beginning of the trace, in exercise tests the steady state phases of the rhythm adjustment were selected for performing the frequency power spectrum analysis by the help of the Fast Fourier Transformation. The main frequencies of the mid and high frequency bands of these spectra and their absolute and relative powers were estimated. In the exercise tests also the power values of the low frequency band were evaluated.

2.2. Effects of voluntary respiratory frequency shifts

In the first experimental set each proband during rest showed three components in his power-spectral density diagramm with maxima at about 0,02, 0,1 and 0,3 Hz. The measured power differed in its absolute values and in its relations betweeen the three bands among the probands. The high frequency band (HF) of the spectrum shifted evidently under the voluntary changes of respiratory frequency (RF). As Tab. 1 demonstrates in one representative case HF moves in concordance to RF

RF:	rest	0.071	0.083	0.100	0.125	0.167	0.250	0.300	0.350	0.400	0.450	0.500
HF:	0.17	-	-	-	-	0.17	0.25	0.3	0.35	0.4	0.45	0.5
P(HF)	1675	-	-	-	-	3896	673	733	499	338	168	188
MF	0.08	0.07	0.08	0.1	0.125	0.1	0.1	0.08	0.09	0.08	0.09	0.09
P(MF)	7109	20374	30715	53234	19379	4642	4774	6836	4067	3194	4166	3078

Tab. 1 Voluntarily fixed respiratory frequency (RF), frequency of mid- (MF) and high- (HF) frequency band maxima and power (P) (arbitrary units) of these maxima

within the frequency range from 0,5 to 0,071 Hz. Under these conditions the absolute power increases with the appproaching of the HF to the midfrequency (MF) band. Below the respiratory frequency of 0,15 both components fuse and their maximal power increases nearly to the tenfold of the sum of the maximal power of both components under resting condition. This summation reaches the largest power values at the frequency of 0,1 Hz, which is the genuine frequency of MF.

2.3. Effects of increasing physical load

In the exercising group of probands the total power diminishes linearly with increasing load from 0,5 to 3,0 W/kg body weight by about 4 orders of magnitude. During the recovery periods power recreates practically completely. Fig. 1 demonstrates these effects in A as in accordance to the SA/HR rhythm diagram from former studies (5) in B.

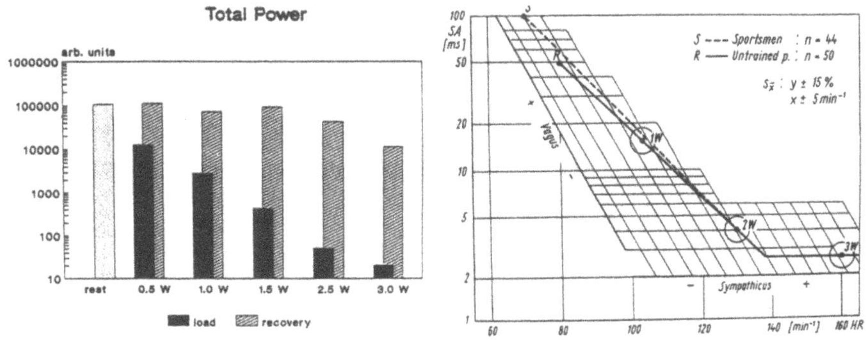

Fig. 1 A Effects of ergometer loading on the total spectral power
1 B Rhythm diagram with SA and HR during physical load of 1, 2 and 3 W/kg

The relative power under these experimental conditions reacts diversily in the three spectral components irrespective of the considerable diminution of total power. A steady decrease of the MF component holding the largest partizipation in rest brings it down till to about 30 % against rest. The low frequency band (LF) increases from a small portion below 10 % in rest up to about 50 % whereas the respiratory HF band shows only a slight diminution to half of its resting part in high load. During recovery phases the resting values are nearly restored. Only the respiratory HF band does not reach its resting values within the period available for recovery after high load (s. Fig. 2.).

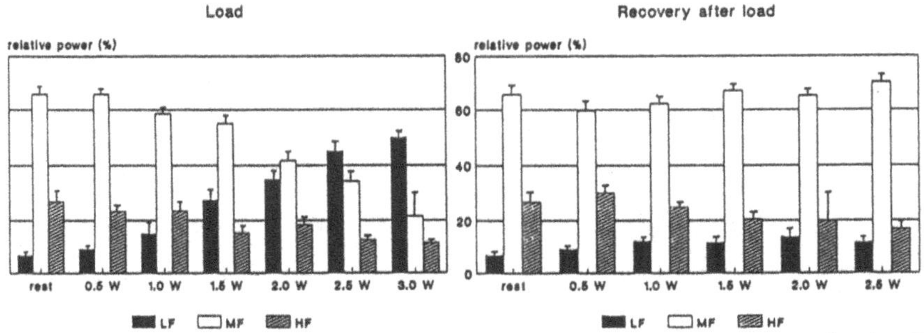

Fig. 2 Relative power of the LF-, MF- and HF-frequency bands of the spectral density during load and in recovery

3. Information about respiratory or exercise conditioned chronotropic reactions of heart rate variability

The voluntary changes of RF clearly reveal the central entrainment effect on the HF band frequency. Near to the MF band a resonance phenomenon may occur. Thus the connection between RF and the HF band becomes evident. Methodical influences of hyperventilation are excluded by getting identical results in using fixed or free tidal volumes and by tests under hypokapnia without remarkable effects [7]. Together with tidal volume depending changes of SA [8] these experiments demonstrate the possible differentiation of central nervous influences on HR-variability affecting the HF band frequency from afferent - efferent mechanisms via baro- or stretchreceptors in the thorax expressed in total power or SA values.

Exercise diminishes total power in the same way as SA. This reflects the central command of ergotropic reactions. The HF component however illustrates the absolute and relative diminution of reflectory influences from respiration. In contrast to recent exercise investigations [9] the retarded HF-recovery after heavy load hints at influences from peripheral metabolic conditions [2] on the setting of the HF-band. Thus central drive and chemo- or metaboreceptive afferents are likely to contribute to the HF band behaviour.

The diminution of the portion of the MF band may be explained by a decrease in the central gain of the baroreceptor reflex with exercise according to [9]. The increase of the portion of the LF band agrees to growing thermoregulatory needs which may influence the activity of vasomotoric reactions.

In summary the different reactions of the 3 spectral components on central or peripheral respiratory, baro- and chemoreceptive or vasomotor influences demonstrate the possibilies of discriminating these afferents by spectral analysis. SA by itself is not able to deliver differentiated informations. SA vs HR allows only the identification of vagal or sympathetic patways.

References

1. E. Schubert, in Advances in Cardiology, (Excerpta Med., Amsterdam 1990) p. 55-58 and J. Electrocardiol. **23**, 280, (1990)
2. E. Schubert, W. Dinter and W. Rielke, in Cardiorespiratory and Motor Coordination, ed. H.-P. Koepchen, (Springer - Berlin 1991) p. 300-306
3. A. Kannenberg and E. Schubert, Pflüg. Arch. ges. Physiol. **420**, Suppl 1, R 87 (1991)
4. E. Schubert, C. Krusche and R. Speda, in Chronobiology and Chronomedicine, ed. G. Hildebrandt (P. Lang - Frankfurt/M. 1987), p. 193-196
5. E. Schubert, Bull. et Mem. Acad. roy. Med. Belg., **136**, 195-206 (1981)
6. S. Akselrod a.o., Science **213**, 220-222 (1981) and Am. J. Physiol. **249**, H 867-875 (1985)
7. A. Patzak a.o., Pflüg. Arch. ges. Physiol. **420**, Suppl 1, R 89 (1992)
8. K. Eckoldt and E. Schubert, Acta biol. et med. germ **34**, 767-771 (1975)
9. R. Perini a.o., Eur. J. Appl. Physiol. **58**, 879-883 (1989)

VECTORCARDIOGRAM AND SIGNAL AVERAGING ECG ANALYSIS IN PATIENTS WITH INFERIOR MYOCARDIAL INFARCTION AND PERI-INFARCTION BLOCK

GOTTI G.,BARDUCCI E.,BORGIONI L.,CATTARINI G.,MAGRIS R.,MASTROBUONI GC.,MORATTI P.,ZILIO G. and PALMIERI M.

Cardiological Dept. - General Hospital - MONFALCONE - Italy

The SA ECG frequently records low-amplitude high-frequency signals (Late Potentials) at the end of the QRS complex in large proportion of pts in the clinical setting of C.H.D. with or without a healed MI and ventricular arrhythmyas. These LP are thought to identifie regions of delayed conduction at the border of the MI in which the mechanism responsible for malignant arrhythmyas can occur.(1)

In particular there is some debate on the presence of LP in pts with inferior myocardial infarction (IMI) and peri-infarction block (PIB), that is in conditions of local parietal block around a MI, where slow conduction ensues.(2-3)

So, if a fragmented and delayed conduction due to parietal block is the ground in which LP are observed, the hypothesis to test could be: if a higher degree of PIB observed at the VCG in pts with IMI may predict the prevalence of LP in the SA ECG.

Material and Method

Fifty (45 m, 5 f) pts, mean age 57.9 $\pm$ 8.9 were studied after an IMI (12-15 days) before hospital discharge with the Frank VCG and a SA ECG (Art System 1200, 25-250 Hz, Noise 0.3 $\pm$ 0.1). We studied: 1) the VCG terminal forces of QRS loop in F and LS planes in the ECG pattern of IMI-PIB and 2) the prevalence of LP in the SA ECG when the PIB is present.

ECG CRITERIA OF IMI WITH PIB

1) Q wave $\geq$ 40 ms or > of the 25% of the QRS height in L_2,L_3,aVF;
2) QRS notching: departure in sign and slope of basic QRS waveform,excluding R wave peack and Q/S nadir;
3) Wide QRS angle with initials and terminal vectors directed in opposite directions ($\geq$ 100°);
4) Wider QRS in L_2, L_3, aVF as opposed to QRS in L_1.(4)

VCG PATTERN IN CASES OF IMI-PIB WITH QRS NOTCHING

VCG evaluation showed in these cases an upward clockwise direction of initial forces due to the inferior necrosis, followed by a terminal delay, and opposition of initial and terminal vectors.

LATE POTENTIALS IN THE SA ECG

According to the criteria of M.B.Simson (5) the LP are present when after the averaging of 200 complexes with a noise of 0.3 ± 0.1 the following are observed:

- QRS duration (QRS D) ≥ 120 ms
- Low Amplitude Signals under 40 μV (LAS 40 uV) ≥ 38 ms
- Root Mean Square vectors amplitude during the last 40 ms (RMS 40 ms) < 25 μV.

Results

Of 50 pts with IMI, 15 (30%) presented the ECG criteria of PIB with an associated notching in the R wave downslope. In our pts the VCG loop delay in the F and LS planes showed: in 15 pts with IMI-PIB the VCG terminal delay was 32-54 ms (mean 40.44 ± 8.7); and in 35 pts without PIB 15-25 ms (mean 19 ± 7.3).

Nevertheless, out of these 35 pts we found that 5 (14.2%)of them presented only a long VCG terminal delay ranging 32-36 ms (mean 33.3 ± 1.2) without a clear notching in the standard ECG, as a marker of conduction defect. The QRS loop analysis in these cases revealed that the loop terminal forces were localized in the left lower quadrant and presented a course along or parallel to the Y axe, as opposed to the terminal forces in pts with QRS notching in whom the closing loop had a couse from the left to the right quadrant before reaching the 0 point. The SA ECG procedure in our pts revealed($p<0.03$):

	IMI-PIB 15 pts	IMI-NO PIB 35 pts
QRS D	127.6 ± 11.5 ms	102.6 ± 13.5 ms
LAS 40	35.6 ± 8.6 ms	22.8 ± 7.6 ms
RMS 40	32.5 ± 1.4 μV	76.5 ± 24.9 μV

As one can see here the pts with PIB had a longer QRS D and LAS 40with a lower RMS 40.

Summarizing, LP were present in 11 (22%) out of 50 pts and in particular: 7 (46.6%) of 15 with ECG criteria of PIB, in 1 (20%) of 5with only evidence of VCG parietal delay without the ECG criteria of PIB , and in 3 (10%) of 30 in the second pts group without PIB.

Conclusions

So, even if our study can be limited by the only approach in the acute phase of the MI without follow-up and the small sample of pts,we can conclude that our findings are in agreement with previous reports showing a relation between IMI-PIB and LP. Furthermore, in our cases the VCG seems superior to the standard ECG in the recording of the QRS delayed terminal forces of depolarization responsible for the presence of the LP in the SA ECG.

References

1. D.L.Kuchar,C.W.Thorburn and N.L.Sammel, Circulation 74,6(1986)1280.
2. B.J.Scherlag,C.G.Gunn,E.J.Berbari and R.Lazzara, Am.J.Cardiol. 55 (1985) 839.
3. M.J.Cowan,R.A.Bruce and D.D.Reichenbach, Am.J.Cardiol. 54(1984)726.
4. D.G.Babbitt,P.F.Binkley and S.F.Schaal, J.Electrocardiol. 24 (1991) 85.
5. M.B.Simson, Circulation 64 (1981) 235.

HEART RATE VARIABILITY AND MAXIMAL EXERCISE CAPACITY IN POST MYOCARDIAL INFARCTION PATIENTS

A. Fazi, A. Florian, F. Bandini; L. Chiodi, R. Vergassola

Department of Cardiology Ospedale S.M. Annunziata Florence, Italy

Abstract

In recent years heart rate (HR) spectral analysis has been proposed as a noninvasive means of investigating autonomic nervous control of the heart. Previous studies proved that, in normal patients, as age increases total spectral power gradually decreases, whereas in chronic congestive heart patients, there is a significant decrease which is independent of the spectral data/age ratio. Moreover, reduced HR variability has been found to be a powerful predictor of mortality in post-myocardial infarction.

Our study aimed at assessing any possible correlation between HR variability and left ventricular ejection fraction (LVEF) and/or exercise endurance in post myocardial infarction (PMI).

Ten male patients were studied 6 to 30 months after myocardial infarction. In all the patients we measured HR variability by spectral analysis, LVEF by radionuclide (99mTC) angiocardiography and exercise endurance by stress testing. There is no significant relation beetween variance of HR and LVEF, whereas there is a significant positive relation between RR variability and exercise endurance: in fact it decreased with decreasing resistance to effort. These results suggest that neural mechanisms underlying HR variability act according to central and peripheral circulatory adjustment.

Introduction

The importance of neurohumoral modulation of cardiovascular function in maintaining a stable hemodynamic balance has been known for some time, as has the fact that this modulation can, at times, contribute to maintaining or worsening congestive heart failure in patients with serious contractile deficiencies, through negative feed-back mechanisms (1).

For some years now, it has been possible to evaluate sympathico-vagal effects on the heart using noninvasive means, and specifically by analyzing oscillations in heart rate fluctuation over time (2,3). These, in fact, are the result of neurovegetative effects on the intrinsic automatism of the sinus node (4).

It has been shown that heart rate variability, evaluated in the time domain (using indices such as standard deviation, variance, etc.) and in the frequency domain (using spectral analyses) correlates weakly yet significantly with the ejection fraction (EF) (5) (reduction in variability with reduction in ejection fraction) so that there is, indeed, a marked reduction among patients with congestive heart failure (6).

Since the autonomous nervous system's effects on the cardiocirculatory system are regulated by influences modulated by cardiac performance as well as stimuli from the peripheral circulation, we intend to assess whether in patients with previous myocardial infarction, the variability indices correlate better with residual physical capacities or myocardial contractility.

Materials and Methods

From the total number of patients, 10 males (mean age 63 ± 5 years) were studied 6 to 30 months after myocardial infarction. Patients with diabetes, thyroid diseases, electrocardiographic evidence of sinus node disfunction or frequent premature beats were excluded.All 10 patients were in sinus rhythm; none were taking drugs that could influence heart rate such as digitalis, betablockers, antiarrythmics or calciumantagonists. Nitrates and diuretics were suspended 36 hours before the tests.
Ejection fraction was measured by technetium myocardial scintigraphy. Heart rate variability was measured in a sound-proofed room, at an ideal and constant temperature betwwen 11:00 a.m. and 12:00 noon, with the patients in a clinostatic position for at least 20 minutes. Electro cardiographic signals were recorded for 600 seconds using a Del Mar Avionics Model 183 CEWS devices. Cardiac rate variance (square of standard deviation) was used as the variability index.
The patients then underwent a maximum stress test using ergometer bicycles. The test was started with a 20 watt load and 20 watt increments every 2 minutes.

Results

The EF in the patients we studied was 41.9% ±12.7 with a minimum of 25% and a maximum of 67%. All the stress tests were negtive and were suspended due to muscle fatigue. The tests lasted from a minimum of 8 minutes (with an 80 watt load) to a maximum of 16 minutes (with a 160 watt load).
Cardiac frequency variances ranged from a minimum of 171 m/sec to a maximum of 1990 m/sec (Table 1). There was no significant correlation between heart rate variance and EF (Fig.1) (r=040, p=n.s.) An excellent exponential correlation was found between variance and stress test duration ($r = 0.93$, $p<0.001$) - ($y = 23.76 * e^{0.29x}$) (Fig. 2).

N.pz.	E.F. (99mTc)	Exercise endurance	Variance (msec)
1 G.G.	38%	15 min.	1990
2 C.A.	57%	10 min.	533
3 P.A.	32%	11 min.	514
4 B.V.	33%	8 min.	207
5 M.F.	35%	8 min.	419
6 R.V.	67%	12 min.	649
7 A.E.	25%	8 min.	171
8 T.E.	42%	10 min.	362
9 V.F.	50%	12 min.	820
10 DL.V.	40%	12 min.	751

Tab. I - Summary of analyzed data

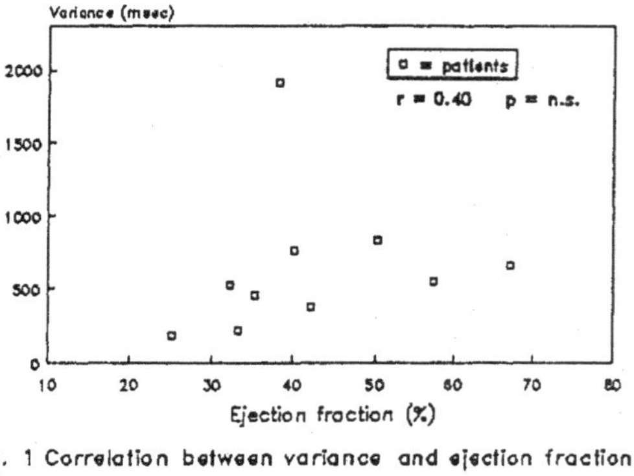

Fig. 1 Correlation between variance and ejection fraction

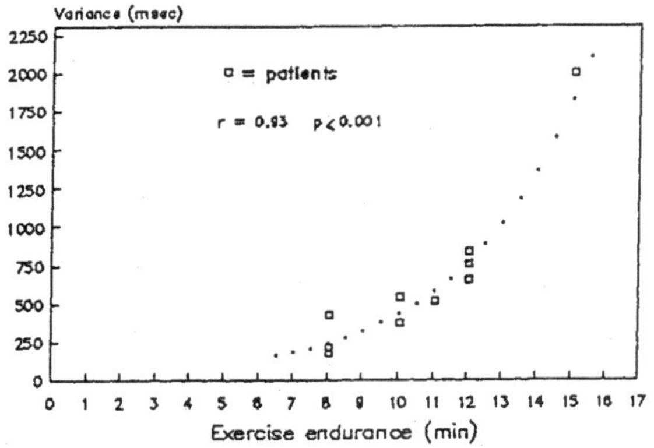

Fig. 2 Correlation between variance and exercise endurance

Discussion

Unlike recent studies (5,7) our results have not revealed any significant correlation between heart rate variability and ejection fraction. This may, in our opinion, be due to the limited number of patients studied.

The striking finding is the excellent correlation between variability and tolerance to stress. This would confirm that the sympathico-vagal interactions on the heart, reflected in the HR variability, also act according to peripheral circulatory adjustments.

Therefore, heart rate variability could be a more complete index as compared to EF when it comes to evaluating an infarction patient's residual capacity, since this method evaluates integrated cardiocirculatory function as it is influenced by the contractility of the myocardium and the effects of the peripheral circulation. This would also explain the enormous sensitivity of variability with respect to the ejection fraction, in predicting mortality after myocardial infarction (5, 8).

These results will have to be confirmed by broader studies and, in our opinion, it will be worthwhile to evaluate variations in the indices of HR variability among patients undergoing postinfarction rehabilitation.

REFERENCES

1. Parker M, Neurohumoral interections and adaptations in congestive heart failure. Circulation 77: 721; 1988.
2. Akselrod S, Gordon D, Ubel FA, Shannon DC, Barger AC, Cohen RJ, Power spectrum analysis of heart rate fluctuation: a quantitative probe of beat-to-beat cardiovascolar control. Science 213: 220; 1981.
3. Pomeran B, Macaulay RJB, Caudill MA, Kuntz I, Adam D, Gordon D,

Kilborn KM, Barger AC, Shannon DC, Cohen RJ, Benson H, Assessment of automatic function in humans by heart rate spectral analysis. Am J Physiol 248: H151; 1985.

4. Machado BH, Brody MJ, Contribution of neurogenic machanism to control of intrinsic heart rate. Am J Physiol 256: R231; 1989.
5. Odemuyiwa O, Malik M, Farrell T, Bashir Y, Poloniecki J, Camm J, Comparison of the predictive characteristics of heart rate variability index and left ventricular Eiection fraction for all cause mortality, arrhythmic events and sudden death after acute myocardial infarction. Am J Cardiol 68: 434; 1991.
6. Casolo G, Balli E, Fazi A, Gori C, Freni A, Gensini G, Twenty-four hour spectral analysis of heart rate variability in congestive heart failure secondary to coronary artery disease. Am J Cardiol 6: 1154; 1991.
7. Saul JP, Arai Y, Berger RD, Lilly LS, Colucci WS, Cohen RJ, Assessment of autonomic regulation in chronic congestive heart failure by heart rate spectral analysis. Am J Cardiol 61: 1292; 1988.
8. Kleiger RE, Miller JP, Bigger JT Jr, Moss AJ and Multicenter Postinfaction Research Group. Decreased heart rate variability and its association with increased mortality after acute myocardial infarction. Am J Cardiol 59: 256; 1987.

ELECTROCARDIOGRAPHY AND HOLTER MONITORING AFTER ANATOMIC CORRECTION OF TRANSPOSITION OF THE GREAT ARTERIES

ANABELA PAIXÃO, MD, CONCEIÇÃO TRIGO, MD, ALBERTO AGUALUSA MD, FERNANDA SAMPAYO, MD, Ph.D.

Serviço de Cardiologia Pediátrica
Hospital de Santa Marta
Rua de Santa Marta
1100 Lisboa Portugal

ABSTRACT

Electrocardiographic changes and rhythm disturbances after anatomic correction of transposition of the great arteries were evaluated. The study group comprised 15 patients who underwent an arterial switch repair from January 1989 to February 1992. Preoperative, early postoperative and follow-up electrocardiograms were reviewed. Outpatient follw-up included 24-hour ambulatory electrocardiographic monitoring. Echocardiography / Doppler provided haemodynamic status information. Mean length of follow-up was 16,7 months. All preoperative electrocardiograms were abnormal. Right ventricular hypertrophy was present in 12. Through the follow-up, 7 patients showed regression to normal pattern. Persistent right ventricular hypertrophy was associated with significant residual lesions or sequelae in 3 patients: 2 with moderate and severe supravalvular pulmonary stenosis and one with large atrial septal defect. The remaining patients had postoperative right bundle branch block. Holter monitoring revealed normal sinus rhythm in all patients. Only one had asymptomatic low-grade supraventricular and ventricular ectopy. Electrocardiogram can reflect haemodynamic status after anatomic correction of transposition of the great arteries. On short term, sinus rhythm is preserved and arrhythmias are not a matter of major concern.

Anatomic correction has evolved as the procedure of choice in most centers for the treatment of complete transposition of the great arteries (TGA)[1]. It has been suggested that the arterial switch repair will prevent the problems associated with the intraatrial repair, including right ventricular dysfunction and cardiac arrhythmias[2-4].

The purpose of this study was to evaluate the postoperative course with respect to electrocardiographic changes and eventual rhythm disturbances in our recent experience with anatomic correction of TGA.

Material and Methods

The study group consisted of 15 patients who underwent anatomic correction of TGA from January 1989 to February 1992 : 10 had simple TGA and underwent primary repair as neonates (range 4-23 days, mean 11.8 ±5.5 days). The remaining 5 patients had TGA with ventricular septal defect (VSD) : 4 underwent primary repair in infancy (range 26 days to 5 months, mean 2.8 ± 1.5 months) and one had a secondary repair at 3 years of age, after a previous pulmonary artery banding.

Electrocardiograms (ECG) obtained in the preoperative period, postoperatively up to one month after surgery and through the follow-up at six month intervals were reviewed. Standard age corrected criteria for chamber hypertrophy and conduction intervals were used[5]. Follow up included two channel 24-hour ambulatory electrocardiographic monitoring in all patients. Echocardiography with pulsed, continuous wave and colour Doppler was used to evaluate haemodynamic status by detecting and quantifying residual shunts, valvular incompetence and anastomotic obstruction. Length of follow-up ranged from 15 days to 3 years (mean 16,7 ± 10 .months).

Results

All patients had some preoperative electrocardiographic abnormality. The most frequent was right ventricular hypertrophy, present in 12. Two infants with TGA and VSD had biventricular hypertrophy and one with simple TGA, only fulfilled criteria for isolated right atrial hypertrophy.

On the early postoperative period only one ECG changed to normal and 3 to right bundle branch block. In the later postoperative period - not less than 6 months after surgery - ECG of 13 patients were analysed. (The two most recently operated patients, one of them with postoperative right bundle branch block were not included.) Seven of those ECG were normal, 3 showed persistent right ventricular hypertrophy and 2 right bundle branch block.

Postoperative haemodynamic abnormalities demonstrated by echocardiography Doppler showed that a normal ECG was consistently associated with a normal or near normal haemodynamic condition (neither large residual shunts at atrial or ventricular level nor transpulmonary gradients in excess of 30 mmHg). Right ventricular hypertrophy was present in 2 patients with moderate to severe supravalvular pulmonary stenosis (transpulmonary gradients of 60 and 80 mmHg respectively) and one with a large residual atrial septal defect (ASD). Right bundle branch block was found in 2 patients: one with no haemodynamic abnormalities, could be related to VSD closure and another one with residual ASD and transpulmonary gradient of 50 mmHg.

Postoperative Holter recordings showed stable sinus rhythm in all patients. Only one child operated on for simple TGA 14 months before had asymptomatic low-grade atrial and ventricular ectopy.

Discussion

The arterial switch operation is now routinely performed in many institutions[1]. Compared with atrial switch operations, the major theoretical advantages are: establishment of the left ventricle as the systemic ventricle and the maintenance of sinus node function[3]. At present time, it appears that few arrhythmias and few electrophysiologic abnormalities occur after the anatomic correction[2].

In our experience, right ventricular hypertrophy decreased rapidly after surgery, in the absence of significant residual lesions or postoperative complications particularly supravalvular pulmonary stenosis. Other groups have observed that abnormalities on the ECG disappeared largely within 3 to 6 moths after surgery in all but those patients who developed pulmonary artery stenosis[3,6,7] and successful surgical relief of right ventricular obstruction was accompanied by reduction in right ventricular forces to the normal range[3].

With respect to arrhythmias, the short and medium term results of the arterial switch operation are highly encouraging[7,8,9]. In our series, no patient had significant rhythm disturbances detected by Holter monitoring although none of those recordings have been obtained immediately after surgery. However, some authors have previously reported that arrhythmias are not completely absent with the arterial switch operation, but significant arrhythmias have been infrequent and limited to the immediate perioperative period; actually, most of them have been transient and benign[4,8].

Conclusions

Our experience supports the view that ECG can reflect haemodynamic status after anatomic correction of TGA and that on short-term, sinus rhythm is preserved and significant rhythm disturbances are usually absent.

References

1. F. M. Lupinetti, E. L. Bove, L. L. Minich, et al. , *J Thorac Cardiovasc Surg* 103 (1992) 421

2. V. L. Vetter and C. S. Tanner, *J Am Coll Cardiol* 12 (1988) 229

3. G. Wernovsky, T. J. Hougen, E. P. Walsh, et al. , *Circulation* 77 (1988) 1333

4. J. E. Deanfield, S. Cullen and M. Gewillig, *Cardiol young* 1 (1991) 91

5. A. Davignon, R. Rautaharju, F. Boiselle, et al, *Pediatr Cardiol* 1 (1990) 123

6. D. Sidi, C. Planché, J. Kachaner, et al. , *Circulation* 75 (1987) 429

7. R. J. M. Klautz, J. Ottenkamp, J. M. Quaegebeur, et al. , *Pediatr Cardiol* 10 (1989) 1

8. R. M. Donato, G. Wernovsky, E. P. Walsh, et al. , *Circulation* 80 (1989) 1689

9. F. S. Idriss, M. N. Ibawi, S. Y. Delcon, et al. , *J. Thorac Cardivasc Surg* 95 (1988) 255

VALUE OF HOLTER STUDY AND LEFT VENTRICULOGRAPHY IN PREDICTING IDIOPATHIC DILATED CARDIOMYOPATHY CLINICAL OUTCOME

Ana Abreu, Helder Pereira, Carlos Catarino, Luisa Branco, Henrique Nunes, Luis Valério, J. M. Gonçalves, R. Gracias, A. Mata Antunes

S. Cardiology, Hospital Sta. Marta
Lisboa, Portugal

ABSTRACT

STUDY OBJECTIVE: Arrhythmic profile of idiopathic dilated cardiomyopathy (DCM) characterization; Evaluation of complex ventricular ectopy and left ventricular failure association; Clinical outcome.
PATIENTS: We studied 20 patients (P) with DCM, 15 males and 5 females, mean age 51,3 +/- 14,4 years (from 17 to 75 years).
METHODS: 24-hours-Holter study and left cardiac catheterization were performed. Patients were followed at the consults.
RESULTS: We detected in the Holter study the presence of ventricular ectopy in 19 P (95%). Nine P had complex ventricular arrhytmias (45%), 10 P had simple ventricular arrhythmias (50%) and 1 P had no ventricular arrhythmias (5%). The mean left ventricular ejection fraction was 28,6 +/- 14,1 (12 to 44%). Two groups were defined based on the severity of left ventricular dysfunction: Group I with 12 P and Group II with 8 P. In Group I, 8 P had complex ventricular ectopy and, in Group II, 1 P had complex ventricular ectopy ($p < 0.05$). Comparing mean left ventricular ejection fraction in the two groups of arrhythmias (simple and complex), 33,9 +/- 12,5% and 22,1 +/- 13,8%, we found out a statisticaly significant difference ($p < 0.05$). After an eight to thirty six months of follow-up, a greater number of cardiac events (mortality, transplant, heart failure aggravation) were detected in the groups of complex arrhythmia and of more severe cardiac dysfunction.
CONCLUSION: We conclude that there is a high frequency of ventricular arrhythmias in this group of patients with DCM. Complex ventricular arrhythmias were more frequently associated to more severe left ventricular dysfunction. The number of cardiac events at follow-up was higher in patients with complex ventricular arrhythmias and in those with more depressed cardiac function.

PURPOSE
The purpose of this study was to define the ventricular arrhytmic profile of a group of patients with DCM; to evaluate the relation of this and the severity of cardiac dysfunction, and to perform the clinical follow-up of these patients.

PATIENTS
We studied prospectively 20 patients (P) with DCM, 15 males and 5 females, mean age 51.3 ± 17.4 years old (17 - 75 years), for a period of 8 to 36 months.
Echocardiographic criteria were used to diagnose of DCM. Specific causes were excluded.

METHODS
All P underwent 24-hours-Holter register. CHF therapy was not interrupted. No patients were on anti-arrhythmic drugs during the study. Ventricular arrhythmias were graded according to modified Lown classification: grades 1 and 2 ("simple arrhythmias"), grades 3, 4 and 5 ("complex").
Left ventricular ejection fraction was determined by contrast angiography. Coronary arteriography was performed to exclude coronary artery disease.

RESULTS
Patients were divided in two groups according to Lown classification: Group A - Lown 0, 1, 2(11 P);Group B - Lown 3, 4, 5 (9 P).
There was no correlation between symptoms and arrhythmias in 95% of the P. Only 1 P refered dyspnea related to nonsustained ventricular tachycardia.
Mean left ventricular ejection fraction (LVEF) was 28.6 ± 14.1% (12-44%): Group I - LVEF < 30% (12 P); Group II - LVEF ≥ 30% (8 P).
There was a significant difference in the frequency of complex ventricular arrhythmias in the two groups of disfunction ($p < 0.05$)(table I)

Table I	Simple arrhythmias (Group A)	Complex arrhythmias (Group B)
LVEF < 30% (Group I)	4	8
LVEF ≥ 30% (Group II)	7	1

Also, comparing LVEF mean values in Group A, 33.9 ± 12.5%, and Group B, 22.1 ± 13.8%, we noticed a statistically significant difference ($p < 0.05$).

FOLLOW-UP
Patients were followed at the consult during a period between 8 and 36 months.

Of the 9 P with complex ventricular arrhythmias, 7 P were taking diuretics, 7 P, ACE inhibitors, 5 P, digitalis, 2 P, nitrates and 3 P, amiodarone. Of the 11 P with simple or without arrhythmias, 8 P were taking diuretics, 3 P, ACE inhibitors, 3 P, digitalis and 2 P, nitrates.
Cardiac events were defined as cardiac death, cardiac transplant and heart failure aggravation (table II).

Table II	Stable patients	Cardiac events
Group A		
(Simple or no arrhythmias)	7	4
Group B		
(Complex arrhythmias)	3	6
Group I		
(LVEF < 30%)	2	10
Group II		
(LVEF ≥ 30%)	8	0

DISCUSSION AND CONCLUSION

Symptomatic DCM has high mortality, 30 to 50% at the first year of symptoms (1,2). Half of the patients dye because of heart failure progression and the other half dye suddenly, probably due to ventricular tachyarrhythmias. In our group of symptomatic DCM patients, the mortality was 30% in a follow-up period of 8 to 36 months.
Previous Holter studies have demonstrated that almost all the DCM patients have ventricular ectopy and aproximately half have nonsustained ventricular tachycardia episodes (2-4). We found out a high frequency of ventricular arrhythmias (95%) and often complex forms (45%). We verified also a significant correlation of complex ventricular arrhythmias and the severity of cardiac disfunction. This controversial relation (2,3,5) had been noticed before (4). In our patients we didn't find any correlation of symptoms and arrhytmias during Holter recording, wich is consistent with prior studies (2,3). It is not definitively established the relation of ventricular arrhythmias complexity and DCM prognosis (1-4), however the majority of studies show a significant association of nonsustained ventricular tachycardia and sudden death (5). Also, some investigators relate the prognosis mostly with the extent of left ventricular failure (6). In the clinical follow-up of our group of patients, we noticed more cardiac events in those with complex arrhythmias, although these patients had also worst ventricular function.
It is not demonstrated uncontroversial benefit of anti-arrhythmic drugs regarding survival in patients with DCM (4). Some authors suggest nevertheless, the use of these drugs, if nonsustained ventricular tachycardia is detected

by Holter (9), specially if the left ventricular ejection fraction is inferior to 40% (3,10). In our patients, only three were on amiodarone because of complex ventricular ectopy, and one died in the follow-up. The impact of vasodilator drugs over ventricular arrhythmias in DCM patients is unknown. Nevertheless, in Consensus (11) there was a decrease in mortality in patients with heart failure (classes III and IV of NYHA) probably because of decrease in the progression of heart failure. In VHEFT-II (12) there was also a decrease in mortality related to the decrease of sudden death.

In conclusion, the incidence of ventricular arrhythmias was high in this group of patients with DCM, with a high percentage of complex ectopy.The complexity of ventricular arrhythmias was related to the severity of ventricular disfunction. In the clinical follow-up more cardiac events were registered in those patients with worst left ventricular function, and complex ventricular ectopy.

BIBLIOGRAFIA

(1) DV **Unverferth**,et al.Factores influencing the one year Mortality of Dilated Cardiomyopathy.Am J Cardiol **54** (1984) 147

(2)SK **Huang**,JV **Meser**, P **Denes**. Significance of Ventricular Tachycardia in Idiopathic Dilated Cardiomyopathy: Observations in 35 Patients. Am J Cardiol **51** (1983) 507.

(3) C S **Meinertz**, T **Hopman**, W **Kasper**, et al. Significance of Ventricular Arrhythmias in Idiopathic Dilated Cardiomyopathy. Am J Cardiol **53** (1984) 902.

(4) C S **Chakko**, M **Gheorgiade**. Ventricular Arrhythmias in Severe Heart Failure: Incidence, Significance and Effectiveness of Antiarrhythmic Theraphy. Am Heart J **109** (1985) 497.

(5)P **Podrid**,J **Wilson**.Should Asymptomatic Ventricular Arrhythmia in Patients with Congestive Heart Failure be Treated? An Antagonists Viewpoint.Am J Cardiol **66**(1990)451

(6) R I **Hamby**. Primary Myocardial Disease: A Prospective Clinical and Hemodynamic Evaluation in 100 Patients. Medicine **49** (1970) 55.

(9) R A **Johnson**, I **Palacios**. Dilated cardiomyopathies of the Adult. N Engl J Med **307** (1982) 1051.

(10)T **Hofmann**, T **Meinertz**,W **Kasper**, et al.Mode of Death in Idiopathic Dilated Cardiomyopathy: A Multivariate Analysis of Prognostic Determinants.Am Heart J **166**(1988)1455

(11) Consensus Trial Study Group. Effects of Enalapril on Mortality in Severe Congestive Heart Failure: Results of the Cooperative North Scandinavian Enalapril Survival Study. N Engl J Med **316** (1987) 1429.

(12) JN **Cohn**, G **Johnson**, S **Ziesche**, et al. A comparison of enalapril with hydralazine-isosorbide dinitrate in the treatment of chronic congestive heart failure N Engl J Med **325** (1991) 303.

VENTRICULAR TACHYCARDIA IDENTIFICATION BY SIGNAL AVERAGED ECG IN TIME AND FREQUENCY DOMAIN

A.Vado,MD, C.Bruna,MD, G.Rossetti,MD and E.Uslenghi,MD.

Cardiology Division, Ospedale S.Croce. CUNEO. ITALY

ABSTRACT

To compare the value of time domain (TD) and frequency domain (FD) analysis of Signal Averaged ECG (SAECG) in identifying patients (pts) with spontaneous sustained ventricular tachycardia (VT), we performed SAECG in 26 normal subjects (GrA), 36 pts with prior myocardial infarction (MI) and VT (GrB) and 32 pts without documented VT in the first year after MI (GrC). TD analysis was performed either at 25-250Hz and 40-250Hz. FD analysis was performed using 120ms data segments starting 20ms before QRS end; Area Ratios (AR) 60-120/0-30 and 30-120/0-30 were calculated for X,Y and Z lead. Mean AR was calculated by algebric mean of each AR from X,Y,Z (MAR1 and MAR2, respectively). TD analysis was not performed in 23 pts (2 in GrA, 8%; 15 in GrB, 41% and 6 in GrC, 18%) because of QRS duration 120ms or the presence of bundle branch block; sensitivity was .61 and specificity .85 at 25-250Hz and .5 and .87 at 40-250Hz. FD analysis was performed in all pts: MAR1 sensitivity was .53 and specificity .78; MAR2 sensitivity was .47 and specificity .76. In conclusion, TD analysis resulted more specific than FD analysis in identifying VT pts; however, almost half of VT pts was excluded from TD analysis.

INTRODUCTION

Non invasive recording of late potentials by signal-averaged electrocardiogram (SAECG) has been used to identify patients prone to ventricular tachycardia (VT) after myocardial infarction. Analysis in time domain developed by Simson (1) is well known and widely used in clinical setting; on the contrary, frequency domain analysis is under evaluation. The purpose of this study was to value the role of selected parameters from frequency domain analysis to properly identify VT patients in coronary artery disease and to compare time domain with frequency domain analysis.

MATERIALS AND METHODS

Definitions and patients

Sustained VT was defined as the spontaneous occurence of VT lasting at least 30 seconds or requiring cardioversion because of haemodynamic compromise.

Patients in this study had a mean age of 54.2±18.8 years and included 79 men and 15 women. We studied three patient groups: group A (GrA) included 26 normal subjects as control group ; group B (GrB): 36 patients with prior myocardial infarction and documented VT ; group C (GrC): 32 patients without documented VT in the first year after the acute myocardial infarction. There was no significant difference in mean age, sex, location of infarct and prevalence of QRS duration more than 120ms between group B and C (table I). Myocardial infarction was classified as anterior or inferior/posterior according to electrocardiographic criteria.

SAECG

Standard 12 lead ECG and SAECG were obtained in all patients on the same day. After careful skin preparation and application of silver chloride electrodes, X,Y and Z lead were averaged by Arrhythmia Research Technology model EPX1200; final noise was $\leq$0.3μV. Analog to digitally converted signals were stored on personal computer file with a sample rate of 1,000Hz.

Time domain analysis: data were filtered by bidirectional band pass Butterworth filter with 25-250Hz and 40-250Hz corners. The three leads were combined in root-mean-square (RMS) vector (filtered QRS;FQRS). The following parameters were analyzed: 1)duration of FQRS; 2)duration of terminal FQRS under 40uV; 3)RMS of terminal 40msec for each filter corners. Normal values for each parameters either at 25 or 40 Hz pass filtering are listed in table II. Time domain analysis was performed only if standard QRS duration was less then 120ms anf if bundle branch block was not present. Late potential was defined as having 2 of three parameters abnormal either at 25Hz(LP25) or 40Hz(LP40) high pass filtering.

Frequency domain analysis: SAECG data were transferred to an IBM compatible computer and analyzed using 120ms data segments starting 20 msec before QRS end for each lead (X,Y,Z); data were not normalized for direct current. After a 4 term Blackmann Harris window function, data were padded with zeros to fill a 512-point array and Fast Fourier transform (FFT) was applied to determine the frequency content. Unsquared data from FFT analysis provided a plot of magnitudo versus frequency. Area ratios (AR) were calculated by dividing area between high and low frequency. The following ARs were evaluated for each orthogonal lead: 60-120/0-30 and 30-120/0-30. Mean AR was calculated by algebric mean of each AR from X,Y,Z (MAR1 and MAR2, respectively).

Statistical methods: standard descriptive statistics were used; a p value of less then .05 was considered significant. Data were analyzed by means of Student's t test, analysis of variance and Fisher exact test when appropriate.

RESULTS

QRS duration more than 120 msec was observed in 23 subjects (24%): 2 in grA (7.6%; 2 bundle branch block), 15 in grB (41%; 6 bundle branch block, 9 non specific intraventricular conduction defects) and 6 in grC (18%; 4 non specific conduction defects and 2 bundle branch block). Myocardial infarction site was anterior in 34, inferior/posterior in 30, both in 3 patients: distribution of myocardial infarction site didn't differ significantly between grB and grC.

Time domain SAECG: Results referred to 71 patients with QRS duration less then 120msec are listed in table III. FQRS duration was significant longer in grB then in grA and grC using 25-250Hz filter (p =.0001) and 40-250Hz (p=.0001). The RMS voltage in the last 40 msec was significant lower in grB than in grA and C at 25-250Hz filter (p=.001) and at 40-250 (p=.001). Duration of potentials under 40uV was significantly longer in grB than in grA and grB using both filter (p=.0001 and p=0.0001).

LP25 was seen in 11/18 of VT patients and normal results in 46/54 of non VT patients: thus sensitivity was .61 and specificity .85. LP40 was seen in 9/18 of VT patients and normal results in 47/54 of non VT patients: thus sensitivity was .50 and specificity .87.

Frequency domain SAECG: Results referred to all the study patients are listed in table IV. Significant difference between groups was seen Mean AR 60-120/0-30 (MAR1, p=.003) and 30-120/0-30

(MAR2,p=.019). The best predictive value was obtained using 1.11 as normal value for MAR1 and 5.3 for MAR2; MAR1 sensitivity was .53, specificity .78; MAR2 showed a sensitivity of .47 and specificity of .76.

DISCUSSION

Sensitivity, specificity and reproducibility of TD analysis of SAECG are well known. The major limitation of TD analysis is the critical definition of the QRS end; therefore patients with bundle branch block or QRS duration more than 120 msec are usually excluded from time domain analysis. In our series of VT patients, up to 41% had a bundle branch block or a QRS duration more than 120msec. Time domain analysis needs complex band pass filters that can be a source of distorsion and artifacts; FFT analysis does not need filters and applies to patients with intraventricular conduction defects.

FFT is a powerful analytic tool in frequency analysis on biological signals. It was applied to SAECG analysis by many authors. Cain at al (3) found a close correlation between VT inducibility and abnormal content in 20-50Hz of the terminal QRS and ST segment. Worley(4) et al using 140 msec window starting at different point, found that location of the window was critical to identify VT patients, but a multivariate analysis failed to show any contribution of FFT to distinguish VT patients. Haberl (5) at al used 120 msec window and showed that increased spectral area between 60-120Hz identified patients with VT. Machac(6) et al. were not able to distinguish VT patients using energy area ratios. Buckingham et al(2) using 140msec window starting 60msec after QRS start, were able to identify patients from spectral plot from 20-50Hz over 0-20Hz; however, stepwise logistic regression showed that parameters from time domain were superior to frequency domain analysis; Pierce (7) et al., using 120msec window and normalized data segment, showed that VT patients had increased spectral area in high frequency. In a previous paper, we compared five area ratios using 120msec window in normal subjects and in VT patients and we showed that only area ratios 60-120/0-30 and 30-120/0-30 differed between the two groups(9).

Limitations of FFT analysis are well known: saturation, need for windowing, lack of any standard in analysis (8). Caution can be used on short data segment when windowing is required: we can recommend to use Blackmann_Harris window on data lenght not less than 100. Use of autoregressive model (MEM, AFD) can help clinician to identify patients with altered frequency content in SAECG with or without spectrotemporal mapping (10).

CONCLUSION

Late potentials can identify delayed ventricular activation that is the substrate for ventricular tachycardia; premature ventricular contraction as the trigger and impaired autonomic tone as favorating factor are also necessary to initiate and sustain this arrhythmia. Patients with old myocardial infartion can, in fact, have late potentials and don't develope clinical VT.

Signal-averaged electrocardiogram can help to identify the substrate for ventricular tachycardia by means of time and of frequency domain analysis. In the present study, TD analysis resulted more specific than FD analysis in identifying VT pts. However, intraventricular conduction defects are frequent in pts with prior myocardial infarction and ventricular tachycardia; thus, FD analysis can be useful in this subset of patients.

TABLE I:

Patients characteristics.

	GrA	GrB		GrC
age(years)	28.1±7.6	65.4±10.0	ns	62.9±10.1
female	12	1	ns	2
MI site				
anterior		17	ns	17
inf/post		15	ns	15
both		3	ns	0
QRS 120msec	2	15	ns	6

TABLE II:
Normal values for time domain analysis

	FQRS	RMS40	LAS40
25-250Hz	114ms	25μV	32ms
40-250Hz	114ms	15μV	40ms

FQRS:duration of the filtered QRS; RMS40:root mean square voltage in the last 40 ms; LAS40: duration of potentials under 40 μV.

TABLE III:
Results:time domain analysis

	GrA	GrB	GrC	p
25-250Hz				
FQRS	100.7±8.7	124.3±17.9	106.4±12.2	.001
RMS40	71.0±38.9	37.3±40.6	54.5±36.1	.001
LAS40	22.5±8.6	37.5±17.4	25.1±13.7	.001
40-250Hz				
FQRS	95.3±16.8	125.6±18.5	104.5±11.8	.001
RMS40	48.5±30.4	20.0±18.4	31.9±17.3	.001
LAS40	27.3±6.8	47.8±18.7	33.1±13.7	.001

See table II for abbreviations.

TABLE IV
Results: frequency domain analysis

	GrA	GrB	GrC	p
MAR1	.7±.9	11.8±27.9	1.4±2.1	.019
MAR2	.5±5.0	37.3±76.4	5.3±7.9	.008

See text for abbreviations.

REFERENCES

1.Simsom MB. Use of signals in the terminal QRS complex to identify patients with ventricular tachycardia after myocardial infarction. Circulation 1981;64:235-242
2.Buckingham TA, Christopher MT, Hertweck D, Janosik DL, Kennedy HL. Signal-averaged electrocardiography in the time and frequency domain. Am J Cardiol 1989; 63:820-825
3.Cain ME, Ambos HD, Witkowski FX, Sobel BE. Fast Fourier transform analysis of signal-averaged electrocardiograms for identification of patients prone to sustained ventricular tachycardia. Circulation 1984; 69:711-720
4.Worley SJ, Mark DB, Smith WM, Wolf P, Califf RM, Strauss HC, Manwaring MG, Ideker RE. Comparison of time domain and frequency domain variables from the signal-averaged eletrocardiogram: a multivariate analysis. JACC 1988;11:1041-1051
5.Haberl R, Jilge G, Pulter R, Steinbeck G. Comparison of frequency and time domain analysis of the signal-averaged electrocardiogram in patients with ventricular tachycardia and coronary artery disease: methodologic validation and clinical relevance. JACC 1988;12:150-158
6.Machac J, Weiss A, Winters SL, Barecca P, Gomes A. A comparative study of frequency domain and time domain analysis of signal-averaged electrocardiograms in patients with ventricular tachycardia. JACC 1988;11:284-296
7.Pierce DL, Easley AR, Windle JR, Engel TR. Fast Fourier transformation of the entire low amplitude late QRS potential to predict ventricular tachycardia. JACC 1989;13:1731-1740
8.Cain ME, Ambos HD, Lindsay BD, Markham J, Arthur RM. Spectral and temporal interrogation of signal-averaged electrocardiograms: the best is yet to come. JACC 1989;13:1741-1743
9.Vado A, Bruna C., Rossetti G, Uslenghi E. Ventricular tachycardia identification by signal averaged ECG in time and frequency domain. New Trends in arrhythmias: 1991;VII:521-523
10.Haberl R, Schels HF, Steinbigler P, Jilge G, Steinbeck G. Top-resolution frequency analysis of electrocardiogram with adaptive frequency determination. Identificarion of late potentials in patients with coronary artery disease. Circulation 1990;82:1183-1192

SLOW UPSTROKE OF THE SIGNAL-AVERAGED QRS COMPLEX IN PATIENTS WITH VENTRICULAR TACHYCARDIA

Kim EM, Katoh T, Tanaka T, Endoh Y, Fujimori H, Kamei S,
Kuroki S, Hayakawa H

The lst Dept. of Internal Medicine, Nippon Medical School, Tokyo, Japan

ABSTRACT

Non-invasive recording of late potential (LP) by signal-averaging technique is useful in predicting ventricular tachycardia (VT) especially in patients with myocardial infarction (MI). However, the rate of positive LP is not high enough to get clinical significance in anterior or anteroseptal MI, since the LP has been masked by QRS complex. The purpose of the present study is, first, to detect local conduction delay even in initial portion of QRS complex and secondly to evaluate the clinical significance of the initial delay in patients with MI. 80 patients of MI were divided into four groups: S(anteroseptal, n=18, including 6 VT), A(anterior, n=22, 7 VT), I(inferior, n=28, 9 VT) and P(posterior, n=12, no VT). 20 non-MI patients were used for control group (C). NEC7T18 was used to record signal-averaged ECG and each 5 msec integral values of filtered QRS complex from the initial upstroke to 60 msec point was measured, so that low value indicates initial delay in ventricular conduction. Integral values of groups S & A were significantly lower than that of group I, P & C. In patients with VT, S shows more delay than A, whereas in patients without VT these differences were not found. In addition, S with VT shows lower integral value than S without VT, however no differences were observed between A with VT and without VT. We conclude that slow upstroke of signal-averaged QRS complex was mainly observed in patients of anteroseptal MI with VT, suggesting the initial conduction delay at ventricular septum may play an important role in the mechanism of VT.

1. Introduction

Non-invasive recording of late potential (LP) by signal-averaged electrocardiographic technique is useful in predicting the occurrence of ventricular tachycardia in patients after acute myocardial infarction[1-4]. Low amplitude, high frequency signals appeared at the end of the signal-averaged QRS complex correspond to slow conduction area and/or inhomogeneity of the refractory period in the ventricle. Thus, the presence of LP indicates that reentry may occur more easily. However, LP appears not frequently enough to get clinical significance in anterior or anteroseptal myocardial infarction, since the LP has been masked by QRS complex. The purpose of the present study is first, to detect local conduction delay even in initial portion of QRS complex and secondly to evaluate the clinical significance of the initial delay in patient with AMI.

2. Patients and Methods

2.1. Patients

The study population consisted of 80 patients admitted to our institution with acute myocardial infarction. Patients were divided into 4 groups. Group S consisted of 18 patients (including 6 VT) with anteroseptal infarction, Group A 22 patients (including 7 VT) with anterior infarction, Group I 28 patients (including 9 VT) with inferior infarction, and Group P 12 patients (no VT) with posterior infarction. All patients underwent signal-averaged electrocardiogram between seven and 14 days after infarction. Studies were done in absence of any antiarrhythmic drugs. Patients with bundle branch block were excluded from the study.

2.2. Signal-averaging technique

Bipolar X, Y and Z leads were digitally recorded, then transferred to NEC7T18 signal processor. Approximately 200 beats were signal-averaged and each averaged lead was digitally filtered using a forward unidirectional bandpass (40-250Hz) filter with a corner frequency of 40Hz to eliminate impulse ringing at the beginning of the QRS complex. Then we measured the root-mean square voltage at the initial portion of QRS complex by 5ms from the upstroke till 60ms.

2. Results

Integral values of Group S & Group A were significantly lower than that of Group I and Group P as shown in Figure 1. In patients with VT, Group S shows more delay than Group A, whereas in patients without VT these differences were not observed as shown in Figure 2 right & left.

In addition, Group S with VT shows significantly lower integral value than Group S without VT as shown in the left panel of Figure 3. But no differences were seen between Group A with VT and without VT.

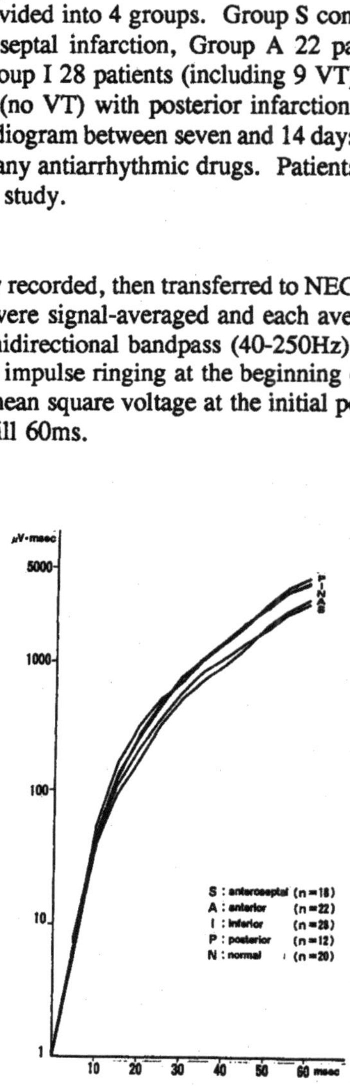

Figure 1. Changes of integral value at the upstroke of signal-averaged QRS complex

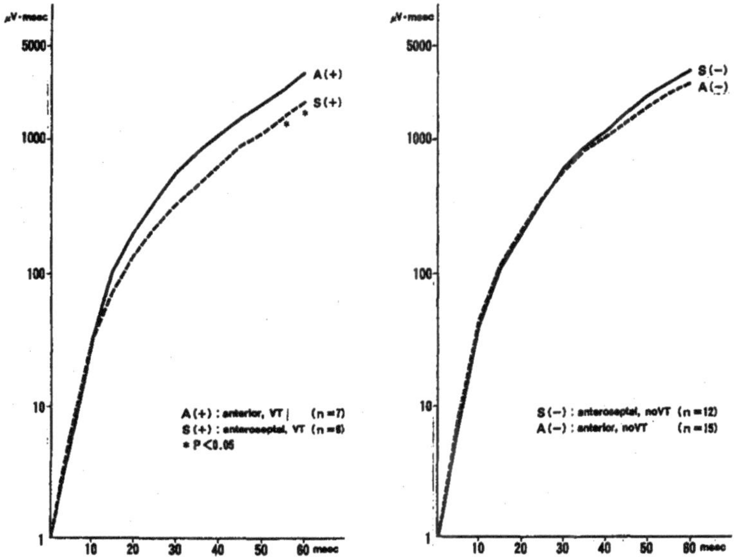

Figure 2. Comparison of initial integral value
—— site of infarction ——

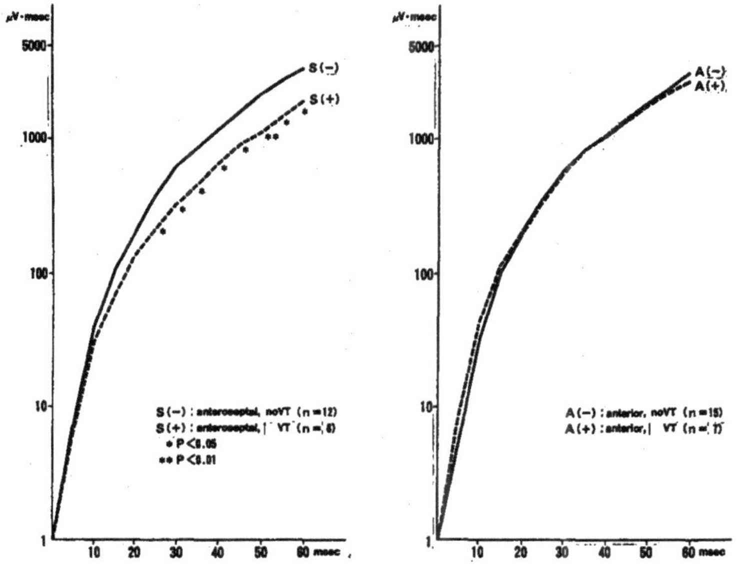

Figure 3. Comparison of initial integral value
—— with and without VT ——

3. Discussion

In this study we found that myocardial infarction causes a reduction of the amplitude in the initial portion of signal-averaged QRS complex. This effect on signal-averaged ECG was mainly noted in patients with anterior or anteroseptal MI, especially in patients with anteroseptal MI who has VT. Since the initial portion of QRS complex may reflect the local activation around septal or paraseptal region, lowering of the upstroke potential indicates the delay or inhomogeneity of conduction through the area.

Thus, we conclude that slow upstroke of signal averaged QRS complex was mainly observed in patients with anteroseptal myocardial infarction who has VT, suggesting the initial conduction delay at ventricular septum may play an important role in the mechanism of VT.

4. References

1. M.B. Simon, W.J. Untereker and S.R. Spielman, *Am. J. Cardiol.* **51**(1983)105.
2. G. Breithardt and M. Borggrefe, *Circulation* **75**(1987)1091.
3. M.G. Kienzle, *Am. J. Cardiol.* **61**(1988)99.
4. M..B. Simon, *Circulation* **64**(1981)235.

DISTRIBUTION PATTERNS OF VENTRICULAR ECTOPIC BEATS AS DETECTED BY HOLTER MONITORING

Gaetano Satullo, Antonino Donato, Santi Mangano, Giuseppe Busà, Giuseppe Paleologo, and Lucio Cavallaro

Servizio di Cardiologia con UTIC, Ospedale Papardo
Ctr. Papardo, 98122 Messina
Italy

ABSTRACT

A regular distribution of ventricular ectopic beats is a relatively common phenomenon known as "concealed extrasystole".

The 24-hours ECGs of 10 pts with highly frequent ventricular extrasystoles have been analyzed looking for significant sequences in their distribution. Five cases (50%) showed an allorhythmic distribution resulting in a prevalent pattern of concealed bigeminy (2n-1) in 3 cases, and concealed trigeminy (3n-1) in 2 cases. The phenomenon showed a dinamic behaviour, alternating the distributions from pattern of concealed bigeminy to concealed trigeminy or less common patterns and viceversa. The evidence of the pure ectopic cycle and mathematically related interectopic intervals in 2 cases, variability of coupling intervals, presence of fusion beats, and/or correlation between post-extrasystolic pause and number of interectopic sinus beats in the remaining 3 cases, strongly suggests the parasystolic origin of the phenomenon.

Ventricular ectopic beats (VEB) often show a regular (allorhythmic) distribution, i.e., manifest after a predictable number of sinus beats (SB). The phenomenon, called "concealed extrasystole", was firstly observed by Schamroth and Marriott in 1963 (concealed bigeminy).[1] Recently other forms of concealed extrasystolic distribution (trigeminy, quadrigeminy, pentageminy, hexageminy) have been reported.[2,3] The phenomenon has been postulated to be due to either modulation of an ectopic ventricular focus[4-7] or ventricular reentry with multilevel exit block.[8]

The 24-hours ECG of 10 patients (selected among the last 100 pts. studied in our division) with more than 2400 VEB/24h, has been analyzed looking particularly for mathematically significant sequences in VEB distribution. The admission criteria were: a) supraventricular impulses exclusevely originating from the sinus node; b) absence of significant sinus arrhythmia; c) absence of complex ventricular arrhythmias (couplets, VT) in the allorhythmic sequences.

According to Nilson,[9] we considered statistically significant sequences containing 10 or more consecutive interectopic intervals (binomial probability, 1/1,024) fulfilling one of the concealed extrasystole formulas (Table III).

Patients's clinical data are showed in Table I.

TABLE I

Case	Age	Sex	Diagnosis
1	33	F	MITRAL REGURGITATION
2	64	M	DILATED CARDIOMYOPATHY
3	12	F	NO ORGANIC HEART DISEASE
4	67	M	HYPERTENSIVE HEART DISEASE
5	58	M	CORONARY ARTERY DISEASE
6	17	M	ARRHYTHMOGENIC RIGHT VENTRICULAR DYSPLASIA
7	76	M	CORONARY ARTERY DISEASE
8	21	M	NO ORGANIC HEART DISEASE
9	55	F	NO ORGANIC HEART DISEASE
10	73	M	NO ORGANIC HEART DISEASE

Table II summerizes the results: 50% of patients (5/10) showed several patterns of concealed extrasystole.

TABLE II

Case	Approved VPCs	Coupling interval	Concealed VPC (%)	Formula
1	4,044	52-68	1.2	2n-1 2n
2	4,972	43-66	0	
3	10,425	32-48	0	
4	2,462	45-70	0.5	2n-1
5	2,421	40-65	0	
6	32,800	35-83	65.2	1/2n 3n-1 2n-1 2n 3n
7	17,269	40-78	45.4	3n-1 2n-1 2/3n 2n 3n
8	12,041	40-73	22.0	2n-1 2n 3n 1/2n
9	9,462	38-108	88.6	2n-1 1/2n 2n
10	9,113	35-72	54.8	2n-1 2n 1/2n 3n 3n+1

In these cases a regular distribution of VEB was evident, resulting in a prevalent pattern of concealed bygeminy (2n-1) in 3 patients, and concealed trigeminy (3n-1) in 2 patients. However, each tracing showed at least 3 different VEB distribution patterns, alternating each other during the 24-hours recording.

The remaining 5 cases did not show any significant distribution. In 2 cases long periods of bigeminy initiated by sudden prolongation of the sinus cycle (secondary extrasystole, rule of bigeminy) was observed. In the remaining 3 cases VEB distribution was absolutely irregular.

DISCUSSION

Concealed distribution of VEB is a phenomenon in whom ventricular extrasystoles regularly manifest after a predictable number of sinus (or dominant) beats. In Table III are listed the formulas corresponding to the concealed VEB distributions observed in the recordings.

TABLE III

	Formula	Number of interectopic sinus beats
Concealed bigeminy	2n-1	1, 3, 5, 7, 9, 11, 13, 15, 17
	2/2n-1	2, 1, 3, 5, 7, 9, 11, 13, 15
	2n	2, 4, 6, 8, 10, 12, 14, 16, 18
	1/2n	1, 2, 4, 6, 8, 10, 12, 14, 16
Concealed trigeminy	3n-1	2, 5, 8, 11, 14, 17, 20, 23
	3n+1	4, 7, 10, 13, 16, 19, 22, 25
	3n	3, 6, 9, 12, 15, 18, 21, 24
	2/3n	2, 3, 6, 9, 12, 15, 18, 21, 24

Analysis of the data indicates that allorhythmic distribution of the ventricular ectopic beats (concealed ventricular extrasystole) is not an uncommon phenomenon, especially in patients with highly frequent ventricular extrasystoles.

Moreover, most cases of this peculiar arrhythmia have a parasystolic genesis. In 2 cases the parasystolic origin was suggested by the presence of a) the "pure" parasystolic cycle, and b) all the classic signs of ventricular parasystole. In the remaining 3 cases the possibility to obtain a phase-response curve from selected strips of the recording strongly suggests the automatic origin (focus) of the ectopic impulses. Moreover, in all the 5 cases manifesting allorhythmic distribution coupling intervals variability was significantly wider ($p<0.005$) than the other cases.

REFERENCES

1. L.Schamroth and H.J.L. Marriott: Concealed ventricular extrasystoles. Circulation 27 (1963) 1043.
2. M.N.Levy, P.Goldman, L.Goldberg:Concealed quadrigeminy and quintageminy. J Electrocardiol 12 (1979) 431.
3. G.Satullo, G.Oreto, F.Luzza, F.Saporito, F.Consolo, L.Schamroth: Concealed ventricular hexageminy. J Electrocardiol 22 (1989) 167.
4. G.K. Moe, J.Jalife, W.J.Mueller, B.Moe: A mathematical modelof parasystole and its application to clinical arrhythmias. Circulation 56 (1977) 968.
5. G.Oreto, F.Luzza, G.Satullo, L.Schamroth: Modulated ventricular parasystole as a mechanism for concealed bigeminy. Am J Cardiol 58 (1986) 954.
6. G.Oreto, G.Satullo, F.Luzza: Concealed ventricular quadrigeminy linked to atrial quadrigeminy: a manifestation of modulated parasystole. J Electrocardiol 20 (1987) 176.
7. G.Oreto, G.Satullo, G.Luzza, L.Schamroth: concealed ventricular bigeminy with exceptions due to time-dependent modulationof an ectopic rhythm. Chest 93 (1988) 647.
8. S.Kinoshita: Concealed ventricular extrasystoles due to interference and due to exit block. Circulation 52 (1975) 230.
9. G.Nilsson, H.Ahlfeldt, T.Ahrén, T.Jonasson: Distribution patterns of ventriculae premature complexes in long-term electrocardiographic recordings and their usefulness in disclosing modulated parasystole. Am J Cardiol 68 (1991) 1045.

LATE POTENTIALS AND VENTRICULAR TACHYCARDIA (SUSTAINED AND NONSUSTAINED) IN PATIENTS WITH SEVERE VENTRICULAR DYSFUNCTION

PEDRO ADRAGÃO, ANTÓNIO VENTOSA
LEONOR PARREIRA, EDUARDA HORTA
DANIEL BONHORST, RICARDO SEABRA-GOMES

Department of Cardiology, Hospital de Santa Cruz
Carnaxide, 2795 Linda-a-Velha (Lisboa), Portugal

1. Introduction

Several studies have proved that after myocardial infarction, late potentials are predictive of the occurrence of clinical sustained ventricular tachycardia, mainly in patients with severe left ventricular dysfunction and/or nonsustained ventricular tachycardia on Holter monitoring [1-10].

The role of late potentials in idiopathic dilated cardiomyopathy have been less studied, but they also seem to be predictive of arrhythmic sudden death [11-12]. Few reports compare late potentials in patients with severe left ventricular dysfunction of ischemic and idiopathic etiologies.

This study reports our preliminary data on evaluation of the prevalence of late potentials and its relation to ventricular tachycardia etiology and characteristics, in a population of patients with severe left ventricular dysfunction and documented ventricular tachycardia.

2. Material and Methods

Patients with documented ventricular tachycardia (3 or more consecutive ectopic beats at a heart rate greater than 110 bpm) were included if they fulfil two other inclusion criteria: 1) left ventricular ejection fraction lesser than 35%, on planimetry of contrast left ventriculography images; 2) diagnosis of ischemic heart disease or idiopathic dilated cardiomyopathy, established by coronary arteriography and left ventriculography.

Two groups were considered, depending on ventricular tachycardia (VT) characteristics: sustained if VT episodes last 30 seconds or more, and nonsustained if not. Sustained ventricular tachycardia group included all patients with clinical sustained ventricular tachycardia studied by electrophysiological study in our laboratory (which started activity some months ago) that met the above criteria. Unsustained ventricular tachycardia group included all patients with this arrhythmia on Holter monitoring and with the other inclusion criteria.

Population selected with this methodology included 28 patients, 54 ± 9 years old (24 men and 4 women). Etiology was coronary artery disease (CAD) in 15 patients and idiopathic dilated cardiomyopathy (IDCM) in 13 patients. Ventricular tachycardia (VT) was sustained (sVT) in 13 patients and nonsustained (nVT) in 15 patients, with an uniform distribution between the 2 etiologies (Table I).

Table I. Population

	sVT	nVT	
CAD	8	7	15
IDCM	5	8	13
	13	15	28

CAD coronary artery disease
IDCM idiopathic dilated cardiomyopathy

Late potentials were detected by high-resolution ECG with signal averaging, using a Mac-VU system from Marquette. Using a filter of 40-250 Hz and a noise level always lesser than 1 μV and in general lesser than 0.4 μV, our criteria for late potentials were the occurrence of two of the following[10]: a) total filtered QRS duration ≥ 120 ms, b) low amplitude (<40 μV) signal duration ≥ 39 ms, and c) terminal 40 ms RMS voltage ≤ 20 μV.

We analysed separately patients with left bundle branch block (LBBB) due to difficulty in using accurate late potentials criteria on this setting[13].

Statistical analysis used the chi-square test.

3. Results

Table II summarizes results. From the 28 patients studied, 14 had positive late potentials criteria, 5 had negative criteria and 9 had LBBB.

Table II
Late potentials prevalence according to ventricular tachycardia etiology and characteristics

	LP -	LP +	LBBB
nonsustained VT	5	7	3
CAD	3	4	0
IDCM	2	3	3
sustained VT	-	7	6
CAD	-	4	4
IDCM	-	3	2

LP late potentials (- absence, + presence);
LBBB left bundle branch block

For the 15 patients with nonsustained ventricular tachycardia, almost half had positive late potentials criteria, one third had negative criteria, and the remaining patients had LBBB. This distribution was different ($p<0.05$) from that observed in the 13 patients with sustained ventricular tachycardia. In this group, all patients had positive late potentials criteria or LBBB (near half of each): there were no patients with sustained ventricular tachycardia and negative late potentials criteria.

Prevalence of late potentials was not modified by etiology of left ventricular dysfunction. For each etiology, near half of the patients had positive criteria, with no significant differences for overall distribution.

4. Discussion

Low-amplitude, high-frequency waveforms and altered frequency components in the terminal QRS complex, usually termed as late potentials, have been object of a large number of studies, due to their reported association with ventricular tachycardia [1-10] and sudden cardiac arrhythmic death [3,4,8,9].

Some technical considerations are needed. The criteria for late potentials that we used have been developed with basis on studies in ischemic patients [10,13]. It is not clarified if they should be the same in other subsets of patients. We used a high-pass filter of 40 Hz, that yields a good cost-benefit compromise. From recommended total filtered QRS criteria [10,13] we used 120 msec, resulting presumably in a better specificity. Adequate criteria for late potentials detection in patients with LBBB have not been developed using time-domain analysis [10,13]. We considered these patients separately. In the future, frequency domain analysis should help the study of this subset of patients.

After myocardial infarction, the risk of ventricular tachycardia or sudden death is increased in patients with late potentials on high-resolution ECG [3,4,8,9], independently from ventricular function data or from complex ventricular arrhythmias [1-6].

Patients with remote infarction and nonsustained ventricular tachycardia have been less studied, but a prospective [14] and some retrospective studies [15-18] suggest also that late potentials could be used for risk stratification and management of patients with nonsustained ventricular tachycardia.

In idiopathic dilated cardiomyopathy, late potentials seem also to be predictive of arrhythmic sudden death [11,12], but more studies are needed to confirm this.

We have studied a selected population of patients with

severe ventricular dysfunction, known as a group prone to sustained ventricular tachycardia and sudden death. The presence of nonsustained ventricular tachycardia seems to increase that risk, mainly in the presence of late potentials, at least in ischemic patients[15-18].

In our "high-risk" patients we found as expected a high prevalence of late potentials. Our preliminary results suggest that late potentials or LBBB are more prevalent in patients with sustained ventricular tachycardia than in patients with nonsustained ventricular tachycardia. This was equally true for ischemic patients, and for idiopathic dilated cardiomyopathy patients, suggesting that late potentials could reflect a common phenomenon - presumably reentry - independently of the etiology of the abnormal characteristics of diseased myocardium.

It is important to emphasise that, in our selected population, all patients with sustained ventricular tachycardia had late potentials or LBBB. The important implication is that, in this small series, the absence of late potentials, excluded the occurrence of sustained ventricular tachycardia (negative predictive value of 100%), suggesting that even on the relatively high-risk group studied, a normal high-resolution ECG can help to restrict the number of candidates to electrophysiologic study, either in ischemic or dilated cardiomyopathy patients.

However larger series and prospective studies are needed to confirm these results, specially in non ischemic patients.

1. ME Cain, D Ambos, FX Witkowski, et al. Circulation **69** (1984) 711.
2. SJ Worley, DB Mark, WM Smith, et al. J Am Coll Cardiol **11** (1988) 1041.
3. DL Kuchar, CW Thornburn, NL Sammel. J Am Coll Cardiol **9** (1987) 531.
4. JA Gomes, SL Winters, D Stewart, et al. J Am Coll Cardiol **10** (1987) 349.
5. JA Gomes, SF Horowitz, M Millner, et al. Am J Cardiol **59** (1987) 1071.
6. TA Buckingham, S Ghosh, SM Homan, et al. Am J Cardiol **59** (1987) 568.
7. BD Lindsay, HD Ambos, KB Schechtman, et al. Circulation **73** (1986) 675.
8. G Breithardt, M Schwarzmaier, M Borggrefe, et al. Eur Heart J **4** (1983) 487.
9. AR Deniss, DA Richards, DV Cody, et al. Circulation **74** (1986) 731.
10. MB Simson. Circulation **85 (supl I)** (1992) I-145.
11. DS Poll, FE Marchlinski, RA Falcone et al. Circulation **72** (1986) 1308.
12. Y Ohnishi, T Inoue, H Fukuzaki. Jpn Circ J **54** (1990) 127
13. Task Force Committee of ESC/AHA/ACC. Circulation **83** (1991) 1481.
14. G Turitto, JM Fontaine, SM Ursell et al. Am J Med **88 (suppl 1N)** (1990) 1-35N.
15. G Breithardt, M Borggrefe, B Quantius et al. Circulation **68** (1983) 275.
16. G Turitto, JM Fontaine, SM Ursell et al. Am J Cardiol **61** (1988) 1272.
17. S Winters, D Stewart, A Targonski, et al. Circulation **78(suppl II)** (1988) II-578.
18. BD Lindsay, HD Ambos, KB Schechtman, et al. Circulation **73** (1986) 675.

EXERCISE-MEDIATED CYCLE LENGTH VARIATIONS IN SINUS PARASYSTOLE

Gaetano Satullo, Antonino Donato, Antonino La Rosa, Antonino Coglitore, Gianni Mobilia and Lucio Cavallaro

Servizio di Cardiologia con UTIC, Ospedale Papardo, Ctr. Papardo, 98100 Messina
Italy

ABSTRACT

Sinus parasystole is the expression of a protected non-dominant sinus pacemaker which is totally independent of the dominant rhythm. The behavior of a regular sinus parasystole during exercise stress test has been studied in a 60-year-old man, undergone the test because of coronary artery disease.

Variability of the parasystolic cycle, and its relation to the basic sinus rate, has been analyzed, resulting an evident concordance. Indeed, effort was able to enhance both the dominant and parasystolic cycle length.

Parasystole is the expression of an automatic focus that is protected from, and thus independent of, the dominant rhythm. The possibility of a parasystolic rhythm originating in the sino-atrial node (sinus parasystole) was first reported by Schamroth in 1967.[1] Five cases of sinus parasystole have been published up to now.[2,3]

This presentation reflects, a case of regular sinus parasystole whose behavior was studied at rest and during exercise stress test. The tracing in Figure 1 was recorded from a 60 year-old-man undergone the test because of Coronary Artery Disease. It is evident the presence of "premature sinus beats". The morphology of these beats (labeled with open circles), indeed, is identical to the "normal" sinus P waves in all the 12 Standard Leads.

In Figure 2 (a continuous recording of Lead V1; 5th minute of the recovery period) is evident the parasystolic origin of the premature sinus beats. The coupling intervals are variable (range:54-76 hundredths of a second) and the interectopic intervals are constantly regular (ranging from 142 to 152 hundredths of a second).

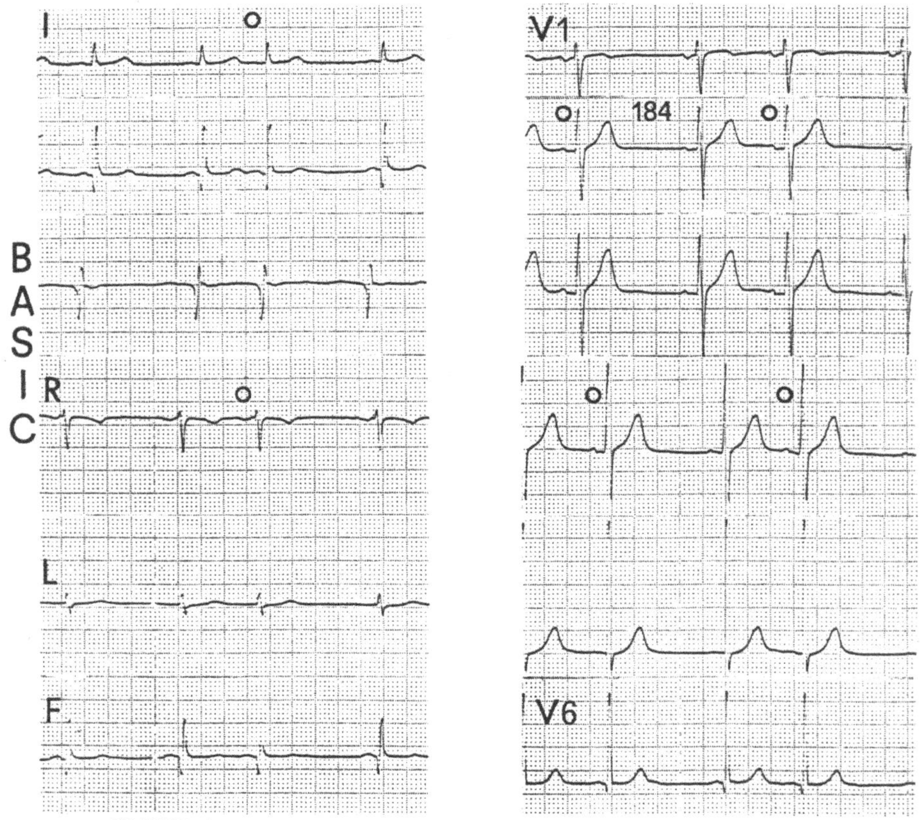

FIGURE 1.

TABLE

Dominant cycle length	Parasystolic cycle length	Step
100	170-184	Basic
84	167-168	Ortho
66	124-132	25W
58	121	50W
52	NO S.Par.	75W
45	NO S.Par.	100W
48	NO S.Par.	1'rec
72	140-152	5'rec

The Table summarizes the behavior of the arrhythmia during exercise stress test.

A significant correlation between the dominant cycle length and the parasystolic cycle length was observed at 25 Watt, 50 Watt, and during the last minutes of the recovery phase.

Effort, indeed, has been able to enhance both the dominant and parasystolic cycle length. For example, when the dominant cycle length was 100 the parasystolic cycle length was 170-184, whereas at dominant cycle length of 66 the parasystolic cycle length was 124-132. At higher heart rates (sinus cycle length < 52) no evident premature sinus beats manifested.

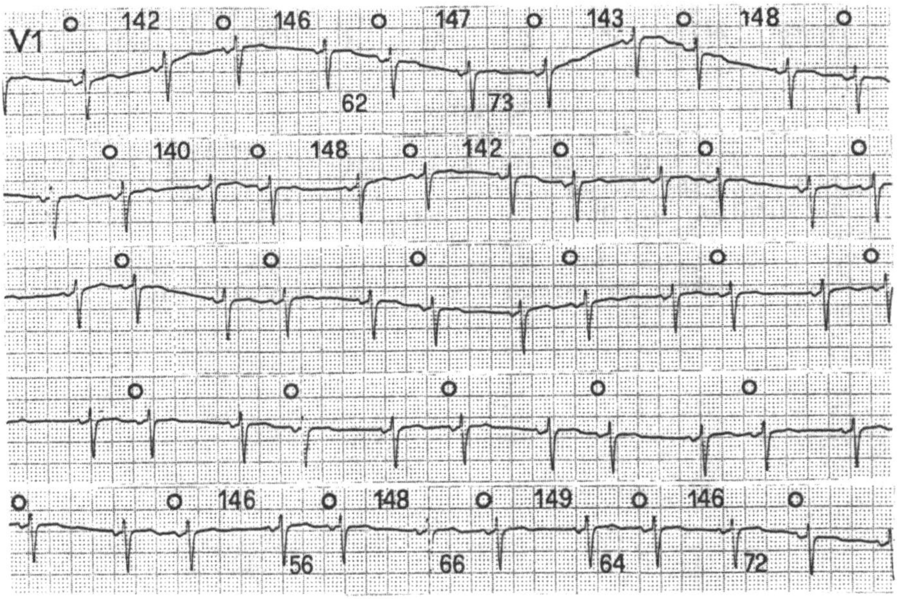

FIGURE 2

DISCUSSION

Diagnosis of sinus parasystole is relatively difficult because there is no difference between the basic sinus P waves and the parasystolic P waves, so that sinus parasystole manifests as an "irregular" sinus rhythm. It is therefore likely that sinus parasystole is somewhat underemphasized, and in several cases a diagnosis of sinus arrhythmia is entertained unless the P-P intervals are carefully analyzed.

The presence of a parasystolic rhythm should be considered in every case presenting as "atypical" or as nonrespiratory sinus arrhythmia, or in the presence of "sinus extrasystoles". Premature sinus beats with variable coupling intervals are the most reliable key to the diagnosis of sinus parasystole, whereas the precise mathematical relationship between the parasystolic P-P intervals is less important; finally, no fusion beats are manifest in sinus parasystole, since both the dominant and the parasystolic sinus impulses result in the same pattern of atrial activation. Although spontaneous daily (circadian) variability of the cycle length, a ventricular parasystolic focus has been already described[4],we report the first clinical evidence of exercise-mediated variability of the sinus parasystolic cycle length.

The exercise-mediated rate variability is wide and it is clearly concordant to variation of the dominant sinus rhythm. The local influence of the neurovegetative stimuli is likely exerted upon both the dominant sinus pace-maker cells and the otherwise protected parasystolic cells, resulting in fastening of their intrinsic rates.

REFERENCES

1. L. Schamroth: Sinus parasystole. Am J Cardiol 20 (1967) 434.
2. J. Jalife, D.C. Michaels, R. Langendorf: Modulated parasystole originating in the sinoatrial node. Circulation 74 (1986) 945.
3. G. Satullo, G. Oreto, F. Luzza, A. Consolo, A. Donato: Sinus parasystole. Am Heart J 121 (1991) 1507.
4. G.A. Lanza, Lucente M., Rebuzzi A.G., Spagnolo A., Dulcimascolo C, Manzoli U: Ventricular parasystole: a chronobiologic study. PACE 9 (1986) 860.

HYPERTENSION IN WELL CONTROLLED DIABETIC PATIENTS — AN ASSOCIATION WITH DIASTOLIC DYSFUNTION

Manuela Fiuza, Armando Pereirinha, José Correia, Bragança Parreira, Rui Duarte, Mário G. Lopes and Fernando de Pádua

INCP, Clínica de Diabetes e Nutrição (Resp:Prof P. Lisboa), Med IV/HSM (Prof F. de Pádua) and CCUL/FML (LA3). Lisbon, Portugal

Abstract

In order to evaluate rhythm/ST segment changes and cardiac function (systolic and diastolic) associated with diabetes, 33 diabetic patients (19 male, 4 female; mean age±SD: 43±12 years), 24 insulin-dependent and 9 non-insulin dependent were studied with 24 hour Holter ECG monitoring (H), 2D Echocardiography (ECHOCG) ans Doppler (PW, CW and colour flow) attending a tertiary hospital. With H rythm profile, heart rate variability and ST segment changes were analised. Systolic function was analised with M and 2D ECHOCG and diastolic function with Doppler. All 4 valves were interrogated for valvular regurgitation. Five (17%) pts had hypertension (3 ID, 2 NID), none had evidence of myocardial infarction or angor, and in 3 pts microalbubinuria was disclosed. All were considered to have a good metabolic control and the duration of the disease ranged from 5.5 to 35 years. None of the patients had significant ST segment changes or arrhytmias, and all presented an adequate heart rate variability to daily activities, showing no autonomic innervation impairment.

Systolic eft ventricular (LV) function was preserved in all patients, and there was no regional motion abnormalities. Diastolic LV function was abnormal in 5 patients all with high blood pressure, with LV hypertrophy, and a lower early to late filling velocity and a higher peak atrial filling velocity (A>E). In 8 (28%) pts, a "physiological" trivial/mild mitral valve regurgitation was detected with colour Doppler. There were no consistent differences between ID and NID pts.

Conclusion: In this population of diabetic patients with a good metabolic control, systolic function as well as autonomic innervation were preserved despite the long standing disease. Only hypertensive patients showed a Doppler pattern suggestive of diastolic abnormalities.

Introduction

Epidemiological studies have clearly demonstrated that diabetic patients are at increased risk for cardiovascular morbidity and mortality (1). The cardiovascular disease associated with diabetes mellitus can involve the small arteries (microangiopathic disease) at all ages, and the large vessels (macroangiopathic disease) of older people.

Hypertension and diabetes is a well known association of two powerful independent risk factors for cardiovascular disease (2). The frequent ocurrence of the two diseases doubles the risk for cardiovascular death as well as cerebral and peripheral vascular disease. Coronary artery disease is the leading cause of death among adult diabetics (almost three times more than in non diabetics) and frequently manifests itself silently and prematurely, as have been demonstrated with exercise stress tests and Holter ambulatory ECG studies (3,4). Diabetic patients also have increased risk of congestive heart failure. In the Framingham population the incidence was four to five times more frequent than in non diabetics, and recent evidence suggests that myocardial dysfunction might develop in the absence of coronary artery disease, hypertension or valvular heart disease. Thus a specific heart muscle disease could be related to diabetes mellitus itself and was named "diabetic cardiomyopathy" (5,6).

Cardiac autonomic dysfunction exists in many diabetic patients and in more than one third is related to the severity of left ventricular dysfunction. These changes in autonomic nervous system result in the presence of tachycardia and a fixed rapid heart rate that is irresponsive to physiological stimuli such as Valsalva manoeuver, carotid sinus pressure and drugs like atropine and propranolol (7,8).

These diabetic related diseases can be detected with non invasive tests, and perhaps diagnosed in a preclinical phase. Therefore, we evaluated with Echocardiography/Doppler studies the left ventricular systolic and diastolic function and with Holter ECG ambulatory monitoring the rhythm and ST changes, a population of metabolically well controlled diabetic patients without overt cardiovascular disease.

Patients and Methods

The study population consisted of 33 consecutive ambulatory diabetic patients, attending a tertiary University Hospital (19 male, 4 female; mean age±SD: 43±12 years), without overt cardiovascular disease. Twenty four were insulin-dependent (ID) with a disease duration of 17±8 years, and 9 patients were non insulin-dependent (NID) in whom the disease duration was 16±10 years.

The design of the study included a baseline evaluation with Echocardiogram (MM and 2D) and Doppler study (pulsed, continuous wave and colour flow) to evaluate the systolic and diastolic left ventricular functions and a 24 hour Holter ECG ambulatory monitoring test, to analyse the rhythm profile and ST segment changes (Table 1). The tests were repeated at six months, one year and then yearly . Only the baseline results are available at this time of the study.

Results

Echocardiographic studies showed that left ventricle systolic function was preserved in all patients, and there were no regional motion abnormalities. In seven patients high blood pressure was disclosed (4 ID and 3 NID): all of them presented with left ventricular hypertrophy evaluated with Echocardiography, as well as, a lower early to late filling velocity and a higher peak atrial filling velocity (A wave > E wave) evaluated with Doppler, suggesting diastolic dysfunction (Figure 1). This pattern was not detected in non hypertensive patients. In 10 pts, a "physiological" trivial/mild mitral valve regurgitation was detected with colour Doppler. There were no consistent differences between ID and NID patients.

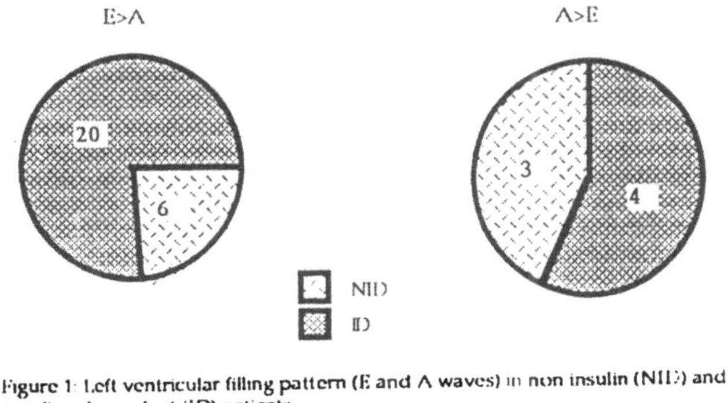

Figure 1: Left ventricular filling pattern (E and A waves) in non insulin (NID) and insuline dependent (ID) patients.

In 24 hour Holter ECG ambulatory monitoring, all patients presented an adequate heart rate variability with daily activities, showing no significative cardiac autonomic dysfunction. Also no significant ST segment changes could be disclosed in this population. With respect to dysrhythmias, 27% of the patients had supraventricular rhythms and 24% ventricular arrhythmias. These dysrhythmias were more prevalent in the hypertensive patients: the supraventricular and ventricular arrhythmias were respectively 71% and 86% (Figure 2).

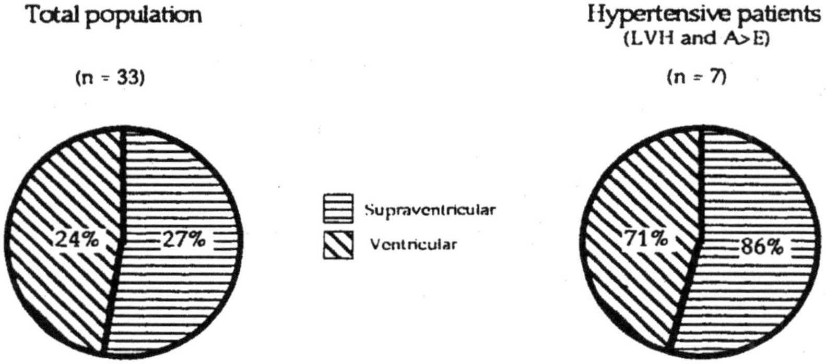

Figure 2: Prevalence of dysrhythmic events in the population under study and on the hypertensive diabetic population. LVH: Left ventricular hypertrophy

Discussion

In our baseline studies of assymptomatic diabetics, only hypertensive patients presented with alterations in left ventricular function and rhythm profile. These alterations of left ventricular relaxation are common in hypertensive patients, specially when associated with left ventricular hypertrophy. This can be seen as an inversion of the left ventricular filling pattern with an A wave greater than E wave (9). Also in these patients the arrhythmic events were more prevalent. This finding was also reported and probably is related to myocardial fibrosis that facilitate reentry mechanisms (10,11). Another contributive factor is diuretic medications, but none of these patients were on diuretics.

No heart rate disturbances were disclosed in these patients. All patients had adequate heart rate variability with daily activities. Cardiac autonomic disturbances are usually present with left ventricular systolic dysfunction which was not the case in our population, however no provocative stimuli was performed.

There were no ST segment significant changes during Holter recordings suggestive of silent ischemia and no patient complained of angina. Probably an exercise stress test should also be performed to disclose myocardial ischemia since no patient complained of significant peripheral vascular disease.

Conclusions

Our findings in a well controlled assymptomatic diabetic population, showed no differences from a non diabetic population. Only the patients with hypertension showed left ventricular hypertrophy with relaxation abnormalities (A wave > E wave in Doppler spectrum), suggestive of diastolic dysfunction.

Eventually only the "good" patients are being selected or probably there is a subgroup of patients in which the good metabolic control can retard the cardiovascular events. Follow-up studies are expected to confirm these baseline findings.

Bibliographic references

1) Kannel WP,McGee DL. *Diabetes and cardiovascular disease. The Framingham Heart Study.* JAMA 1979; 241: 2035-8

2) The Working Group on Hypertension in Diabetes: *Statement on hypertension and diabetes mellitus. Final report.* Arch Intern Med 1987; 147: 830

3) Herlitz J, Malmberg K, Karlson BW et al: *Mortality and morbidity during a five year follow-up of diabetics with myocardial infarction.* Acta Med Scand 1988; 224:31

4) Langer A, Freeman MR, Josse RG et al: *Detection of silent myocardial ischemia in diabetes mellitus.* Am J Cardiol 1991; 67: 1073-8

5) Senevineratne BIB: *Diabetic cardiomyopathy.* British Med J 1977, 1:1444-6

6) Kannel WB, Hjortand M, Castelli WP; role of diabetes in congestive heart failure. Am J Cardiol 1974; 34: 29-34

7) Roy T, Peterson HR, Snider HL et al: *Autonomic influence on cardiovascular performance in diabetic subjects.* Am J Med 1989; 87: 382

8) Smith SA: *Reduced sinus arrhythmia in diabetic autonomic neuropathy: diagnostic value of an age related normal range.* British Med J 1982; 4: 1599

9) TakenaKam K, Sakamoto T, Amano K et al: *Left ventricular filling determined by Doppler echocardiography in diabetes mellitus.* Am J Cardiol 1988; 61: 1139

10) Fiuza M, Pinto F, Dias E et al: *Ventricular dysrhythmias in ambulatory hypertensive patients: how important is left ventricular echocardiographic pattern ?* Advances in Electrocardiology (ed. Antalóczy Z). Excerpta Medica 1990, 339-42.

11) Mclenachan JM, Henderson E, Morris KL et al: *Ventricular arrhythmias in patients with hypertensive left ventricular hypertrophy.* N Engl J Med 1987; 317: 787

PART VI

Ischemic Heart Disease including Exercise Testing

VCG DATA CLASSIFICATION OF IHD USING PROBABILISTIC EXPERT SYSTEM

VALOVÁ DAGMAR
Institute of Physiological Regulations
Czechoslovak Academy of Sciences
Prague, CSFR

and

DRŠKA Z., KALOŠ M., MÁLKOVÁ A.
Institute of Physiological Regulations
Czechoslovak Academy of Sciences
Prague, CSFR

ABSTRACT

This paper deal with our experiences with utilization of probabilistic expert system for VCG classification of myocardial infarction. Correct classification of studied groups was found equal to 85.8% for healthy subjects, 86.5% for patients with posterior m.i., 80.8% for patients with anterior m.i. and 100.0% for patients with anteroseptal m.i.

1. Introduction

One of the most important features of expert systems is the ability to deal with uncertain knowledge. For solution of VCG signal interpretation problem we choose the probabilistic expert system, because the uncertainty is expressed by probability distribution and the result diagnoses admit more possibilities with different weights. It exhibits other suitable properties, which has been described in previous papers. [3,4]

The classification of VCG was chosen because of the well evaluating original system of quantitative parameters and also because larger amount of data supplied with results of complete cardiological diagnoses have been investigated.

2. Materials and Methods

In diagnostic problem solution the dimension decreasing without information lost plays often significant role, because the redundant description of information makes the decision algorithm to be worse and the computing time to be too long. This data reduction was the aim of system KARDIO, the result of which is diagnostic characteristic set. This system was developed by Laufberger, Drska, Král, Novák [1,2] and tested on great number of patients and healthy subjects.

This set of data should be subdivided into two groups:
1. local characteristics - describe 13 points on the module, velocity and curvature curves. Some of them can be seen on figure 1.:

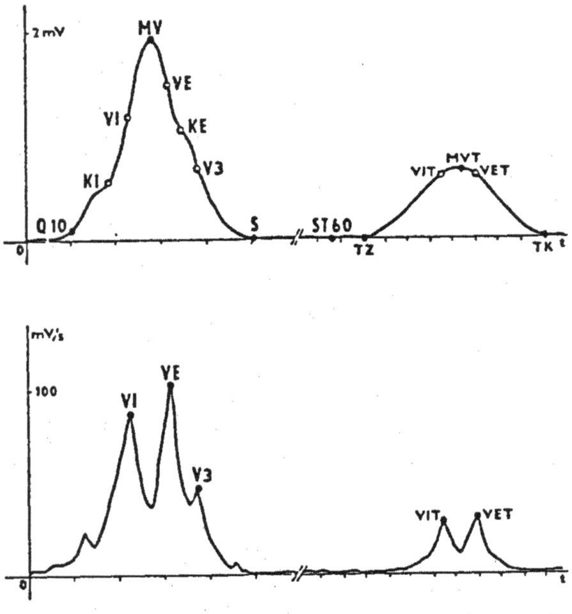

Fig.1: Local characteristics describe significant points
a) on the module b) on the velocity /2/

Q,S	= the beginning and the end of QRS;
MV	= maximal module during QRS;
TZ,TK	= the beginning and the end of T-wave;
MVT	= maximal module during <TZ,TK>;

VI,VE = local max. velocity closely appeared before and after MV;
V3 = local max. velocity during < VE+1,S-1>;
VIT, VET = local max. velocity during <TZ,MVT>,<MVT,TK >;
KI,KE = max. curvature during < Q+3,VT>, < VE,S >;

2.The interval characteristic are:

1. Parameters of the QRS (T) mean plane i.e. of plane fitted to QRS (T) spatial curve during <Q,S> (<TZ,TK>) interval and the parameter of nonplanarity;
2. Spatial distribution of the VCG curve area and time expressed by octant share (in % of the whole area);
3. Mean values of module, velocity and curvature during <Q,S>, <S,TZ>, <TZ,TK> intervals and their durations;

Described parameters offer from diagnostic problem point of view more objective information than visual evaluation of digitized VCG signal. And also their quantitative form is very useful.

For solution of VCG signal interpretation problem we choose upper mentioned probabilistic expert system. We applied this expert system on followed groups of subjects: a group of 76 healthy subjects (H), a group of patients with old myocardial infarction subdivided into followed subsets: 107 patients with anterior (MIA) and 35 patients with anteroseptal (MIAS) and 112 patients with posterior infarction (MIP). The VCG data of all these groups were recorded at rest. These data files were subdivided into two groups: files for creating the knowledge base and testing files. (see table 1.)

Table 1: Number of subjects in studied groups

	knowledge base	testing file
Healthy	41	35
MIP	60	52
MIA	65	52
MIAS	0	35

3. Results

Correct classification for healthy subject is equal to 85.8%, for patients with posterior old myocardial infarction to 55.8%, for patients with anterior infarction to 71.2% and for patients with anteroseptal infarction to 94.3%. (see table 2.)

Results of dichotomizing classification (of two classes:the first one is class of healthy subjects and the second one is the class of all types of old myocardial infarction) for healthy subject is equal to 85.8%, for patients with posterior old myocardial infarction to 86.5%, for patients with anterior infarction to 80.8% and for patients with anteroseptal infarction to 100.0%.

Table 2: Summary of VCG classification of studied groups by probabilistic expert system (in %)

	B	H	MIP	MIA
H	5.7	85.8	2.8	5.7
MIP	7.7	5.8	55.8	30.7
MIA	17.3	1.9	9.6	71.1
MIAS	0.0	0.0	5.7	94.3

B = common background (Subject belogs to this group when the probabilistic expert system is not able to decide for classification to any other group - its knowledge base is given as a mean of all other groups knowledge bases.)

4. Conclusion

It was then proved, that chosen probabilistic expert system is suitable for VCG interpretation problem solution and the significant contribution to other cardiology interpretation problem could be expected.

In the next study we would like to verify this result on larger amount of data, which has been measured yet.

5. References

1. Drška,Z., Král,V., Novák V.,*In: Neue Ergebnisse der Electrokardiologie II.* Ed: E.Schubert,(Jena, Gustav Fischer Verlag 1974) p. 263-265.
2. Drška,Z., Poláková,M., Drozen,D., Král,V., *Annales de Cardiologie et d'Angiologie*,(1990), 30,4, p. 199-201.
3. Grim J.: *Proceedings of 10th Prague Conference on Information Theory.*(Prague 1986).
4. Valová D., Drška Z. , Málková A., *In: Electrocardiology '91 World Scientific Publishing Co Pte Ltd, Singapore.* printed.

COMPARISON OF ELECTROCARDIOGRAPHY, VECTORCARDIOGRAPHY AND ANGIOGRAPHY FOR THE DETECTION OF MYOCARDIAL SCARS IN SINGLE VESSEL CORONARY HEART DISEASE

Ute Reckers
Medical clinic, Department of Cardiology, University Münster, Germany.

and

Jutta Jahnel, Betty Brisse
Medical clinic, Department of Cardiology, University Münster, Germany.

ABSTRACT

Non invasive detection of CHD by myocardial scars and/or wall motion abnormality was analyzed in patients (n=54, mean age of 53,9 ± 7,3 (SD) years, 46 males, 8 females) with single vessel disease and 26 normals (mean age of 47,1 ± 12,3 (SD), 14 males, 12 females).

Methods: Patients (n=54) with single vessel coronary heart disease, 12-lead ECG, Frank VCG (500 Hz), cine: 30° RAO LV-angiography, 16 hemiaxial and 16 radial diameters.

Results: LAD-obstruction: Sensitivity of ECG 65%, VCG 94%, anterior wall motion abnormality in 45% (hemiaxial) 52% (radial diameter). LCX-obstruction: Sensitivity of ECG 60%, VCG 95%, dorso-inferior wall motion abnormality in 42% (hemiaxial) and 44% (radial diameter).

Conclusion: 1. VCG is superior to ECG for the diagnosis of myocardial scars in LAD-obstruction; in LCX-disease the difference in sensitivity increases by 40%. 2. Wall motion analysis by hemiaxial and radial monoplane method with 40-50% positive results is a specific but not very sensitive method.

1. Introduction

The reliability of ECG and VCG in patients with typical myocardial infarction has been studied several times. It has been pointed out that the sensitivity of the 3 dimensional recording is superior to the standard ECG in detecting small scars and posterior or multiple defects.[5,8,9]

But this did not lead to clinical concequence. Under clinical conditions ECG and exercice ECG are performed and there is often a discrepancy between anamnestic ischemic episodes, the scars seen by the ECG and the functional disturbance of the LV, shown by angiography.

Regarding the literature, up to 25% of ischemic episodes remain silent and sometimes lead to non-specific symptoms. Invasive methods in these patients cannot be indicated. As a consequence early signs of CHD cannot be verified in this cohort.

On the other hand angiography in patients with clinical signs of CHD sometimes reveals normal coronary arteries or only minor changes of the vessels, but major changes of LV wall motion and pump function. It can be assumed, that muliple small events led to this late stage of the myocardial disease. Both problems are espacially evident with CHD in women.

The following study compared the clinical sensitivity of the ECG, VCG and LV wall motion analysis for LV-scars in correlation with CHD.

2. Patients and Methods

A comparative study was performed in 54 consecutive patients with angiographically proved single vessel CHD, 46 males, 8 females, mean age 53,9 years (s = 7,3) and 26 healthy controls, 14 males, 12 females, mean age 47,1 years (s = 12,3) with angiographically normal coronary arteries. Patients with bundle branch block were excluded.

In all of them standard ECG (12 lead), Frank VCG (500 Hz)[2] and LV-angiography were performed. The VCG was recorded by a polaroid photo of the 3 dimensional deflection of the cathod ray oscillograph, one with the continous slope and a second one with interruptions every 2 msec, leading to small arrow like bits, demasking the forward direction of the complex. Infarction criteria were used according to Csapo[1] for ECG and Lichtlen[7] for VCG.

Left ventricular angiograms in 30 degree right anterior oblique projection were obtained by standard methods. The frame of the endsystolic and enddiastolic LV-volume were defined by manual method and digitized by a computer tablet. Regional wall motion abnormalities were assessed as follows: the length axis connected the apex and the midpoint of the aortic valve plane; it was intersected by 2 equidistant short axes perpendicular to the length axis. Each of these segments of the length axis was again intersected by 2 equidistant short axes. The resulting 8 diameters were analysed as 16 hemiaxes, 8 anterior and 8 infero-posterior segments.

From the midpoint of the long axis, radial diameters were also connected to the afore mentioned coordinates of the endsystolic and enddiastolic frame. Systolic shortening of a segment was calculated as the difference of the diastolic and systolic distance divided by the diastolic value. A deviation of 10% of the mean of controls had to be exceeded for abnormal values.

3. Results and Discussion

The detection of myocardial scars by ECG is of limited sensitivity and specifity, as could be shown by several studies. In our patients with single vessel CHD 65% positiv results were seen in LAD-obstruction and only 60% with LCX-disease.

The VCG detected scars in 94% (LAD) to 95% (LCX). No false positivs could be detected in our controls. (figure 1,2)

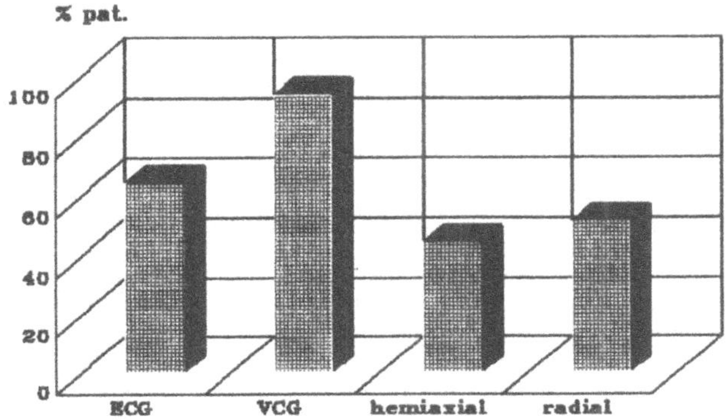

figure 1: ventral and septal LV-scars

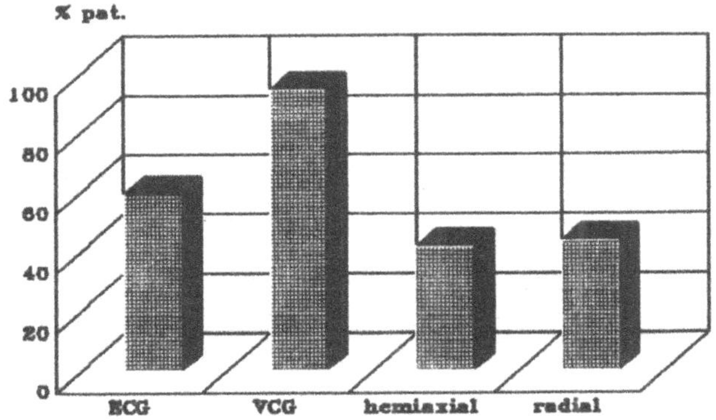

figure 2: dorsal and dorso-inferior LV-scars

This difference of sensitivity in LAD-disease may be due to the better resolving power of the VCG and the possibility to discriminate small defects and abnormal velocity of depolarisation, not identified by the ECG.

This interpretation is further verified by the sensitivity of only 45% (hemiaxial) and 52% (radial) measuring wall motion abnormality. The results show that only about half of the patients with LAD-obstruction essencially those with LAD-occlusion or at least 70% obstruction have scars and or ischemic areas large enough to be detected by this wall motion analysis.

Another 40-45% have smaller defects or abnormalities of depolarisation only seen by VCG. Therefore the VCG may offer the chance to detect CHD much earlier and to stimulate prevention of complications.

Concerning the results of the LCX-disease wall motion analysis of the 30° RAO-projection cannot be expected to be as effectiv as in LAD-disease, because the region of the marginal branch cannot be seen by this projection.[3,4,6] Wall motion of the dorso-inferior part of the posterior region, however could be measured. This method as well as the ECG is not very sensitiv in LCX-disease; the indirect and summed up information can be improved in as much as 40% of this group by VCG. These results are in aggreement with former studies of our clinic and show the advantage of the 3 dimensional recording method with high resolution[8].

4. Conclusions

In single vessel CHD the detection of myocardial scars by ECG, VCG and wall motion analysis of the LV shows a different sensitivity of the 3 methods. Concerning all coronary vessels the overall sensitivity of the ECG and wall motion analysis is similar; ECG 63%, wall motion 65% (hemiaxial) 79% (radial) positiv results. The VCG is superior with 96%. Correlation of the 3 methods is better in detecting ventral and septal scars; for the dorsal and dorso-inferior region VCG is superior. Myocardial scars not leading to ECG changes and wall motion abnormalities can be detected by VCG only. Non-invasiv screening methods may thus lead to an earlier and more sensitive diagnosis of CHD and give a better base for preventive and therapeutic procedures.

1. G. Csapo in *Konventionelle und intrakardiale Elektrokardiographie* (Ciba Geigy, Wehr/Baden 1980)
2. E. Frank, *Circ.* **13** (1956) p.737-49
3. H. Gelberg, B.H. Brundage, S. Glantz, W.W. Parmeley, *Circ.* **59** (1979) p.991-1000
4. M. Gottwick, W. Frimmel, G. Staemler, B. Winkler, M. Schlepper, *Zeitschr. f. Kardiol.* **69** (1980) p.692
5. W. Gray , M. Corbin, Y. King, M. Dunn, *Br. Heart J.* **34** (1972) p.1163-69
6. R.F. Leighton, A.D. Nelson, P. Brewster, in *Ventricular Wall Motion*, ed. U. Sigwart, P.H. Heintzen (Stuttgart, New York, Thieme 1984) p.99-106
7. P.R. Lichtlen, *Klinische Vektor-Elektrokardiographie*, ed. (Berlin, Heidelberg, New York, Springer 1967)
8. H. Portheine in *Aktuelle Probleme der Vektorkardiographie*, ed. R. Wenger (Thieme, Stutgart 1968) p.216-225
9. J.W. Starr, G.S. Wagner, V.S. Behar, A. Waltson J.C. Greenfield, *Circ.* **49** (1974) p.829-36

PARDEE T WAVE FROM 1920 TO 1992:
An STT Marker for Coronary Artery Disease

Michael M. Laks, M.D., Monica Kraft, M.D., and William J. French, M.D.
Harbor-UCLA Medical Center, Torrance, California 90509

ABSTRACT

In 1920 Harold Pardee showed that ST segment elevation followed by T wave inversion in the electrocardiogram is associated with the presence of severe coronary artery disease. The criteria of a Pardee T wave were defined as minimal ST segment elevation of the onset to midpoint greater than or equal to 0.02 mV above the baseline followed by a T wave inversion greater than or equal to 0.06 Mv in one of the precordial leads V1-V6. Using ECL computer language to program the computerized ECG system both retro-spective and prospective analysis revealed a correlation between the presence of the Pardee T wave and significant coronary artery disease. The overall incidence of the Pardee T wave was 15%. The study is limited by a small sample size and by excluding many patients. However, the excluded patients had high risk factors for coronary artery disease such as left ventricular hypertrophy, a history of previous myocardial infarction, bundle branch block, older age, hypertension, cardiovascular disease and peripheral vascular disease. Consequently, the estimate of the incidence of the Pardee T wave should be higher. The Pardee T wave is concluded to be an early and probably frequent marker for coronary artery disease. This study suggests that the use of a computerized ECG program system is a valuable tool to identify patients at risk for coronary artery disease.

Introduction: Coronary artery disease (CAD) remains the number one cause of mortality of middle-aged men in the United States. An unknown number of patients remain asymptomatic with significant CAD. Many of these latter patients suffer from the ravages of silent ischemia which may result in an acute myocardial infarction or sudden death. Thus, there has been a great emphasis on the development of simple, safe and inexpensive noninvasive cardiac tests that could recognize patients with severe CAD who are at high risk of developing angina, acute myocardial infarction or sudden death. ECG, radionuclide and exercise echo stress testing are relatively more sensitive in detecting the presence of CAD but are expensive and often inconvenient to perform. Overlooked in the rush to use more sophisticated cardiac studies have been the resting, 12-lead electrocardiogram, even though the electrocardiogram is frequently a useful marker of severe CAD. In 1920 Harold Pardee from New York Hospital did a simple post mortem ECG correlation study of patients with and without CAD[1]. He discovered that 36% of the patients with atherosclerotic heart disease had T wave and ST segment changes which he called the coronary T wave. Other patients without CAD who had valvular heart disease and chronic fibrous myocarditis did not have these ECG changes. In the paper published in the American Society for Clinical Investigation, Harold Pardee described the coronary T wave as follows: "The significant feature is the presence, in one or more leads, usually one, of a downward, sharply peaked T wave with an upward convexity of the ST interval." Throughout my training and professional life I was taught that an ECG change called the Pardee T wave was diagnostic of CAD. I was always curious as to the validity of this entity. Therefore, as our group was facile in writing programs into an ECG computer system utilizing Hewlett-Packard ECL language, I decided in 1980 to program the computer to diagnose these ST and T wave changes which I have been calling the Pardee T wave[2]. The Pardee T wave consists of: The ST segment onset and midportion elevated 0.02 Mv above baseline and a negative T wave 0.06 mV in any precordial lead V1-V6. In addition, the R wave progresses normally with no Q wave > 30 msec (Fig. 1).

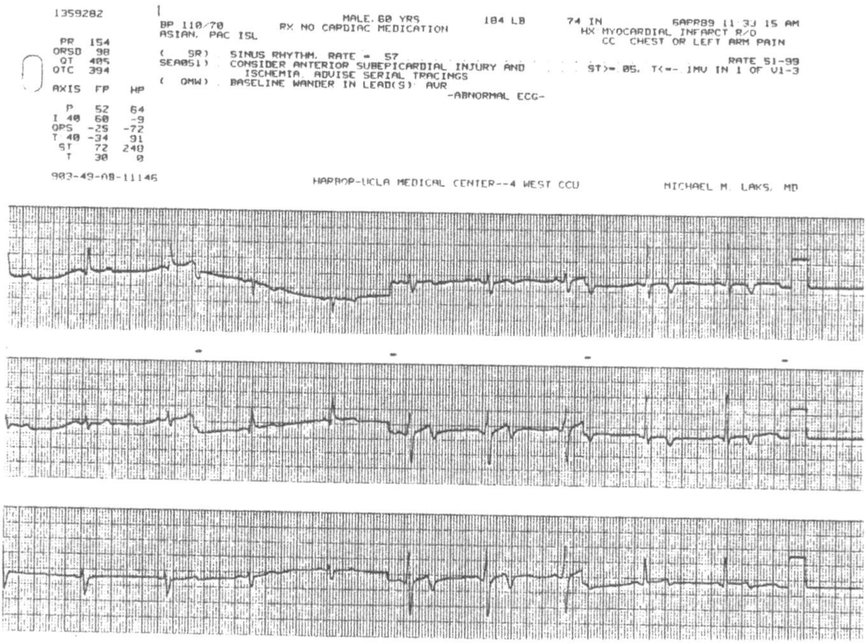

Figure 1: An example of an ECG with Pardee T waves. Note the anterior ST elevation at least 0.05 mV at the onset followed by T wave inversion ≤ -0.1 mV.

We hypothesized that the Pardee T wave may be a frequent and early marker of CAD and performed the Pardee T study retrospectively and prospectively. Our goals were: (1) to correlate the computerized ECG program with the location and severity of CAD. (2) to determine the incidence and clinical significance of the Pardee T wave in a hospital-based population.

Methods: In the retrospective portion of this study, the population consisted of 225 consecutive patients who had undergone cardiac catheterization for suspected CAD. These ECGs were screened by our ECG computer for the presence of Pardee T waves. Of 225 patients screened, 15 patients had Pardee T waves on ECG and no evidence of LVH, MI or BBB. The results of the cardiac catheterizations were: 6 (40%) had significant left main obstruction > 50% stenosis; 4 (27%) had > 70% obstruction and 5 (33%) had significant mid or distal LAD obstruction. Thus, all patients had significant CAD with either left main or LAD obstruction. None of the patients without CAD had Pardee T waves.

A prospective analysis of the presence and significance of Pardee T waves was carried out using the computer program "Datasearch." ECG criteria for the Pardee T wave were programmed to have the ECG computer retrieve ECGs on a daily basis from a hospital-based population of patients admitted through the Emergency Department during a 3-month period. Patients with life-threatening non-cardiac disease (such as cerebrovascular accident, sepsis and terminal malignancy) were excluded because it was inappropriate to pursue a further cardiac evaluation.

Results and Discussion: From our emergency department, a total of 129 ECGs was retrieved over a 3-month period out of a total of 890 ECGs done, resulting in an overall incidence of the Pardee T wave of 150/1000 or 15%. Of these 129, 25 patients were not hospitalized decreasing the number to 104. There were 63 patients whose ECGs fulfilled criteria for LVH, 17 patients had ECG criteria for myocardial infarction and 10 patients had BBB, resulting in 14 patients (with pure Pardee T waves, resulting in a stand-alone incidence of the Pardee T wave of 15/1000 or 1.5%.

Of these 14 patients, 9 underwent cardiac catheterization. Six of these 9 patients had significant LAD lesions defined as > 50% obstruction, 2 patients had significant RCA lesions, and 1 patient's cath was entirely normal. However, this patient had a history of hypertension; thus, her chest pain and Pardee T wave may be explained on the basis of diastolic dysfunction due to ventricular hypertrophy. Of those patients who underwent noninvasive cardiac evaluation using thallium exercise treadmill testing or exercise echocardiography, 2 had abnormal tests. Of the normal tests, 2 had normal thallium studies and 1 had normal exercise echocardiography. Of importance, because 2 of these patients had systemic lupus erythematosus, they still may have had occult CAD. Thus, 71% or 10 of these 14 patients had significant CAD as determined by cardiac catheterization and exercise testing.

To update the incidence of the Pardee T wave at our hospital, we used a computer program which we developed called Program Optimizer that automatically accumulates the statistics on all ECG statements from electrocardiograms performed in our hospital. As shown below, from 9:31 a.m. February 11, 1991 to 6:57 a.m. May 26, 1992 we analyzed 47,918 ECGs.

PROGRAM OPTIMIZING MODULE
Harbor-UCLA Medical Center Modified Program: <890221.0908>
Criteria Version 50
FEB 11, 1991 9:31 AM TO MAY 26, 1992 6:57 AM
\# ECGS READ
TOTAL 47918

The program prints out in columns the correct statements, correct but modified, added by the physician, added and modified and deleted by the physician. This collection is done automatically and continuously during the ECG editing process.

					FALSE -				FALSE +	
	CORRECT		CORRECT BUT		ADDED BY		ADDED AND		DELETED BY	
STATEMENT	STATEMENT		MODIFIED		PHYSICIAN		MODIFIED		PHYSICIAN	
	#	%	#	%	#	%	#	%	#	%
ANTERIOR ST ELEV										
SEA021	1343	95.5	0	0.0	26	1.8	0	0.0	38	2.7
SEA02L	0	0.0	0	0.0	1	100.0	0	0.0	0	0.0
SEA11	177	94.7	0	0.0	7	3.7	0	0.0	3	1.6
SEA11L	33	94.3	0	0.0	1	2.9	0	0.0	1	2.9
SEA025	74	96.1	0	0.0	1	1.3	0	0.0	2	2.6
SEA23L	1	25.0	0	0.0	0	0.0	2	50.0	1	25.0
TOTAL	1628	95.0	0	0.0	36	2.0	2	0.0	45	3.0

The total number of Pardee T waves was 1,666 statements (the correct plus false negatives). The number of Pardee T wave statements (1,666) in the anterior leads divided by the total number of ECGs (47,918) results in an incidence of 35 per 1,000 or 3.5% of Pardee T waves in our general hospital population from February 11, 1991 to May 26, 1992. From the same time period, if the inferior waves (not shown) are added to the anterior lead Pardee T waves, the incidence increases to 5.2%. Consequently, the Pardee T wave is frequently found in a general hospital population and, as expected, was more frequent in the emergency department with an incidence of 15%, where patients have a higher incidence of chest pain. As a personal note, in our hospital we discover at least 2 new ECGs with the Pardee T wave every day!

Limitations of the Study: A limitation of this study is the small sample sizes in both the retrospective and prospective portions of the study. Although more data will be necessary to confirm the significance of this entity, the incidence of the Pardee T wave as a marker for CAD is probably higher since we excluded many Pardee T wave patients with high risk factors for CAD such as LVH, bundle branch block, older patients, hypertension, cerebrovascular disease and peripheral vascular disease. The 2 patients with systemic lupus erythematosus (SLE) probably had significant cardiac involvement in the form of myocarditis or coronary arteritis which may not be evident on exercise thallium, ECG or echocardiographic testing[3,4]. Thus, the incidence of heart disease in patients with Pardee T waves is probably greater than 70% and closer to 90%.

In conclusion, the Pardee T wave on the anterior leads of the ECG is a significant marker of CAD. The computerized ECG appears to be a valuable noninvasive technique to identify patients with Pardee T waves. At our hospital, because our house physicians have been made aware of the significance of the Pardee T wave, we have two expressions: "The patient with a Pardee T wave is not having a Party" and "Be specific and you will be terrific!" because a slight ST and T wave change can specifically diagnose ischemia using the Pardee T wave ECG criteria.

We owe a debt of gratitude to the insight of Dr. Harold Pardee for his description of the coronary T wave which he correctly stated has both diagnostic and prognostic significance in defining a group of patients with severe CAD. This landmark observation of Pardee was similar to that of Prinzmetal who also related the ECG changes to the post mortem heart. I was a high school student working in the laboratory when I observed with Mike Prinzmetal the patients at post mortem with normal coronary arteries who during life had marked ST segment elevations. Both Pardee's and Prinzmetal's observations were from simple pathologic and ECG correlations. I predict that the Pardee T wave will have the same impact on ECG diagnosis of ischemia as Prinzmetal's ST elevation has had on the diagnosis of coronary artery spasm. Thank you, Dr. de Padua, for giving me and our ISCE members the opportunity to present our current studies of the diagnostic value of the ECG in heart disease.

References

1. H.E.B. Pardee, Arch. Intern. Med. **26** (1920) 244.
2. M.M. Laks, M. Kraft, W.J. French, Computers in Cardiology **(1991)** 365.
3. N.E. Doherty and R.J. Siegel, Am. Heart J. **110** (1985) 1257.
4. C.J. Homcy, R.R. Liberthson, J.T. Fallon et al., Am. J. Cardiol. **49** (1982) 478.

ELECTROCARDIOLOGIC PATTERNS OF LEFT VENTRICULAR WALL MOTION ABNORMALITY IN ISCHEMIC HEART DISEASE

MÁLKOVÁ A.
Institute of Physiological Regulations, Czechoslovak Academy of Sciences, FN Bulovka, 180 85 Prague 8, CSFR

and

POLÁNKOVÁ M., DRŠKA Z., VALOVÁ D., JEBAVÝ P., NIEDERLE P., KALLMÜNZER B.
Institute of Physiological Regulations, Czechoslovak Academy of Sciences, FN Bulovka, 180 85 Prague 8, CSFR

ABSTRACT

New electrocardiologic features, derived from maps, characterizing left ventricular regional wall motion abnormality in ischemic heart disease were studied.

Mapping was performed in 60 patients with ischemic heart disease. Integral maps of Q wave and QRS and ST-T intervals were calculated. Isochronous maps of ventricular activation time and maps of Q wave asynchronous potential minima were determined. Left ventricular contraction abnormality detected by left ventricular angiography was evaluated by a point score and expressed as an index of asynergy. Number of coronary artery branches with significant narrowings was determined. Using quantitative parameters from maps multiple stepwise linear regression was performed.

Relationship between data from maps and index of asynergy corresponded to multiple correlation coefficient r=0.63 (p=0.01) in the whole group of patients, relationship between these parameters in the group of patients with present left ventricular contraction abnormality was expressed by r=0.82 (p=0.01).

Relationship between data from maps and number of coronary artery branches with significant stenosis corresponded to r=0.68 (p=0.01) in the group of patients with positive result of coronary angiography.

1. Introduction

The aim of this study was the next step of quantitative evaluation of body surface potential maps in patients with ischemic heart disease.[1]

Further we tried to judge the significance of studied electrocardiologic parameters by comparison with results of other diagnostic methods.

2. Methods

Mapping was performed using PC aided ECG diagnostic system Cardiag. Standard 12-lead electrocardiograms, vectorcardiograms using Frank lead system and matrix of 80 electrocardiograms for mapping were recorded simultaneously on sitting patient.[2]

A group of 60 patients with ischemic heart disease was investigated, 43 men and 17 women of mean age 51.2 years. 28 patients underwent Q myocardial infarction, 15 of them have had anterior and 13 posterior myocardial infarction. 19 patients underwent non Q myocardial infarction and 13 patients were treated for angina pectoris without history of myocardial infarction.

Integral maps of Q wave, QRS and ST-T interval were evaluated with the aim of measured data reduction with observation of their information contents. Isochronous maps of ventricular activation time and maps of Q wave asynchronous potential minima were determined.

Left ventricular angiography and coronary angiography were performed in all of patients. Regional wall motion of left ventricle was evaluated by a point score using these parameters: extent of asynergy determined in 10 segments of left ventricle, degree of asynergy evaluated by a 4 degree scale and index of asynergy expressed as a product of extent and degree of asynergy.[3]

Number of coronary artery branches with significant stenosis or occlusion was defined.

For the next step we tried to quantify the significance of coronary artery disease using an arbitrary defined index. Stenosis less than 50 % of artery diameter was evaluated by a half of point, stenosis equal or more than 50 % by 1 point, stenosis equal or more than 75 % by 2 points, 90 % stenosis by 3 points and occlusion by 4 points. The total individual index was calculated by points addition, for a single coronary branch only the most significant stenosis was considered.

Relationship of quantitative parameters from maps to parameters obtained by other diagnostic methods was studied using multiple stepwise linear regression.

3. Results

In the whole group of investigated persons relation between electrocardiologic patterns from maps and index of asynergy detected by left ventricular angiography was expressed by multiple correlation coefficient 0.63. In the group of patients with present left ventricular wall motion abnormality this relationship was expressed by coefficient 0.82 and in the group of patients with old Q myocardial infarction correlation coefficient was equal to 0.84. All multiple correlation coefficients were statistically significant on the level 0.01.

In the group of patients with old Q myocardial infarction significant relationship between map parameters and ejection fraction was proved (correlation coefficient 0.70).

In the whole group of investigated persons only open relationship of map data to number of significantly damaged coronary arteries was found out (multiple correlation coefficient 0.41). In the group with positive coronary angiography finding correlation coefficient 0.68 was obtained.

In the whole group of investigated persons open relation of map data to significance of coronary artery disease expressed by described index was discovered (correlation coefficient 0.54), that is supposed to be influenced by data of patients without significant coronary stenosis. In the group of persons with positive coronary angiography finding the correlation was expressed by coefficient 0.71. In the group of patients with old Q myocardial infarction and significant coronary stenosis the correlation coefficient was equal to 0.80.

For evaluation of relationship between map parameters and features of regional wall motion abnormality the most important patterns were: minimum potential value obtained from integral map of Q wave and minimum potential value from integral map of ST-T interval.

For estimation of significance of coronary artery damage the most important electrocardiologic parameters were: minimum potential values from integral maps from the first 30 or 40 ms of QRS, minimum potential value from QRS integral map and minimum potential value from integral map of 35 msec interval from the J point.

4. References

1. A. Málková, D. Valová, Z. Drška and M. Poláňková, in *Abstracts of XVII International Congress on Electrocardiology* (Florence, 1990) p. 153.
2. A. Málková, M. Poláňková, Z. Drška and D. Valová,

in *Electrocardiology 1991,* ed. J. Jagielski (World Scientific Publishing Co Pte Ltd, Singapore, 1992) in press.
3. A. Málková, D. Valová, Z. Drška and M. Polánková, in *Electrocardiology 1989,* ed. Z. Antaloczy (Elsevier Science Publishers B.V., Amsterdam, 1990) p. 149-152.

ECG OF ISCHEMIC HEART DISEASE IN THE THROMBOLYTIC ERA

X.Viñolas, X.García-Moll, J.García, J.Guindo, A.Bayés de Luna.
Hospital Sant Pau. Cardiology Department. Universitat Autonoma Barcelona.
Avda. San Antonio Mª Claret 167. 08025 Barcelona. Spain.

ABSTRACT

The most characteristics ECG signs of reperfusion include the reduction of the ST elevation, the appearence of accelerated idioventricular rhythm and premature ventricular contractions. Although they are markers of reperfusion their predictive value for patent coronary artery is low. Coronary angiography performed during acute or subacute phase of myocardial infarction has allowed us to better understand coronary anatomy responsible for the ECG changes during myocardial infarction. During an inferior myocardial infarction ST depression in right precordial leads ussually is due to a mirror image, but when ST depression is greater than 3 mm and persists after 6 hours, left anterior descending artery involvement must be suspected. When ↓ST V2/↑ST VF < 0.5 a right ventricular infarction must be suspected. Presence of ST depression in lead I suggests that the right coronary artery is involved and ST ascent in this lead suggests an involvement of the left circumflex. During anterior myocardial infarction, the presence of ST depression in inferior leads is usually observed in proximal lesions of a short left anterior descending coronary artery that does not wrap the apex. On the other hand ST elevation in these leads can be explained by an inferior ischemia caused by a long left anterior descending artery that wraps the apex, or in less cases due to the involvement of another artery (ischemia at a distance).

Electrocardiographic changes induced by thrombolytic therapy

The most characteristics electrocardiographic signs of thrombolysis include the reduction of the ST segment elevation and the appearance of acelerated idioventricular rhythm.

Using the surface electrocardiogram, the time course of ST elevation is considered to be a good non-invasive predictor for reperfusion, but not very specific[1]. During bipolar recording with Holter technique, sudden changes in the ST segment were found to be specific for reperfusion, but occured in only one-third of reperfused patients[2]. In the course of evolving myocardial infarction[3] patency of the infarct-related artery was associated with marked decrease in R and T waves in infarct leads, but less evident changes were found in presence of occluded artery. The differences in Q wave and ST segment between groups with occluded and patent infarction related artery were not statistically significant. Thus evident reduction in R and T waves during acute infarction may indicate infarct-related artery patency rather than infarct progression. The ST-segment changes recorded by serial VCG has been used to demonstrate succesful reperfusion[4].

In patients undergoing thrombolytic therapy accelerated idioventricular rhythms and/or single and repetitive premature ventricular contractions often occur, but they are not specific markers for reperfusion[5] The frequency of idioventricular rhythms was not related to any clinical variable, including maximal creatinine phosphokinase level, ST segment changes and type or number of disease vessels. Specificity improve markedly without a decrease in sensitivity when idioventricular rhythms occur frequently (>30 episodes/hour) or were observed for >3 consecutive hours[2]. In some series the incidence of runs of clinical ventricular tachycardia in reperfused patients is very high compared with non reperfused, and attains their maximum late after the beginning of thrombolysis[2]. There is no evidence that the two parameters (ST-changes and reperfusion-induced ventricular arrhythmias) predict each other. Despite all these findings, in the individual patient, the ST changes and reperfusion arrhythmias do not have high positive predictive value to accurately predict patency of the occluded artery. The most promising results seem to be obtained with dynamic QRS-ST vectorcardiographic monitoring[4].

There are also other electrocardiological characteristics in thrombolized patients: 1) the surface ECG using Silvester scoring Las more limitations to estimate infarction size[6] than in non thrombolized patients. 2) There is less incidence of malignant ventricular arrhythmias and markers of sudden death (PVC, late potentials, ejection fraction, heart rate variability) than in non thrombolyzed patients. What is most important, is that the prognostic value of these markers as predictors of sudden death is lower (except for heart rate variability) than in non-thrombolized patients[7]. Further large scale trials are needed to confirm these results.

Significance of the ST segment changes in reciprocal leads

From a clinical stand point, there are two basic zones of the heart affected by a myocardial infarction; inferoposterolateral zone (right coronary artery or circumflex coronary artery occlusion) and anteroseptal zone (left anterior descending coronary artery occlusion). The extension of infarct can be limited to one part of a zone (e.g. inferior wall), or extend to other part of the other zone (e.g. the anteroseptal zone + the inferior wall if the left anterior descending coronary artery wraps the apical area).

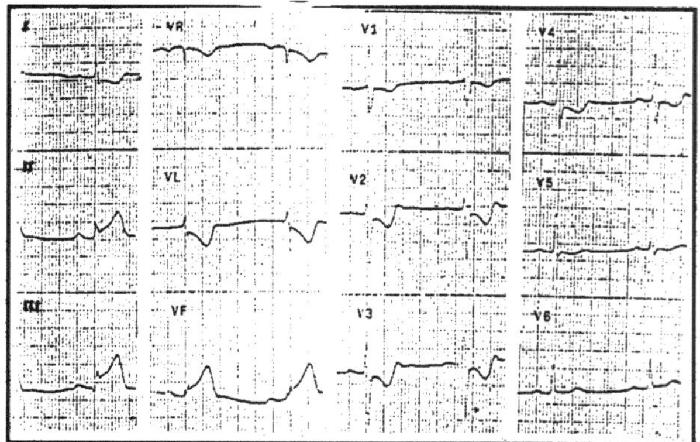

Figure 1.

The performance of coronary angiography during thrombolytic therapy in the acute phase of a myocardial infarction has made it easier to understand ECG-angiogram correlation . This information based on the elevation and depression of the ST segment on surface ECG provides an opportunity to assess myocardial infarction extension and predict the coronary artery occluded. A review of this correlation in the cases of acute infarction of inferior wall (ST ascent in leads II, III, VF) and anterior or anteroseptal wall (ST ascent in leads V1-2 to V3-4) is described in this section.

Acute inferior myocardial infarction (ST ascent in leads II, III, VF). 1 - Presence of evident ST segment depression in right precordial leads (fig 1). ST segment depression in the right precordial leads is observed in the 50-70% of patients with inferior myocardial infarction. It is usually the mirror image of the inferior ST elevation and is caused by inferoposterior or posterolateral ischemia. It is not usually caused by an occlusion of the left anterior descending coronary artery. When ST depression is greater than 3 mm and persists after 6 hours, this would make involvement of left anterior descending coronary artery more likely (ischemia at a distance). In conclusion depression of the ST segment is often seen in leads V_1-V_3 if there is a significant inferior myocardial infarction and is usually a mirror image of ascent of ST in leads II, III, VF.

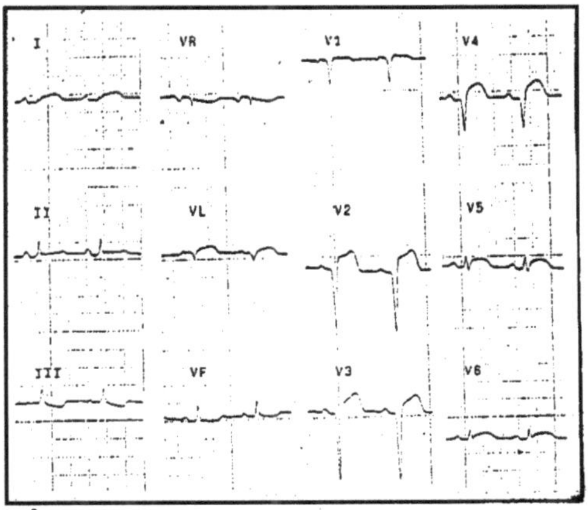

Figure 2.

2 - Presence of slight ST depression, normal ST, or elevated ST segment in right anterior precordial leads. Slight ST depression or normal ST in leads V_1-V_2 can be considered as a normal morphological pattern seen in small inferior myocardial infarction (1-2 mm ST elevation in leads II, III and VF). It does not have the same significance if important elevation of the ST segment in the inferior leads exists. In these cases when the descent of the ST segment in V1-2 is slight (↓ST V_2 / ↑STVF < 0.5) or if the ST segment is normal or elevated in leads V_1 - V_2, one should consider a right ventricular (RV) infarction[8]. The possibility of associated anterior infarction might be suspected only if a new Q wave is appearing in follow-up in precordial leads.

Therefore in patients with inferior myocardial infarction (ST elevation in leads II, III and VF) who have a slight ST descent or normal ST segment in V_2, right ventricular infarction should be considered and probably the artery occluded is the proximal right coronary artery. A significant ST depression in $V_{1\text{-}3}$ in association with inferior myocardial infarction is usually due to extension of inferior wall infarction to the posterior wall (inferoposterior involvement). In these patients, occlusion involves probably the distal right coronary artery or the left circumflex artery.

3 - Circumflex versus right coronary artery occlusion. Knowledge of the coronary artery involved in inferior myocardial infarction (right coronary or circumflex artery) can be predicted by lead I[9]. Presence of ST depression in this lead indicates that this lead faces the tail of the injury vector which points toward the injured zone (in this case right ventricle). Therefore the injured vector is directed to the right, (opposite to 0°, the place of positivity of lead I) and consequently a descent of ST will be seen in lead I. If this finding is seen the right coronary artery is usually the culprit vessel (fig 1). A normal or slight ascendent ST segment in lead I indicates that the injury vector is directed to the left towards 0° and suggests that the occlusion involves the left circumflex artery that is placed more in the left side. In this latter case a relatively tall R wave in V_1 is frequent, and is caused by associated posterior necrosis.

B) Acute anterior myocardial infarction (ST ascent in lead V1-2 to V3-4). 1. Presence of ST depression in leads II, III and VF (fig 2). This depression is the mirror image of an anterior myocardial infarction. It is more frequently observed in proximal lesions of a short left anterior descending coronary artery that does not wrap the apex[8]. There is therefore no concomitant inferior ischemia.

2. Normal or near normal ST or ST elevation in II, III and VF (fig 2). These morphologies can be explained by an inferior ischemia caused by a long left anterior descending coronary artery that wraps the apex, and induces ischemia of the inferior wall. Occasionally associated ischemia detected in inferior leads is due to a lesion involving other than anterior descending coronary artery (ischemia at a distance). In the hyperacute phase of myocardial infarction due to proximal occlusion of a long left anterior descending coronary artery, a pattern of ST depression in leads II, III and FV may be observed. Nevertheless this pattern disappears after 2-3 days when ST ascent in V_1-V_3 still persists.

We have described the most frequent ST changes, usually "ups and downs" of ST, that occur in the acute phase of infarction. A simultaneous ST segment ascent in both anterior and inferior leads, occurs specially when a great dominance of an artery exists (i.e. long descending anterior coronary artery that wraps the apex) or when an artery supplies blood to the myocardium of other area through collaterals.

REFERENCES

1.- Krucoff MW, Green CE, Satler LF et al. Non-Invasive detection of coronary artery patency using continous ST-segment monitorization. Am J Cardiol 1986;57:916-922.

2.- Zahender M, Utzolino S, Furtwängler A et al. Time course and interrelation of reperfused-induced ST changes and ventricular arrhythmias in acute myocardial infarction. Am J Cardiol 1991;68:1138-1142.

3.- Clements IP, Christian TF, Gibbons RJ. Serial electrocardiograms as indicators of patency of the infarct-related artery. JACC 1992;19:303A.

4.- Dellborg M, Topol EJ, Swedberg K. Dynamic QRS complex and ST segment vectocardiographic monitoring can identify vessel patency in patients with acute myocardial infarction treated with reperfusion therapy. Am Heart J 1991;122:943-948.

5.- Miller F, Krucoff M, Satler L et al. Ventricular arrhythmia during reperfusion. Am Heart J. 1986;112:928.

6.- Christian TF, Clements IP, Behrenbeck T et al. Limitations of the electrocardiogram in estimating infarction size after reperfusion therapy for myocardial infarction. Annals Int Med 1991;114:264-270.

7.- Farrell T, Bashir Y, Polionecki J et al. The effects of thrombolysis on risk stratification for arrhythmic events in post infarction patients. JACC 1991;17:17A.

8.- Lew AS, Laramee P, Shah PK et al. Ratio of ST segment depression in V2 to ST segment elevation in VF: An aid to early diagnosis of concomitant right ventricular involvement during inferior myocardial infarction. Am J Cardiol 1986;57:1047-1051.

9.- Bairey CN, Shah PK, Lew AS et al. Electrocardiographic differentiation of occlusion of the left circumflex vs. right coronary arteries as a cause of inferior myocardial infarction. Am J Cardiol 1987;60:456-459.

EXERCISE PERFORMANCE BY GENDER AND AGE IN MITRAL VALVE PROLAPSE SYNDROME

Silva E., Telles E., Esteves M., Almeida G., Lutucuta S., Duarte L., Sousa J., Vagueiro C. and Amram S.
S. Cardiologia, Hospital Santa Maria, Lisbon, Portugal

ABSTRACT

Exercise perfomance in patients with Mitral Valve Prolapse Syndrome (MVPS) is stillcontroverse. Fifty patients with MVPS were submitted to Exercise Stress Testing. Results were compared to that of the normal control group. Concerning to mean-exercise duration, heart rate and blood pressure evolution during the test, differences were found between the two populations more clearly in female. However, the stricking difference was the absense of the linear inverse correlation between age increasing and exercise duration in female with MVPS contrary to male MVPS and the normal people.

1. Introduction

There is general acceptance that patients (P) with MVPS have low exercise tolerance, but this has not been supported by large clinical trials. Also, women appear to have an improvement in symptoms with increasing age, contrary to men, but, to our knowledge, there are no studies supporting these data.

2. Material and Methods

Fifty P with MVPS from an out- patient clinic of an Universitary Hospital were studied: 18 male (mean-age 57.61 ± 10.35 years) and 32 female (mean-age 45.94 ± 8.21 years).

Patients were refered because of complaints from a symptomatologic complex, including: palpitations, atypical chest pain, exercise intolerance and dizziness.

Diagnosis of Mitral Valve Prolapse (MVP) was made by cardiac auscultation and both M-mode and two-dimensional echocardiography. Mitral Valve Prolapse Symdrome was considered when there was coexistence of MVP and one or more symptoms. Left ventricular function, both sistolic and diastolic, evaluated by two dimensional echocardiography and by radionuclide ventriculography, was normal in all the patients. Cardiac Doppler detected mild mitral regurgitation in 8 patients.

No one had other cardiac disease or sistemic illness.

A sex-and age-matched control group consisted of 36 normal subjects, 18 male (mean-age 56.0 ± 12.79 years) and 18 female (mean-age 46.06 ± 11.49 years).

There were no significant differences in exercise training between the two groups.

MULTILEVEL EXERCISE TESTING was performed by all the patients and the normal control group, on an upright bicycle ergometer. Nobody was under therapeutics for, at least, one week at the time of the test. A modified Astrand protocol was used, beginning at a workload of 30 Watts and charge increasing in 30 Watts every 3 min., at 60 rotations per minute.

3. Results

In the group of the MVPS exercise was stopped owing to physical exhaustion in 49 patients and because of non-sustained ventricular tachycardia in one patient whose rest electocardiogram was normal. No one had chest pain.

Rest ECG showed infrequent monomorphic ventricular premature beats in 11 P. Slight ST depression was present in 16 P, 14 in DII, DIII and aVF, and 2 P in V4-V5. There was no significant increase in the number of ventricular premature beats during exercise in 49 P. Ventricular repolarization abnormalities seen in the ECG of 16 P normalized in 11 and remained identical in 5. When rest ECG was normal (34 patients) there was no appearance of ST or T abnormalities with stress test.

In the control group, everyone stopped exercise owing to physical exhaustion. There were neither arrhythmias nor ventricular repolarization abnormalities in this group.

3.1. Mean Exercise Duration

In MVPS group, mean exercise duration was 7'23" ± 3.16 for total group. According to gender, it was 10'44" ± 2.36 for male and 5'30" ± 1.43 for female.

In control group, the total duration was 9'57" ± 3.15. For male it was 12'04" ± 2.57 and, for female, 7'50" ± 1.55.

The differences in mean exercise duration between the two groups were significant for the total group and for female ($p < 0.001$). Fig. 1.

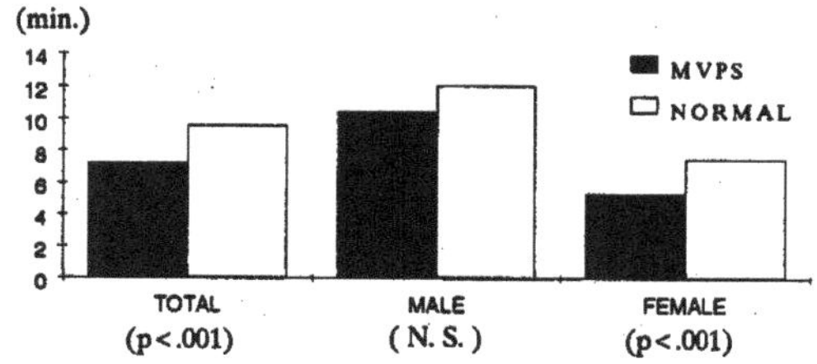

Fig. 1 - Mean Exercise Duration

Mean exercise duration was analized according to age increasing in both male and female. It was found a progressive decrease with increasing age in male with

MVPS and in the control group, but not in female with MVPS. Fig. 2, 3.

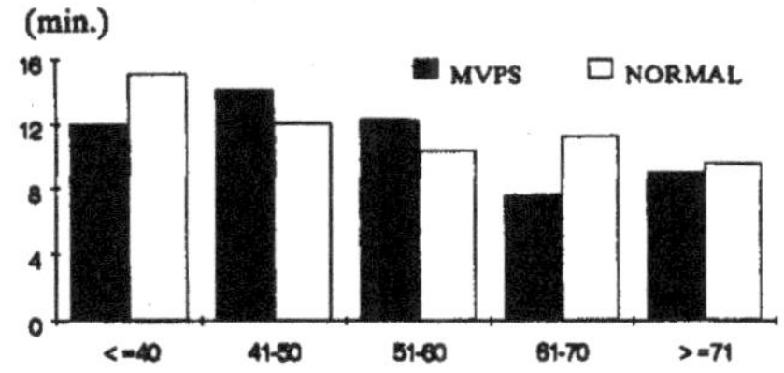

Fig. 2 - Exercise Duration - Male

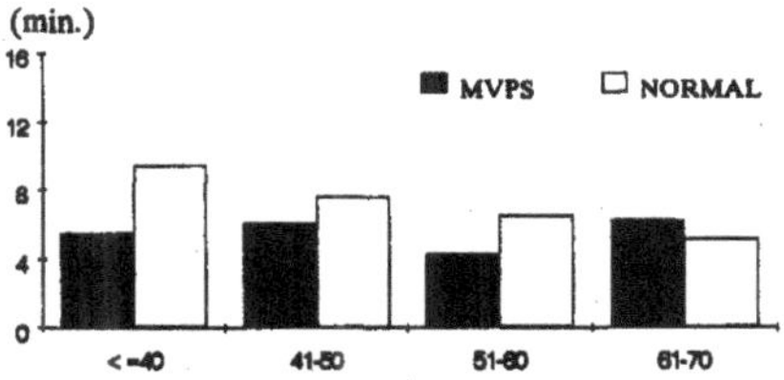

Fig. 3 - Exercise Duration - Female

3.2. *Heart Rate Evolution*

During exercise, heart rate was trendly but not significantly lower in the male MVPS than in the control group, being similar to the control in the female MVPS. During the recovery period it was persistently lower in the patients with MVPS, the difference being significant at 6 p<0.01 (male), p<0.001 (female). Fig. 4, 5.

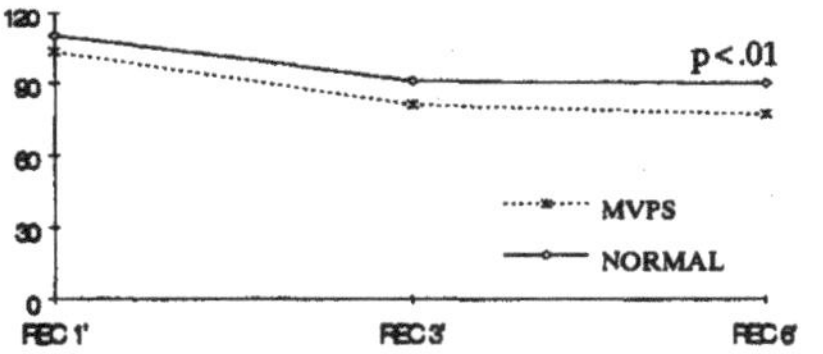

Fig. 4 - Heart Rate - Male

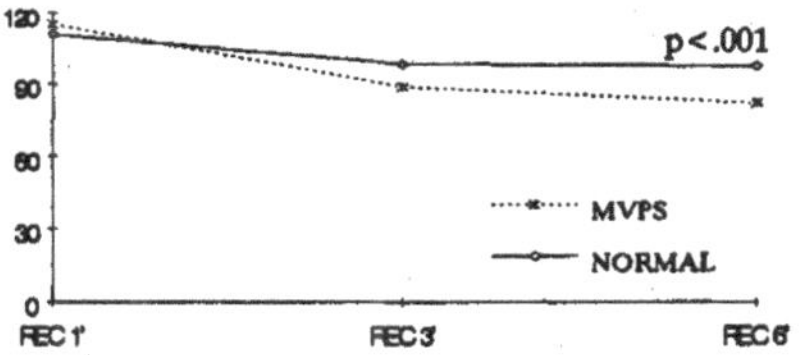

Fig. 5 - Heart Rate - Female

3.3. *Blood Pressure Evolution*

In male, sistolic and diastolic blood pressure had no significant differences between MVPS and the control group, except in the last stages achieved, when sistolic blood pressure was significantly lower in patients with MVPS (p<0.05). Fig. 6.

Female with MVPS had sistolic and diastolic blood pressure significantly lower, at all the stages, than did the female of the control group. Fig. 7.

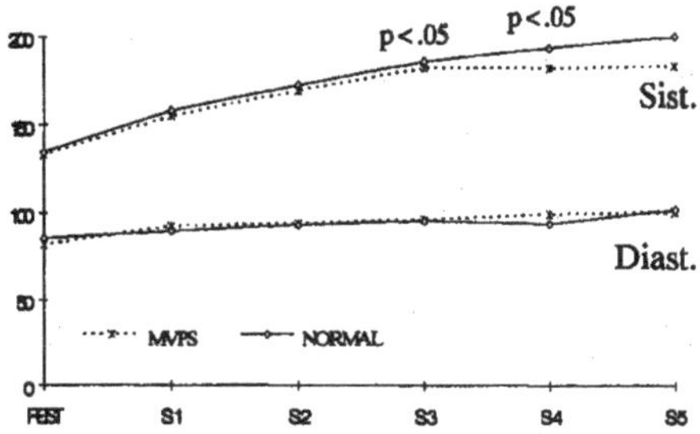

Fig. 6 - Blood Pressure - Male

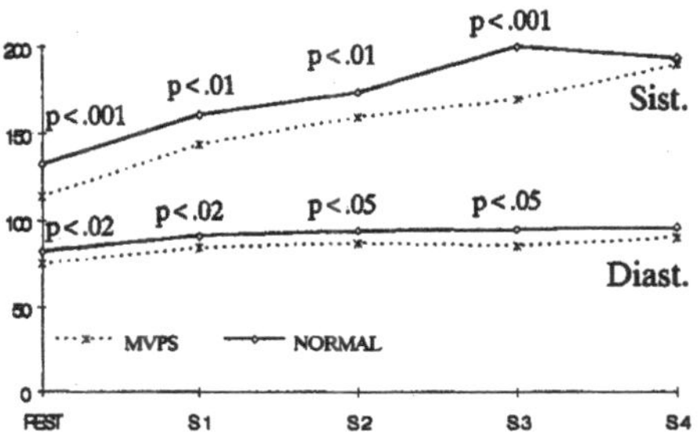

Fig. 7 - Blood Pressure - Female

4. Discussion

Our results are in agreement with that of other authors concerning to exercise tolerance, both exercise duration and maximal workload achieved, which are reduced in patients with MVPS when compared to age- and sex-matched normal control subjects. Patients with MVPS have a normal response to supine exercise but fail to increase end diastolic and stroke volume significantly during upright exercise. Impaired left ventricular preload is an important factor and inadequate venoconstriction may contribute for it. This fact could be related with some singularities found in the present study: blood pressure, both sistolic and diastolic, was significantly lower in female patients with MVPS than in the control group, although heart rate evolution was identical in the two populations. Also not described is the absence of diminution of exercise capacity with increasing age in women, contrary to men, which supports a better clinical course of MVPS in female. It can be postulated that the hormonal changes and weight gain frequent in older women, decrease the ventriculo-valvular disproportion with improvement of Mitral Valve Prolapse.

It remains to be explained the significant difference in heart rate between patients and the normal control group subjects, in the late recovery period, which did not exist in the pre-exercise period.

In conclusion, in the present study, female with Mitral Valve Prolapse Syndrome were a clearly identified sub-population when compared to men with MVPS and the control group.

5. Selected References

C. F. Wooley: The mitral valve prolapse syndrome, *Hosp. Pract.* JUNE, (1983) 163-74.

F. A. Gaffney, R. L. Huxley, P. Nicod et al.: Abnormal cardiovascular regulation in mitral valve prolapse symdrome (MVPS) during exercise, *Circulation* **64** Suppl 4 (1981) 248.

W. A. Pocock: Mitral leaflet billowing and prolapse, in *Perspectives* on the mitral valve, ed J. Barlow (F. A. Davis Co, Philadelphia, 1987).

M. B. Higginbotham, K. G. Morris, R. E. Coleman et al., Sex related differences in the normal cardiac response to upright exercise, *Circulation* **70** (1984) 357-66.

L. R. Poliner, G. J. Dehmer, S. E. Lewis et al. : Left ventricular perfomance in normal subjects: a comparision of the responses to exercise in the upright and supine positions, *Circulation* **62** (1980) 528-34.

ERGOMETRIC AND ANGIOGRAPHIC SIGNIFICANCE OF ST SEGMENT RECOVERY TIME DURING STRESS TESTING IN STABLE ANGINA

Ana Abreu, Rui Ferreira, Helder Pereira, Luis Valério, Henrique Nunes, José Serra, Mário Ferreira, J. M. Gonçalves, A. Mata Antunes

Serviço de Cardiologia, Hospital of Santa Marta, Lisboa, Portugal

Abstract

In order to evaluate the ergometric and angiographic significance of the ST segment depression recovery time, we studied 82 patients (P), 12 females and 70 males, mean age 58 +/- 11 years, who had a positive stress test for coronary artery disease and who also underwent coronary arteriography. Positive stress testing was defined as ST segment depression (>= 1 mm at 80 msec of Jpoint). Onset of ST segment depression (on ST), maxymal ST segment depression (max ST), recovery time of ST segment depression (rec ST), number of METS (METS), variation of double product (var DP), number of diseased coronary vessels (N cor ves), degree of coronary stenosis (% sten) and rest ejection fraction (EF), were evaluated. Two groups were defined based on rec ST: Group I, rec ST <= 3 min (62 P); Group II, rec ST > 3 min (20 P). Max ST was similar in the two groups. METS and var DP was greater in Group I but without statistical significance. On ST was earlier in Group II (3 vs 3.98 min; $p < 0.05$). There was no difference in EF or in the N cor ves, however the severity of coronary stenosis (% sten >= 90%) was greater in Group II ($p<0.001$). In conclusion, P with longer ST rec time had an earlier on ST and showed a tendency for achieving lesser number of METS and smaller Var DP. Also, despite no significant difference in the extension of coronary artery disease was found, these P had more severe coronary stenosis.

Introduction

Exercise testing has been used for long to provide the diagnosis of coronary artery disease (1-5). It is now fundamental to evaluate the use of electrocardiographic variables in predicting the severity of coronary artery disease.

Purpose

The purpose of our study was to evaluate the ergometric and angiographic significance of the ST segment depression recovery time.

Population

We studied retrospectively 82 consecutive patients (P), 12 females and 70 males, mean age 58+/-11 years old, with stable angina, who had a positive stress test for coronary artery disease and who were submitted to coronary arteriography. Myocardial infarction patients were excluded.

Methods

All patients performed treadmill stress testing, according to Bruce protocol. The following parameters were analised on ST segment depression (on ST), the maxymal ST segment depression (max ST, the recovery time of ST segment depression (rec ST), the number of METS (METS) and the variation of double product (var DP). Positive stress testing was defined as ST segment depression (>= 1mm at 80 msec of J point).
Coronary arteriography and contrast left ventriculography were performed. We evaluated the number of diseased coronary vessels (N cor ves), degree of coronary stenosis (% sten) and rest ejection fraction (EF). Seventy percent or greater coronary stenosis were considered significant.

Results

Regarding the stress testing, we defined two groups based on the recovery time of ST segment depression: Group I, with rec ST <= 3 min, including 62 P and Group II, with rec ST > 3 min, including 20 P. Our results were the following:

	Group I	Group II	p
Var DP	18482 +/- 37	17276 +/- 4254	0.13
METS	6.2 +/- 2.4	5.6 +/- 2.3	0.15
On ST	3.98 +/- 2.1	3.0 +/- 1.9	0.03
Max ST	1.89 +/- 0.9	1.8 +/- 0.68	0.3

METS, var DP and max ST, were greater in Group I, but without statistical significance. On ST was earlier in Group I (3 min vs 3.98; $p < 0.05$).
In respect to left ventriculography, 27 P had normal left ventricular systolic function (20 P in Group I and 7 P in Group II) and 55 P had depressed funtion.
There was no significant difference in the frequency of patients with abnormal function in Gsoup I and II (32% vs 35%, repesctively $p > 0.05$).
Coronary artery disease was distributed in single-vessel disease (Group I-17 P; Group II-4 P); double-vessel disease (Group I-12 P; Group II-4 P); and triple-vessel disease (Group I-12 P; Group II-4 P). There was no significant difference in the mean number of affected vessels in the two groups (1.7 vs 1.95, respectively; $p > 0.05$). The severity of coronary stenosis was defined as the percentual luminal reduction and patients were distributed as following:

Stenosis severity	<50%	50-70%	70-90%	>90%
Group I	10	20	25	7
Group II	0	3	7	10

Severe coronary lesions were significantly more frequent in Group II ($p < 0.001$).

Discussion

In our group of stable angina patients, we could identify by stress test, two subsets of patients with ST segment depression, one with earlier recovery after discontinuation of exercise, and another with late recovery (after 3 min). Not surprisingly, patients with longer recovery time had a significant earlier onset of ST segment depression and showed a tendency, although insignificant, for achieving fewer METS and a smaller double-product variation. Unespectedly, patients with earlier recovery had greater ST segment depression, although no significant.
Regarding coronary arteriography, some authors (6) have found a relation between late ST segment recovery and the prevalence of double and triple vessel disease. On the contrary, in the present study there was no significant difference in the number of vessels affected in the two groups, although the cutpoint for recovery time was at 3 and not at 8 minutes.
It is frequently thought that the earlier the ischemic changes appear, the later they persist in the postexercise phase and the more severe the coronary disease present. Patients with later recovery time had more severe coronary stenosis than those with earlier recovery, which is in accordance with some investigators (7). These authors in another study declared that despite prolonged ischaemic postexercise ST segment depression had been related to more severe coronary stenosis it had no prognostic implications (8).

Regarding rest left ventricular ejection fraction, this was similar in P with earlier and later recovery time, as in a previous study (7). We could speculate that if exercise ejection fraction had been determined, it might have been higher in P with earlier recovery time, however this remains to be determined.

Conclusion

In conclusion, patients with longer ST segment recovery time had an earlier onset of ST segment depression and showed a tendency for achieving lesser METS and a smaller variation of double-product. Also, despite no significant difference in the extension of coronary artery disease was found, these patients had more severe coronary artery stenosis.

References

1. GP **Robb**, HH **Marks**. *Postexercise electrocardiogram in arteriosclerotic heart disease: its value in diagnosis and prognosis.* JAMA, **200** (1967) 918.
2. TW **Mattinghy**. *The postexercise electrocardiogram: its value in the diagnosis and prognosis of coronary arterial disease.* Am J Cardiol, **9** (1962) 395.
3. RA **Bruce**, JR **McDonough**. *Stress testing in screening for cardiovascular disease. Bull NY Acad Med,* **45** (1969) 1288.
4. DR **Redwood**, SE **Epstein**. *Uses and limitations of stress testing in the evaluation of ischaemic heart disease.* Circulation, **46** (1972) 1115.
5. AA **Katus**. *Exercise electrocardiography recognition of the ischaemic response, false positive and negative patterns.* Am J Cardiol, **33** (1974) 721.
6. N. **Goldschlager**, A **Selzer**, K. **Cohm**. *Treadmill stress tests as indicators of presence and severity of coronary artery disease.* Annals of Internal Medicine, **85** (1976) 277.
7. JC **Kaski**, S **Gavrielidis**, G **DiBona**, A **Galassi**, G **Pupita**, F **Crea**, A **Maseri**. *Clinical significance of prolonged ST segment depression after exercise testing in chronic stable angina.* J Am Coll Cardiol, **15** (1990) 45-A.
8. JC **Kaski**, P **Mure**, P **Burton**, S **Gavrielidis**, D **Tousoulis**. *Prolonged ischaemic ST segment depression after exercise testing in patients with chronic stable angina is not associated with adverse prognosis.* Eur Heart J, **13** (1992) 116.

PROGNOSIS SIGNIFICANCE OF MYOCARDIAL ISCHEMIA DETECTED BY EARLY EXERCISE TESTING AFTER SUCCESSFUL CORONARY ANGIOPLASTY

H. Pereira, A. Abreu, L. Patrício, L. Branco, H. Nunes, M. Pitta, J. Quininha, J. Ramos, M. Ferreira, L. Figueiredo, J.M. Gonçalves.

Cardiology Sercice - Santa Marta Hospital
1100 Lisboa - Portugal

ABSTRACT

In order to assess the incidence and prognostic importance of silent and symptomatic myocardial ischemia detected after successful coronary angioplasty 59 patients were studied by early exercise testing. All patients were followed for an average of 18 months (4-37). During exercise 2 patients (3,4%) had chest pain without ST-segment change, 14 (23,7%) had abnormal exercise induced ST-segment depression (≥ 1 mm) without chest pain, 6 (10,2%) had both exercise - induced chest pain and ST-segment depression (group 1). Thirty-seven (62,7%) had a normal exercise test with no chest pain (group 2). The groups were similar in what refers to age, sex, history of previous myocardial infarction. Mutually exclusive cardiac events were class III angina and aditional revascularization. There were no cardiac deaths or nonfatal myocardial infarction during follow up. The rate of cardiac events in groups 1 and 2 were different (45,5% vs 10,8% p <0,001). In conclusion, we may say that exercise-induced myocardial ischemic episodes early after successful coronary angioplasty are predictive of an unfavorable prognosis.

Restenosis after successful percutaneous transluminal coronary balloon angioplasty (PTCA) occurs in 25-35% of patients within the first 6 months after the procedure[1]. This study was aimed to evaluate the prognostic significance of chest pain and ST changes by early treadmill exercise testing after successful PTCA.

METHODS

The study group consisted of 59 patients (pt), 48 men and 11 women, aged 54,2 years (27-76), who underwent successful elective percutaneous transluminal coronary angioplasty (PTCA). All pt had a positive exercise test for myocardial ischemia before angioplasty. They were followed during a mean period of 18 months (4-37). Twenty one patients had a previous myocardial infarction. Patients were divided in 2 groups according to the results of the exercise test. Group 1 consisted of 22 pt (37,3%) with abnormal exercise test: 14 pt (23,7%) who had exercice-induced ST-segment depression ≥1 mm without chest pain, 2pt (3,4%) who had exercice-induced chest pain without ST-segment changes and 6 pt (10,2%) who had both chest pain and abnormal ST-segment response. Group 2 consisted of the remainder 37 pt (62,7%) who had neither ST-segment changes nor angina during the exercise test. Age, sex and the frequency of prior myocardial infarction were similar in the two groups.

Exercise Testing: a symptom limited exercise test was performed using the Bruce protocol at an average of 6 days after PTCA (maximum 10 days).

At the time of the test, 88% pt were receiving calcium antagonists, 10% were taking ß-blockers and 37% long-acting nitrate theraphy. Beta-adrenergic blocking agents were stopped 72h before the test. Abnormal exercise electrocardiogram was defined by horizontal or downsloping ST-segment depression ≥ 1 mm measured at 80 ms after the J point.

Coronary Angiography and Angioplasty: selective coronary arteriography was performed by Judkins technique. Ninety-two percent of the patients had 1-vessel disease and 8% had 2-vessel disease. Successful PTCA was defined as dilatation of all attempted lesions by > 30% and achievement of < 50% average diameter narrowing without in-hospital complications (acute myocardial infarction, need for coronary bypass grafting or death).

Follow-up: all patients were followed for an average of 18 months (range 4 to 33) months by clinic visit. Cardiac events were classified as death, nonfatal myocardial infarction, need for an additional revascularization (including coronary by-pass revascularization or repeat PTCA) and recurrent angina (Class III C.C.S.).

RESULTS

Exercise test: the maximum exercice workload achieved by pt in group 2 was significantly greater than group 1 (9,5 min vs 6,7 min, respectively; p < 0,05). Both groups attained similar maximum heart rate and systolic blood pressure.

Prognosis: the incidence of cardiac events in group 2, 10,8%, was significantly lower than in group 1, 45,5% (p< 0,001).

Figure 1 shows higher cardiac event rate in group 1 compared with group 2. There were no cardiac deaths or nonfatal myocardial infarction in both groups.

Comparing the subsets of abnormal stress testing with the normal group we found out the occurrence of cardiac events in 5 of the 6 pt with chest pain and ST changes (83,3% vs 10,8%; p< 0,0005). On the contrary, in the silent ischemia subset (14 pt) the frequency of events was not significantly different from the normal group (35,7% vs 10,8%; NS).

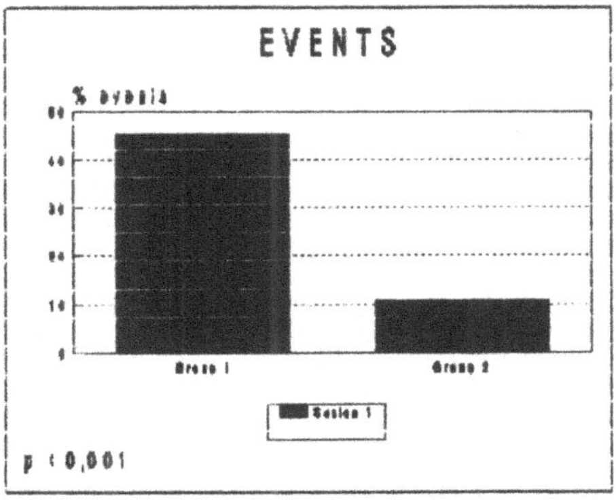

Figure 1

DISCUSSION

Restenosis after successful PTCA occurs in 25-35% of patients within the first six months after the procedure[1]. Early treadmill exercise is frequently performed during the first month after PTCA to assess the result of the revascularization procedure and to assess future changes in exercise test. Our study shows that patients with abnormal test were later found to have cardiac events, in particular in patients with chest pain and ECG changes.

The results of our study are consistent with those of Tamini et al[1] who found that an early positive test correlates with future restenosis, whose process begins as early as 3 days after PTCA. As a possible pathophysiologic mechanism they hypothetised that early positive testing could partly be due to vasoconstriction[2,3] resulting from the vessel wall damage leading to platelet adhesion and aggregation with release of vasoconstriction substances[4,5]. In our study silent ischemia was not predictive of unfavorable prognosis, in spite of the reports by others investigators[6] were symptomatic and silent ischemia induced by early treadmill exercise were predictive of cardiac events, particularly in patients with multivessel disease and incomplete revascularization[6,7]. In the present study only 8% of the pt had multivessel disease and the revascularization was always considered complete.

Thallium-201 scintigraphy has been used to stratifie subsets at high and low risck for late restenosis, however the ideal timing for its performance remains controvercial[8,9,10].

REFERENCES

1. W. McBride, R. Lange, L. Hillis. Restenosis after successful coronary angioplasty. *N Engl J Med* 1988;318:1734-7

2. H. El-Tamimi, G. Davies, D. Hackett, G. Fragasso, F. Crea, A. Maseri. Very early prediction of restenosis after successful coronary angioplasty: anatomic and functional assessment. *JACC* 1990;15:259-64

3. T. Fischel, G. Derby, T. Tse, M. Stadius. Coronary artery vasoconstriction routinely occurs after percutaneous transluminal coronary angioplasty. *Circulation* 1988;78:1323-34

4. D. Faxon, T. Sanborn, C. Haudenschild. Mechanism of angioplasty and its relation to restenosis. *Am J Cardiol* 1987;60:5B-9B

5. J. Lamb, J. Chesebro, L. Badimon, V. Fuster. Serotonin and thromboxane A2 receptor blockade decrease vasocontriction but not platelet deposition after deep arterial injury (abst). *Circulation* 1986;74(suppl II):II-97

6. U. Deligonul, M. Vandormael, L. Younis, B. Chaitman. Prognostic significance of silent myocardial ischemia by early treadmill exercice after coronary angioplasty. *Am J Cardiol* 1989;64:1-5

7. U. Deligonul, M. Vandermael, Y. Shah, K. Galan, M. Kern, B. Chaitman. Prognostic value of early exercice stress testing after successful coronary angioplasty: Importance of the degree of revascularization. *Am Heart J* 1989;117:509-514

8. R. Hardoff, A. Shefer, S. Gips, A. Merdler, M. Flugelman, D. Halon, B. Lewis. Predicting late restenosis after coronary angioplasty by very early (12 to 24 h) Thallium-201 scintigraphy: Implications with regard to mechanisms of late coronary restenosis. *JACC* 1990;15:1486-92

9. H. Hecht, R. Shaw, H. Chin, C. Ryan, S. Stertzer, R. Myler. Silent ischemia after coronary angioplasty: Evaluation of restenosis and extent of ischemia in asymptomatic patients by tomographic Thallium-201 exercice imaging and comparison with symptomatic patients. *JACC* 1991;17:670-7

10. W. Breisblatt, F. Weiland, L. Spaccavento. Stress Thallium-201 imaging after coronary angioplasty predicts restenisis and recurrent symptoms. *J Am Coll Cardiol* 1988;12:1199-1204

QRS DURATION AS A MARKER OF ISCHEMIC BURDEN AFTER MYOCARDIAL INFARCTION

Pedro Abreu, Marisa Trabulo, António Ventosa,
Victor Gil, N.Lobo da Costa, R.Seabra-Gomes

Department of Cardiology - Santa Cruz Hospital
Carnaxide - Portugal

1.Introduction

QRS score defined either by amplitude, duration or ratio of the electrocardiographic waves has been established for the evaluation of the myocardial infarction size and related residual left ventricular function[1-5]. Thallium 201 scintigraphy, has also been used to improve that relation in patients surviving myocardial infarction[6].

Improvement of diagnostic ability in detection of residual ischemia by reinjection of Thallium 201 after myocardial infarction, has been suggested, and this technique could also help us in defining which segments a well succeded revascularization could contribute for a recovery of ventricular function[7].

It is accepted that when we compare Thallium reinjection with redistribution, we can obtain an improvement of about 30%, in diagnosis of viable myocardium[8,9].

The question we would like to answer is if there is any chance for the diagnosis of myocardium viability using an easy and fast analysis of the electrocardiogram in patients after myocardial infarction.

2.Main purpose

The main purpose of this study was to relate QRS duration, with the extent of myocardial perfusion defects, evaluated by stress and reinjection Thallium 201 scintigraphy.

3.Study population, material and methods

For this, 32 patients, 29 males and 3 females, with a mean age of 51.5 +/- 11.1 years have been studied.

All the patients had previous myocardial infarction, anterior in 18 patients, inferior in 11, lateral in one and combined (anterior plus inferior) in 2 patients.

QRS was mesured manually, in Q wave myocardial infarction in the Q wave longest duration lead, and in non-Q wave myocardial infarction in the QRS longest duration lead. All patients with bundle branch block were excluded.

Concerning QRS duration, patients were divided in two groups: A, with QRS greater than 80 msec. (10 patients), and B, with QRS lesser or equal to 80 msec. (22 patients).

There were no differences between the two groups related to age, sex, previous angina or stress testing parameters.

On Thallium 201 scintigraphy, myocardial perfusion was assessed semi-quantitatively, after stress and after reinjection, and the myocardium was divided into five segments - septal, anterior, lateral, inferior and apical. Afterwards, a perfusion score was cálculated for each segment, ranging from zero (no perfusion) to four (normal perfusion), resulting in a global score of one to twenty.

4.Results

1) When QRS had a normal duration, 19 patients had a perfusion score equal or greater than 11 points, and there were only 3 patients with a perfusion score lesser than 11 points; 2) on the other hand, in the 10 patients with an enlarged QRS, 7 had a perfusion score lesser than 11, and only 3 patients had a score equal or greater than this value ($p<0.01$).

This difference was enhanced when perfusion score was calculated with reinjection. 3) the reinjection allows a reduction of the perfusion score to 10 points; 4) the number of patients with an enlarged QRS, and perfusion score lesser than 10 points, was 7, while in group B, only one of the 22 patients had normal QRS duration and perfusion score lesser than 10 points ($p<0.001$).

Results concerning myocardial infarction site, show statistically significant differences only in the anterior infarction group. Therefore, after stress, in group A (enlarged QRS), there were 11 patients with perfusion score lesser than 11 points, and only 2 patients with score equal or greater than 11, against the group with normal QRS duration (group B), where only one patient had perfusion score equal or greater than 11 ($p<0.01$). Also in this group, reinjection allows diminishing the calculated perfusion score to 10 points. Although there were similar results in enlarged QRS group, there were almost no patients with a perfusion score lesser than 10 (1 versus 12 patients, $p<0.001$).

5.Discussion

It has been possible to relate QRS score with myocardial infarction size, evaluated by CK level, and with residual left ventricular function after myocardial infarction[5]. On the other hand, it has been accepted that these relations were more clear for anterior myocardial infarction, when compared with other localizations[2,3]. Nevertheless, presence of Q waves in the ECG (necrosis waves) seems to have no clear relation with the absence of myocardial viability at this segments, as has been shown in a study with the positron emission tomography (PET)[10].

Recent studies show a great similarity of results in detection of viability when PET is compared with reinjection Thallium 201 scintigraphy[11].

Our study, by a simple analysis of the electrocardiogram, give us some interesting data. By the QRS duration, we can make an approach to myocardium viability in patients with previous myocardial necrosis.

We think that the explanation for this phenomena, particulary in anterior myocardial infarction, relates to a greater amount of myocardium assessed by Thallium 201 scintigraphy, corresponding to the left anterior descending artery, almost always the anterior myocardial infarction related artery.

6.Conclusions

These results suggest that by a simple and easy analysis of the ECG, an enlargement of the QRS greater than 80 msec, in the absence of bundle branch block, could be a marker of ischemic burden, evaluated by reinjection of the Thallium, after anterior myocardial infarction.

7.Bibliography

1.G.S.Wagner, C.J.Frye, S.T.Palmeri, S.F.Roark, N.C.Stack, R.E.Ideker, F.E.Harrel, R.H.Selvester. Circulation **65** (1982) 342.

2.S.F.Roark, R.E.Ideker, G.S.Wagner et al. Am J Cardiol **51** (1983) 382.

3.R.E.Ideker, G.S.Wagner, W.K.Roth, D.R.Alonso, S.P.Bishop, C.M.Bloor, J.T.Fallon, G.J.Gottlieb, D.B.Hackel, H.R.Phillips, K.A.Reimer, S.F.Roark, W.J.Rogers, R.M.Savage, R.O.White, R.Selvester. Am J Cardiol **49** (1982) 1604.
4.S.T.Palmeri, D.G.Harrison, F.R.Cobb, K.J.Morris, F.E.Harrel, R.E.Ideker, R.H.Selvester. N Engl J Med **306** (1982) 4.
5.H.J.Eisen, B.Barzilai, A.S.Jaffe, E.M.Geltman. Am Heart J **115** (1988) 993
6.N.L.DePace, A.Hakki, A.S.Iskandrian. Am Heart J **107** (1984) 1210.
7.H.Ohtani, N.Tamaki, Y.Yonekura, I.Mohiuddin, K.Hirata, T.Ban, J.Konishi. Am J Cardiol **66** (1990) 394.
8.D Kayden, S Sigal, R.Soufer, J.Mattera, B.Zaret, F.Wackers. J Am Coll Cardiol **18** (1991) 1480.
9.V.Dilsizian, T.Rocco, N.Freedman, M. Leon, R.Bonow. N Engl J Med **323** 3 (1990) 141.
10.R.Brunken, J.Tillisch, M.Schwaiger, J.Child, R.Marshall, M.Mandelkern, M.E.Phelps, H. Schelbert. Circulation **73** (1986) 951.
11.R.Bonow, V.Disizian, A.Cuocolo, S.L.Bacharach. Circulation **83** (1991) 26.

ELECTROCARDIOGRAPHIC DIAGNOSIS OF ISOLATED CIRCUMFLEX CORONARY ARTERY DISEASE: RELATION BETWEEN CHANGES DURING EXERCISE TEST AND CORONARY ANGIOPLASTY

Pedro Abreu, José Baptista, Teresa Real, R.Seabra-Gomes

Department of Cardiology - Santa Cruz Hospital
Carnaxide - Portugal

1.Introduction

The diagnosis of circumflex (CX) coronary artery related myocardial infarction seems to be a very difficult using the acute phase ECG analysis[1,2]. The great variability of this ECG changes could be related to anatomic localization of CX, but also with its phisiologycal behavior[3]. Coronary angioplasty (PTCA), with transient occlusion of the coronary flow, could be an interesting model to evaluate ECG changes during acute phase of myocardial infarction[4-6].

It is recognized the lower diagnostic ability of the exercise test analysis when one vessel disease is concerned[7-9]. Also whenever thre is a positive exercise test, the ST changes appear related to the same leads, independently of the involved vessel.

2.Main purpose

The main purpose of this study was to evaluate and relate the ECG changes during exercise test and PTCA, in patients with isolated CX coronary disease.

3.Study population, material and methods

Of the patients submited to PTCA in our Hospital where selected those with isolated CX coronary disease, who has been submited previoulsly to exercise test.

There were 28 patients, 25 males and 3 females, with mean age of 51+/-10 years.

ECG changes were defined whenever there were ST deviation equal or greater than 1 mm (80 msec. after J point). During exercise test and PTCA, all the patients had continuos electrocardiographic recording in the 12 classic leads.

It were also analysed the previous clinical and angiographyc profile, such as myocardial infarction (defined by ECG criteria, by the presence of Q waves), PTCA site, vessel patency and coronary circulation dominance.

Of the 28 patients, 13 had previous myocardial infarction evidence (1 antero-septal, 7 inferior and 5 lateral). Concerning angiographyc caracthreristics, PTCA was performed in proximal CX in 7 patients (the vessel was occluded in 2), in distal CX in 13 patients, with 4 occlusions, in obtuse marginals (OMs) in 6 patients (in 2, the vessel was occluded), and lastly in a combination of CX and OMs in 2 patients, both with occluded vessels. Coronary circulation was considered as rigth dominance in 21 patients and left in 4 patients.

4.Results

Nineteen patients had electrocardiographic changes during the PTCA, and 26 patients during stress test, but of these only 6 patients (+/-20%) had similar ECG changes.

Leads V4-6, were the most frequently involved during both PTCA and exercise test.

When PTCA was concerned, inferior leads and aVL were also important. In the exercise test, V2-3 and inferior leads, were the most frequently involved, after V2-4.

No electrocardiographic changes were seen in lead D-I.

The involvement of V4-6 leads, were more frequent in exercise test (23 patients - 82%) being ST elevation in 9% and ST depression in 91% - $p<0.001$. In PTCA 16 patients (57%) had ECG changes in these leads, with similar distribution of ST changes.

With regard to V2-3 leads, there were changes in 10 and 4 patients in the exercise test and PTCA respectively. In the exercise test, ST was always depressed. During PTCA one patient had ST elevation.

If we analysed the inferior leads, ECG changes were more frequent during PTCA (11 patients - 40%), being in 73% ST elevation, against only 5 patients in the exercise test, 4 of which with ST depression.

Concerning lead aVL, there were ECG changes in 9 patients, 6 of them during PTCA, and the remaining during exercise test. All of them had ST depression.

The relations of electrocardiographic changes with clinical parameters and angiographyc data, evidence that the PTCA site and the fact of the vessel being previously occluded, was related to less frequent electrocardiographic changes during both, PTCA and exercise test.

5.Discussion

As we have seen in a previous study, there is a great variability in electrocardiographic changes that occur during the isolated CX artery angioplasty[6].

This phenomena also occurs when there is a CX infarction. Several causes have been advanced to explain this fact, but the anatomic localization at the artery is the most accepted[3].

In this study the relation between changes during PTCA and during exercise test, give us some interesting data. First, the low percentage of similarity between both situations, not so much because of their localization, but specialy because of differences in ST changes.

Possibly that fact, reflects the difference between abrupt coronary flow interruption, that mimics myocardial infarction, and a progressive reduction in coronary flow that enables the progressive adaptation of the myocardium to the changes in coronary flow, frequently seen during the exercise test[10].

Also the localization of the involved vessel is not coincidental.

The exercise test is not the best way to evaluate the localization of the involved vessel, because most of the time, ST changes are seen in left precordial and inferior leads[7-9].

Nevertheless we want to reinforce the importance of lead D-I to evaluate CX coronary artery disease, because also in the exercise test we couln't find any change in that lead.

6.Conclusions

The authors underline the great impredictability of the electrocardiographic changes when circumflex coronary artery is involved, and the low similarity of those changes when using two different methods such as exercise test and coronary angioplasty.

This shows the dificulty in diagnosing circumflex coronary artery disease. Nevertheless it is important to notice that there are no praticaly changes in lead D-I, and that this fact can be important to the diagnosis.

7. Bibliography

1. R.M.Fuchs, S.C.Achuff, B.A.Grunwald, F.P.Yin, L.C.Griffith. Circulation **66** (1982) 1168.
2. C.N.Bairey, P.K.Shah, A.S.Lew, S.Hulse. Am J Cardiol **60** (1987) 456.
3. B.L.Huey, G.A.Beller, D.L.Kaiser, R.S.Gibson. J Am Coll Cardiol **12** (1988) 456
4. N.B.Wagner, D.C.Sevilla, M.W.Krucoff, K.S.Peiper, K.L.Lee, R.D.White, K.M.Kent, R.Renzi, R.W.Selvester, G.Wagner. Am J Cardiol **63** (1989) 1208.
5. M.Dellborg, H.Emanuelsson, M.Riha, K.Sweedberg. Coronary Artery Disease **2** (1991) 43.
6. P.Abreu, J.Baptista, T.Real, R.Seabra-Gomes. 10 (1992) **16** XIX Congress on Electrocardiology (abstract book)
7. M.H.Ellestad. Stress Testing. Principles and practice (Philadelphia, F.A.Davis Co, 1986) 316
8. D.A.Weiner, C.H.Mc Cabe, T.J.Ryan. Am J Cardiol **46** (1980) 21
9. V.Gil, A.Ventosa, R.Seabra-Gomes. **31** (1991) XVIII Congress on Electrocardiology (abstract book).
10. K.L.Gould, G.W.Hamilton, K.Lipscomb, J.L.Ritchie, J.W.Kennedy. Am J Cardiol **34** (1974) 557.

ACCURACY OF DETECTION OF MYOCARDIAL SCARS IN CORONARY HEART DISEASE (CHD) BY ECG, VCG AND ANGIOGRAPHY IN PATIENTS WITH MULTIPLE VESSEL DISEASE

Jahnel, J.
Medical Clinic, Department of Cardiology, University of Münster, Germany

and

Reckers, U. and Brisse, B.
Medical Clinic, Department of Cardiology, University of Münster, Germany

Patients with two- or three-vessel disease show a high incidence of typical, abnormal electrocardiographic signs. In order to evaluate the additional clinical value of vectorcardiographic data of these patients, we analysed registrations of 110 patients (8 females, 102 males, mean age 54 years) with angiographic evidence of predominantly proximal stenosis (≥ 50 %) of the RCA, RCX and RIVA.
The contraction analysis of laevocardiogramms was performed in RAO-position by 16 hemiaxial and radial diameters method. Myocardial contraction patterns were compared with results from 26 patients without wall-motion abnormalities and without CHD.
68 % (69 %) of patients with two- (three-)-vessel disease showed contraction abnormalities, 70 % (68 %) ECG potential defects and 100 % (97 %) VCG myocardial scars.

We concluded that VCG has a higher sensitivity in detection of myocardial scars than ECG. VCG is a useful, additional, non-invasive method for diagnosing myocardial defects in CHD.

1. Aim of the study

Generally it is no problem to diagnose acute myocardial infarction, many authors have shown the relations between ECG-changes and infarct localisation[1]. While some classical infarction patterns correspondend to ECG-criteria others do not.
If patients have the typical symptoms of angina pectoris without any changes in 12-lead-ECG or during exercise-ECG, it is much more difficult to diagnose coronary heart disease.

Likewise it is possible not to recognize silent myocardial infarction in the ECG. VCG differs from ECG only in the method of display of the electrical field generated by the heart. While the ECG reflects the changes in time and amplitude best, the VCG adds the important dimension of recognition of direction in time. It has been suggested that VCG is particularly useful in detection of myocardial infarction. Exact determination of myocardial infarction is only possible by angiography, but as a non-invasive method VCG might be superior to ECG[2,3].

We performed a retrospective clinical study on 110 patients with angiographic evidence of predominantly proximal stenosis of two or three vessels in order to evaluate the additional clinical value of vector-cardiographic data.

These patients underwent ECG and VCG and cardiac catheterisation with left ventriculography.

Patients were excluded if one of the following conditions was present: permanent arrhythmias, bundel branch block, hypertrophy, acute myocardial infarction, heart failure, large left ventricular aneurysmas.

The group with angiographic evidence of two-vessel disease included 41 patients, 3 females and 38 males, mean age 55 years.

The group with angiographic evidence of three-vessel disease consisted of 69 patients, 5 females and 64 males, mean age 54 years.

The control-group was composed of 26 patients, 12 females and 14 males, mean age 47 years, without angiographic changes.

2. Methods

Ventriculography was recorded in RAO position.

Coronarangiography was performed using Judkins technique. A computer analysis was performed according to contractions abnormalities (akinesia, dyskinesia and hypokinesia)[4].

The length-axis of the heart was divided into three equidistant areas, 16 perpendicular axes were chosen for analysing the heart contraction in the anterior-septal and the posterior-dorsal region.

Coronary artery stenosis was determined $\geq$ 50 % for the following arteries:

left anterior descending, left circumflex and right coronary artery.

Standard 12-lead-ECG was recorded and manual measurements were made from the Q and R wave[4].

The vectorcardiogramms were recorded (using the FRANK lead system) with an oscilloscope and a camera.
VCGs were recorded with 500 Hz either as a continuous loop or interrupted every 2 msec.
The following parameters were measured:
- amplitude of the 10-msec-vector and the 15-msec-vector
- maximal QRS magnitude[5].

3. Results

In two and three vessel disease proximal stenosis (71 and 61 %) predominated. Distal stenosis occurred less frequently (21 and 26 %). High graded stenosis of > 70 % exceeded moderate stenosis in 81 and 89 % of our cases.
The contraction analysis demonstrated significantly more wall-motion abnormalities by the radial method (73 and 96 %) than by hemiaxial method (21 and 25 %).

Patients with two vessel disease had evidence of myocardial scars in the inferior and dorsal region evaluated by ECG in 29 % and by VCG in 12 % of our cases. Combined defects were detected in 5 % with ECG and in 34 % with VCG (fig 1).

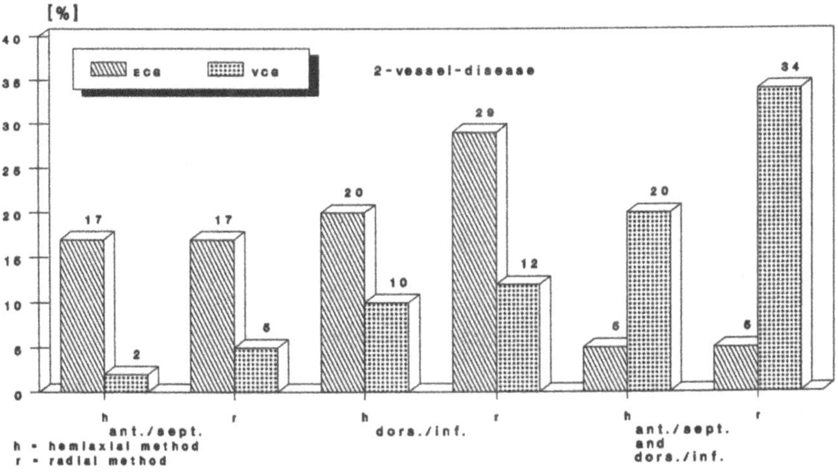

fig 1: wall-motion-abnormalities (a-, dys- and hypokinesie) and ECG- or (VCG) scars

The results of patients with three vessel disease demonstrated the superiority of VCG-methods especially in detection of myocardial scars in combined regions (fig 2).

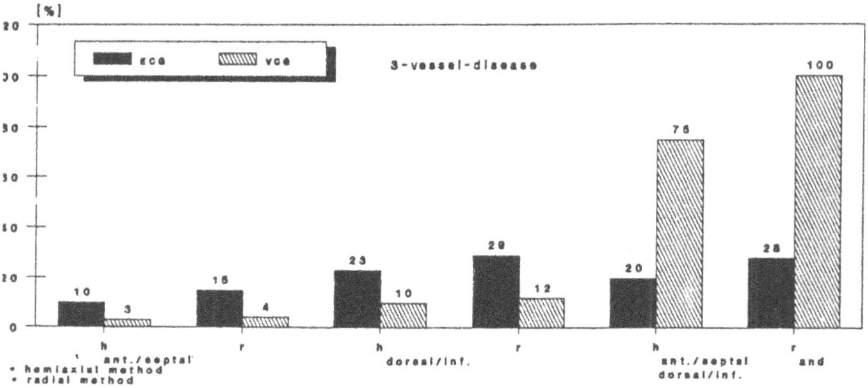

fig 2: wall-motion-abnormalities (a-, dys- and hypokinesie) and ECG- (or VCG) scars

4. Conclusions

The detection frequency of myocardial scars in two and three vessel disease varies for ECG, VCG and wall-motion analysis. In anterior and septal infarction the three methods are comparable.

For the posterior region and combined defects VCG is superior. The addition of VCG to none-invasive screening methods may lead to an earlier and more precise detection of CHD in dorsal and multiple vessel disease.

References

1. N. Treese, R. Erbel, T. Pop and J. Meyer, *Dtsch.med.Wschr.* **117** (1992), 789-794
2. E. Braunwald, *Heart disease* (2. edition, W.B. Saunders Company, Philadelphia, 1984), 205-232
3. H. Portheine, R. Wenger (ed.), *Aktuelle Probleme der Vektorkardiographie* (Georg Thieme, Stuttgart, 1968) 216-225
4. H. Roskamm, H. Reindell, *Herzkrankheiten* (Springer, Berlin, 1989), 195-218 and 329-366.
5. P.R. Lichtlen, *Klinische Vektorkardiographie* (Springer, Berlin, 1969), 9-119.

INDIVIDUAL DIFFERENCES IN THE CONTROL OF HEART RATE DURING EXERCISE

D. ROMBERG E. SCHUBERT
Institute of Physiology, Humboldt-University,
Berlin-1040, Hessische Str. 3-4, Germany
and
H. CAMMANN G. UHLMANN
Institute of Medical Mathematics, Humboldt-University,
Berlin-1040, Schumannstr. 20-21, Germany

ABSTRACT

To assess individual differences in the heart rate control of normal subjects during mild exercise we used a least-squares fits of heart rate (HR) for the function HR = a*exp(b*t) and a time-series analysis technique that extractes the heart rate variability (HRV) in the frequency band of 0.2 - 0.8 Hz as a marker of the vagal tone. Depending on the coefficient b the subjects were classified in group A (exponential increase of HR) and group B (linear increase of HR). The majority (n=36) of the investigated students shows an exponential increase (|b| = 0.18) of HR during mild exercise (0.07 W/kg body weight). In 33 of these subjects HRV decreases synchronously in an exponential manner. Subjects (n=14) with a distinct linear increase of HR (|b| = 0.12) show a corresponding linear decrease in HRV in response to mild exercise. The differences between both groups may be due to the individual autonomic balance and training level in the subjects.

1. Introduction

The Heart rate (HR) is known to increase above resting levels with both static and dynamic exercise in normal humans. According to the change of HR during a mild exercise testing on a cycle ergometer we observed on principle two different groups of normal subjects (Fig.1) : In the subjects of Group A the increase of HR due to exercise follows an exponential course with a distinct steady state. In contrast, the subjects of the group B show a mainly linear increase in their HR without a steady state. Because HR represents a combination of sympathetic and parasympathetic activity, an interpretation of these differences by analysing the HR only is impossible.

To determine the influence of the parasympathetic activity on the cardiac chronotropic regulation we ascertained the heart rate variability (HRV) in the frequency band of 0.2 - 0.8 Hz as a marker of the vagal tone.[1]

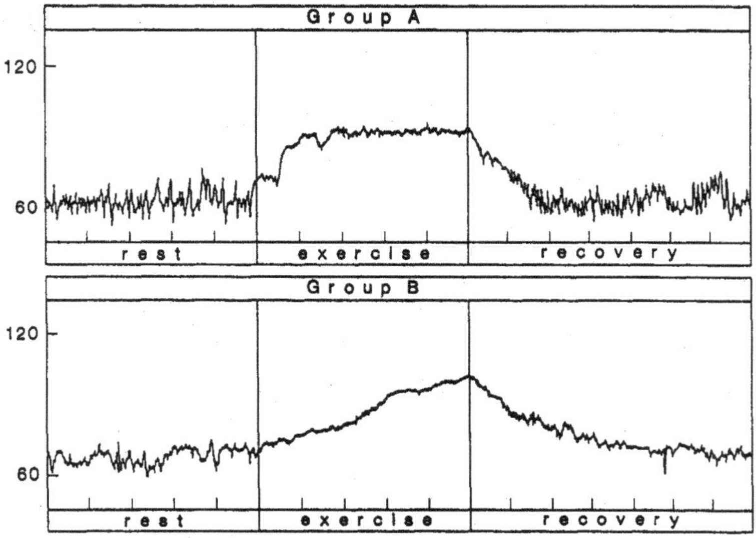

Fig.1:
Typical examples for changes of HR (in beats/min).
Group A : exponential increase with a distinct steady state
Group B : linear increase without a steady state

2. Methods

Subjects. The exercise tests were performed on 35 healthy male students ranging in age from 19 to 24 years (mean: 21 yr.) without physical training.

Testing. After 5 minutes of rest, the students exercised in a sitting position on a cycle ergometer for 5 minutes at a mild work load of 0.07 Watt per kilogram of body weight. The recovery period was observed for 7 minutes.

Signal analysis. The R-R interval duration of successive heart beats was determined from the ECG lead CM5 by a hardware based QRS-peak-detector. To extract the HRV in the 0.2-0.8 Hz frequency band the smoothed time-series of R-R intervals was processed with a digital band-pass filter. From the filtered R-R time-series the HRV was calculated as the mean difference of 15 successive time intervals.

Mathematical analysis. For the classification of the HR-rate control during exercise the least-squares fits for an exponential function of the form $HR = a*\exp(b*t)$ were computed. The coefficients a, b and the correlation coefficient r were estimated for each subject. Depending on the coefficient b the students were classified in group A ($|b| \geq 0.15$) and group B ($|b| < 0.15$).

3. Results

The majority (n=36) of the investigated students shows an exponential increase (|b| = 0.18 - group A) of the HR during exercise (Fig.2). In 33 of these subjects the HRV decreases synchronously. During recovery both HR and HRV follow an exponential decline to the rest level (Fig.3). Subjects with a distinct linear increase of the HR (|b| = 0.12 - group B) show a corresponding linear decrease in the filtered HRV in response to exercise. In 12 subjects of this group also linear changes of the filtered HRV can be observed during the recovery.

Fig.2:
Coefficients (a,b) for least-squares correlation of HR to the function HR = a*exp(b*t).

number	exponent b (mean ± SD) exercise	recovery
36	0.18 ± 0.04	0.12 ± 0.03
14	0.08 ± 0.02	0.06 ± 0.02

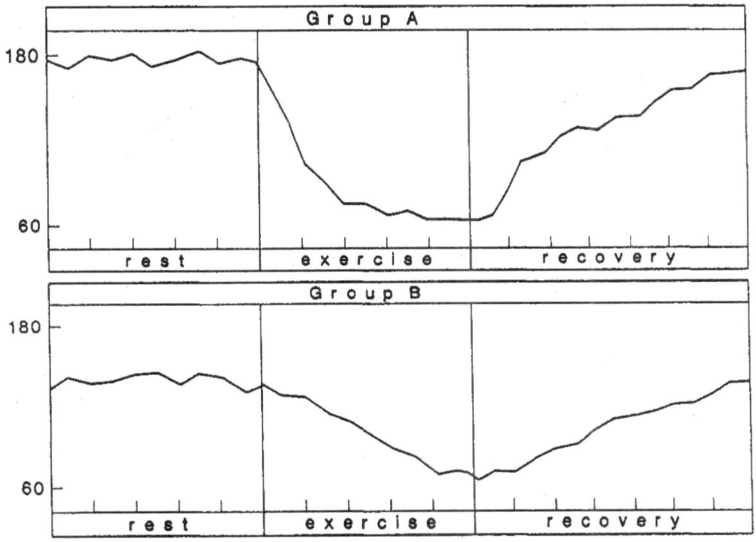

Fig.3:
Filtered HRV (in ms) for a representative subject of group A and B. The changes in HR of this subjects are shown in Fig.1.

4. Discussion

The changes in HR are mediated primary by the sympathetic and parasympathetic system.[3,4] In previously reports [5,6] we found distinct individual differences in the increase of HRrate during exercise. The statistical analysis which we used to quantify the beat-to-beat HRV cannot distinguish between the sympathetic and parasympathic activity. In the present study we apply a time-series analysis technique that evaluates the HRV of the vagal-influenced 0.2 - 0.8 Hz frequency band.[1] In contrast to the power spectral analysis techniques the digital band-pass filter is not limited by the stationarity of the HR patterns. The filter technique therefore allows one the measurement of rapid changes in cardiac vagal activity rather than steady-state events.

The analogous course in the exercise-induced changes of heart rate and filtered HRV of both groups (A and B) corroborate previous findings that the HR increase, associated with mild-intensity exercise, results exclusively from a decrease in the parasympathetic activity.[7,8] A dominance of the vagal reactivity was also described for the recovery after mild exercise.[9]

In a simplified model the differences in the HR control is explained by individual transfer functions for the central autonomic regulation (Fig.4). The transfer functions T_S and T_P represent the form and depth of the modulation of the vagal and sympathetic efferent tone for a given state of afferent and central activity. In low-level exercise the vagal drive is influenced especially by the efferent outflow of the motor cortex (tractus corticospinalis).[10] The character of the vagal transfer function T_P is expressed by the exponential (group A) and linear (group B) changes of the filtered HRV during mild exercise. The differences in T_P may be due to the individual autonomic balance and training level in the students.

In patients with cardiovascular pathology the evaluation of the transfer function T_P in response to well-characterized autonomic interventions should be useful in the assessing of the autonomic regulation in these patients. In particular, individuals with heart diseases often have impaired vagal control of the heart and this reduction in the parasympathetic activity increases the likelihood of dying suddenly.[11] The described method therefore can be valuable in the identification of patients particularly at risk of dying suddenly.

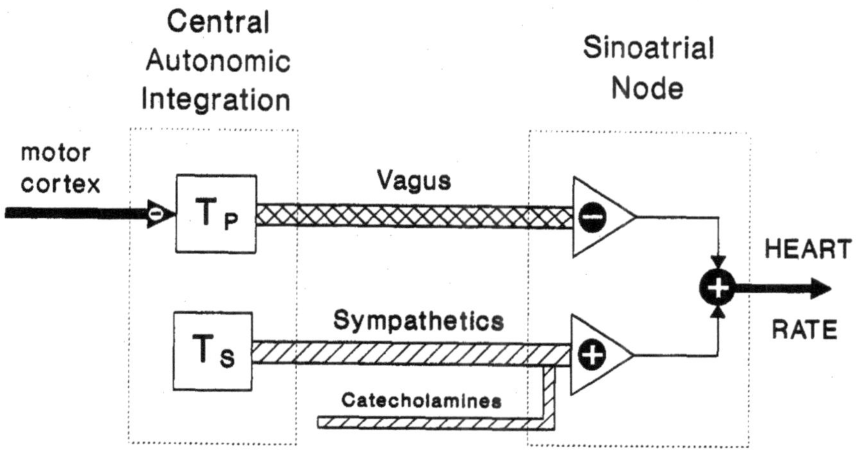

Fig.4:
Simplified model used to represent the modulation of vagal efferent activity during mild exercise.

T_P : parasympathetic transfer function
T_S : sympathetic transfer function

5. References

1. S.D. Akselrod et al., *Science* **213** (1981) 220
2. B. Pommeranz et al., *Amer J Pysiol* **248** (1985) H151
3. H.L. Stone et al., *Fed Proc* **44** (1985) 2271
4. G.B. Billmann et al., *Amer J Physiol* **258** (1990) H896
5. E. Schubert et al., in *New Frontiers of Electrocardiology*, ed. F. de Padua (RSP, Wiley & Sons, Chichester, 1981)
6. E. Schubert, in *Progress in Electrocardiology*, ed. P.W. Macfarlane (Pitman Med., Tunbridge Wells, 1979)
7. B.F. Robinson et al., *Circ Res* **19** (1966) 400
8. M.F. Pagini et al., *Circ Res* **59** (1986) 178
9. W.M. Savin et al., *J Appl Physiol* **53** (1982) 1572
10. R.M. Berne, *Physiology* (Mosby, St.Louis, 1988)
11. G.B. Billmann et al., *Circulation* **66** (1982) 874

DIAGNOSIS OF ISCHEMIA AFTER MYOCARDIAL INFARCTION: EXERCISE ECG VERSUS STRESS-REDISTRIBUTION THALLIUM SCINTIGRAPHY

ANTÓNIO VENTOSA
JOÃO CALQUEIRO, JORGE FERREIRA
VICTOR GIL, RICARDO SEABRA-GOMES

Instituto do Coração and
Department of Cardiology, Hospital de Santa Cruz
Carnaxide, 2795 Linda-a-Velha (Lisboa), Portugal

1. Introduction

Ischemia detection after myocardial infarction has important implications on the management of patients and in the selection of candidates to surgery or angioplasty.

The aim of this study was to evaluate the accuracy of exercise ECG and stress-redistribution thallium scintigraphy in the diagnosis of ischemia after a Q-wave myocardial infarction.

2. Material and Methods

In this retrospective study we included patients evaluated after a Q-wave myocardial infarction with stress-redistribution thallium scintigraphy after treadmill exercise test, and with selective coronary arteriography. We excluded patients on digitalis and patients with left bundle branch block, hypertensive response or other conditions that would compromise ST-segment analysis.

The population included 100 patients with a mean age of 52 ± 10 years, 93 men and 7 women. Infarct localization was anterior in 52 patients, inferior in 46 patients and lateral in 2 patients. Twenty six patients had received thrombolytic therapy.

Exercise tests were performed on a Quinton-4000 treadmill, using Bruce protocol (with or without Sheffield modification), with a target heart rate of at least 85% of predicted. A 2 mCi bolus of thallium chloride was given 1 minute before the end of exercise. Test was considered positive in the presence of ST-segment depression (80 ms after J point) ≥ 1 mm if horizontal or downsloping or ≥ 2 mm if upsloping. The occurrence of typical angina in the absence of ST criteria was also noted. In the absence of ST criteria or angina, test was considered negative if target heart rate was reached, and inconclusive if not.

Tomographic acquisitions (SPECT) begun 10-15 minutes after end of exercise and 3-6 hours after, using a digital gamma camera Siemens-Orbiter with 75 photomultiplier tubes, a single 1/4 in NaI crystal and a LEAP collimator. SPECT used a 180° orbit with 32 views of 40 seconds.

We reconstructed oblique slices and performed a visual analysis on short axis and horizontal and vertical long axis views. Perfusion was classified in 5 segments (septal, anterior, apical, lateral and inferior) according to perfusion in stress study (grades 0 to 4). By stress-redistribution comparison, perfusion defects were classified as totally reversible, partially reversible or not reversible.

On coronary arteriography 54 patients had multivessel disease, including 35 with 2-vessel disease, 18 with 3-vessel disease and 1 with left main involvement. Forty patients had significant disease in only 1 vessel, and in 3 patients, coronary arteries were considered normal, despite their documented infarct and the presence of perfusion defects. For subsequent analysis, these patients were classified as having single-vessel disease.

3. Results

Perfusion was considered normal in 3 patients (all with relatively small Q waves and with 1-vessel disease). In 16 patients, all perfusion defects were irreversible. In 81 patients perfusion defects had some reversibility, including 40 patients with reversible perfusion defects and 57 with partially reversible perfusion defects.

Exercise ECG was considered negative in 22 patients and inconclusive in 29 patients. ST criteria were present in 39 patients (15 of which had also angina). Angina occurred without ST criteria in 10 patients.

Comparing single with multivessel disease (Table I),

Table I. Thallium reversibility and exercise ECG results in single-vessel and multivessel disease

	SingleVD n=46	MultiVD n=54
Thallium scintigraphy		
Reversibility of PD	70%	91%
PD in remote areas	-	52%
Exercise ECG:		
Negative	31%	15%
Inconclusive	39%	20%
ST criteria	26%	50%
Angor (no ST)	4%	15%

VD vessel disease, PD perfusion defects

we found thallium perfusion defects with reversibility in 70% of single-vessel disease patients and in 91% of multivessel disease patients. In multivessel disease, thallium disclosed perfusion defects in remote areas in 52% of patients.

ST criteria on exercise ECG were present in 26% of single-vessel disease patients, and in 50% of multivessel disease patients, while angina without ST criteria was present in additional 4% in single-vessel disease and 15% in multivessel disease. Exercise ECG was negative or inconclusive in 70% of single-vessel disease and 35% of multivessel disease.

Table II summarises the analysis of the detection of ischemia by exercise test, in this series. For this purpose, we considered ischemia as the occurrence of perfusion defects with reversibility on thallium scintigraphy.

Table II. Diagnosis of ischemia (reversibility of thallium perfusion defects) by treadmill exercise test

	SingleVD n=46	MultiVD n=54	Total n=100
Sensitivity (%)	31/35	51/67	43/54
Specificity (%)	86/79	60/60	79/74
(+) predictive value (%)	83/79	93/94	90/90
(-) predictive value (%)	35/34	11/16	25/27
Accuracy (%)	48/48	52/67	50/58

Results expressed as xx/yy where xx denotes ST criteria alone and yy denotes occurrence of ST criteria or angina on treadmill exercise test
VD vessel disease, (+) positive, (-) negative

ST criteria were 31% sensitive for single-vessel disease and 51% sensitive for multivessel disease, with good specificity and positive predictive value, but with a very low predictive value of a non positive test: 65% if single-vessel disease patients and 89% of multivessel disease patients without ST criteria on exercise test had ischemia on thallium scintigraphy. Overall accuracy was around 50%. If we considered positiveness of exercise test as the presence of ST criteria or angina, there would be some improvement in sensitivity, in special in multivessel disease (35% in single-vessel disease and 67% in multivessel disease), but still with high rates of false non-positive tests.

4. Discussion

Prognosis of patients surviving acute myocardial infarction depends, besides ventricular function, on the extent of ischemia and viability in infarcted-related as well as remote myocardial areas [1-5]. The value of classic electrocardiographic analysis of exercise tests in the identification of high-risk patients is well established [3,6-9].

The wide use of thrombolytic therapy in acute myocardial infarction and the increasing availability of non surgical revascularization, by PTCA, has enlarged, since some years ago, the need for a more accurate detection and quantification of ischemia after myocardial infarction, with particular emphasis in the selection of an intermediate-risk group of patients that might not be detected by conventional exercise test, but would still obtain significant benefit from revascularization.

Myocardial perfusion scintigraphy with thallium-201 after exercise became in recent years the most widely used method of accurate detection, localization and quantification of ischemia, with high ability of identifying subgroups of patients with significant risk of developing cardiac events [10-20].

We intended in this series to analyse the performance of conventional exercise test in the detection of ischemia after myocardial infarction. Patients were studied after discharge, including a large majority of patients with an intermediate risk, based on classic risk stratification. The exercise test which clinical and electrocardiographic features were analysed was, in every patient, the same that was used for the thallium scintigraphy.

We detected perfusion defects with reversibility (total or partial) in the large majority of patients (81%), even in single-vessel disease (70%). Thrombolytic therapy, to which half of the patients had been submitted is without doubt one of the main responsibles for this high rate of ischemia.

We analysed exercise test results based on ST criteria or on angina without ST criteria separately in single-vessel and in multivessel disease. Besides the well known low sensitivity of exercise ECG in single-vessel disease, we can conclude that exercise test has good predictive value when positive. The consideration of angina without ST criteria may be important, in special because it results in a significant improvement in sensitivity in multivessel disease, although with a small decrease in specificity in single-vessel disease. The high rates of false non positive exercise tests, even when considering only multivessel disease, suggests that scintigraphic tomography with thallium or other perfusion agents should be considered in every patient with negative or inconclusive exercise test, if revascularization is being considered.

1. EH Schuster, BH Bulkley. N Engl J Med **305** (1981) 1101.
2. AS Maisel, S Ahnve, E Gilpin, et al. Circulation **71** (1985) 211.
3. MR Starling, MH Crawford, GT Kennedy, et al. Am J Cardiology **46** (1980) 909.
4. GS Roubin, PJ Harris, L Bernstein, et al. Circulation **67** (1983) 743.
5. SE Epstein, ST Palmeri, RE Patterson. N Engl J Med **307** (1982) 1487.
6. The TIMI Study Group. N Engl J Med **320** (1989) 618.
7. RF DeBusk, HC Kraemer, E Nash, et al. Am J Cardiol **52** (1983) 1161.
8. P Theroux, DD Waters, C Halphen, et al. N Engl J Med 301 (1979) 341.
9. FM Weld, K-L Chu, JT Bigger Jr, et al. Circulation 64 (1981) 306.
10. JW Deckers, P Fioretti, RW Brower, et al. Am Heart J **113** (1987) 90.
11. P Fioretti, RW Brower, ML Simoons , et al. J Am Coll Cardiol **8** (1986) 40.
12. DD Waters, X Bosch, A Bouchard, et al. J Am Coll Cardiol **5** (1985) 1.
13. P Fioretti, RW Brower, ML Simoons, et al. Am J Cardiol **55** (1985) 1313.
14. DA Weiner, TJ Ryan, CH McCabe, et al. J Am Coll Cardiol **12** (1988) 595.
15. RS Gibson, GJ Taylor, DD Watson, et al. Am J Cardiol **47** (1981) 1010.
16. RE Patterson, SF Horowitz, C Eng, et al. Am J Cardiol **51** (1983) 361.
17. RS Gibson, DD Watson, GB Craddock, et al. Circulation **68** (1983) 321.
18. J Hung, ML Goris, E Nash, et al. Am J Cardiol **53** (1984) 1221.
19. JP Smeets, P Rigo, V Legrand, et al. Cardiology **68 (supl 2)** (1981) 67.
20. RD Abraham, SB Freedman, RF Dunn, et al. Am J Cardiol **58** (1986) 423.

MYOCARDIAL PATHOLOGY OF PATIENTS WITH POSITIVE EXERCISE STRESS TEST BUT NORMAL CORONARY ARTERIOGRAMS

Hiroaki Kawano, Sachio Kawai, Ryhozo Okada
Research Laboratory for Cardiovascular Pathology, Juntendo University School of Medicine,
2-1-1 Hongo, Bunkyo-ku, Tokyo 113, Japan

and

Koichi Yokoyama, Takao Araki, Tamio Miura, Toshikazu Goto
Internal Medicine, Yamagata Prefectural Central Hospital,
7-17 Sakura-cho, Yamagata-city, Yamagata 990, Japan

ABSTRACT

To investigate the myocardial pathology of patients with positive exercise stress test, but angiographically normal coronary arteries and normal left ventricular function, an endomyocardial biopsy study was performed on 8 patients, who consisted of 3 males and 5 females with ages ranging from 35 to 61 years (mean:51 years). From the pathological findings, 3 cases of simple anoxia, 4 cases of catecholamine-related myocarditis and 1 case of mixed characteristics were differentiated. Simple anoxia, which was characterized by vacuolization and perinuclear halos of myocytes, may have resulted from a microcirculatory disturbance in the myocardium. Catecholamine myocarditis showing disarray and hypertrophy of myocytes, may have been related to catecholamine-excess or hypersensitivity. The two conditions showed some difference in the incidence of chest pain and positive rate in ^{201}Tl scintigraphy.

Likoff et al.[1] first described patients with angina pectoris, ischemic-type electrocardiographic response to exercise and a normal coronary angiogram. In 1981, Opherk et al.[2] reported that such patients had a reduced coronary dilatory capacity and ultrastructural changes of the myocardium. More recently, Cannon et al.[3] explained this condition by suggesting that it was angina caused by a reduced vasodilator reserve of the small coronary arteries, and proposed the term "microvascular angina" to account for the specific disease.

Materials and Methods

Eight patients, including 3 males and 5 females, ranging in age from 35 to 61 years (mean: 51 years), were selected as subjects, based on the criteria of a positive exercise stress test, but angiographically normal coronary arteries and a normal left ventricular function. The clinical features of the patients are shown in Table 1. Three patients had symptomatic chest pain, 2 patients had hypertension, 1 patient had hyperlipidemia, and 2 patients were diagnosed as having borderline diabetes mellitus by 75-g oral glucose tolerance test. Ergonovine test was performed on 4 of 8 patients, and none showed spasm. Multiple small specimens of the left ventricular myocardium from each patient were obtained using a transcatheter endomyocardial biopsy technique. The specimens were fixed by formalin immediately after sampling, and embedded in paraffin in the usual manner. After cutting at 5-μm-thick sections, the thin slices were stained by hematoxylin-eosin (H-E), azan, and PAS methods.

Table 1. Clinical and Pathological Features of Patients

Pt. No.	Sex	Age (yrs)	Chest pain	HT	HL	CAG, LVG, UCG	Ergonovine Test	^{201}Tl Scinti.	Ht	Dis	Vac	PH	Fib
1	F	42	+	–	–	N	negative	n.p	+	+	–	–	I
2	F	50	–	–	–	N	negative	N	–	–	+	+	L
3	F	58	–	+	–	N	n.p	RD	–	–	+	+	L
4	F	59	+	+	–	N	negative	n.p	+	+	–	–	L
5	F	60	+	+	+	N	n.p	N	+	+	+	+	L
6	M	35	–	–	–	N	negative	N	+	+	–	–	I
7	M	44	–	–	–	N	n.p	RD	–	–	+	+	L
8	M	61	–	–	–	N	n.p	RD	+	+	–	–	I

F: female, M: male, HT: hypertension, HL: hyperlipidemia, N: normal, n.p: not performed
RD: redistribution, Ht: hypertrophy, Dis: disarray, Vac: vacuolization,
PH: perinuclear halo, Fib: fibrosis, L: loose, I: irregular

Results

The clinical and pathological features of 8 patients are summarized in Table 1. From the pathological findings, Cases No. 2, 3 and 7 showed a characteristic combination of vacuolization, perinuclear halo and absence of hypertrophy of myocytes, which is expression of simple anoxia in the myocardium, as well as spotty replacement and loose interstitial fibrosis and a small amount of macrophage infiltration (Fig.1). On the contrary, Cases No. 1, 4, 6, and 8 showed a combination of hypertrophy and disarrangement of myocytes, spotty replacement and irregular interstitial fibrosis and a small amount of lymphocyte infiltration, which suggested catecholamine myocarditis (Fig.2). Case No. 5 had lesions showing both anoxia and catecholamine-related characteristics. The simple anoxia group consisted of 2 males and 1 female and showed a positive redistribution of ^{201}Tl exercise scintigram which suggested ischemic myocardial condition in 2 of the 3 cases. The catecholamine-related group consisted of 2 males and 2 females and showed chest pain in 2 of the 4 cases. One mixed case was female and had chest pain. None of the 8 cases showed occlusive lesions in the small vessels.

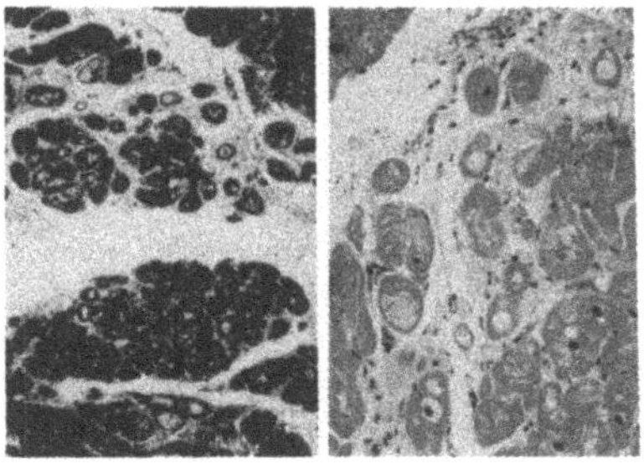

Fig.1 Photomicrographs of myocardium of the simple anoxia type (No. 3 case). (left; azan stain, ×100, right; H-E stain, ×200) The left picture shows edematous loose interstitial fibrosis. The right picture shows vacuolar degeneration and perinuclear halos in the myocytes.

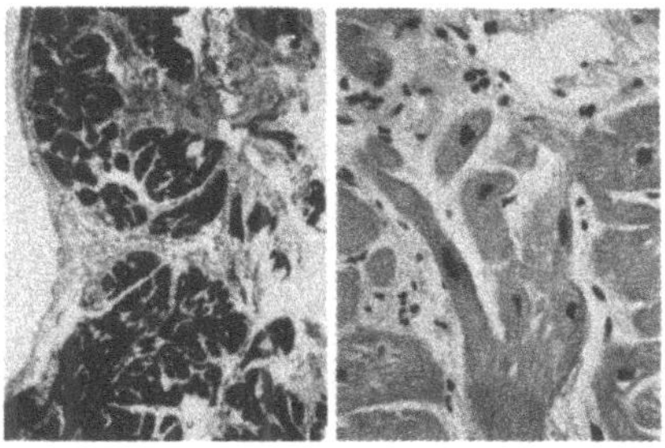

Fig.2 Photomicrographs of myocardium of the catecholamine-related type (No. 1 case). (left; azan stain, × 100, right; H-E stain, × 400) The left shows irregular tigh tfibrosis. The right shows hypertrophy and disarrangement of the myocytes, and a few lymphocytes.

Comments

Our study suggests that so-called syndrome X contains 2 categories of pathological lesions in the myocardium. One is simple anoxic change of myocytes, which could be related to the microcirculatory disturbance already mentioned by Strauer et al.[4], though smallness of the specimens might have been impossible to reveal microvascular abnormality. The other category consisted of catecholamine-related changes, which were almost identical with those of animal experiment using repetitive low dose catecholamine injections.[5] The characteristic lesions might have resulted from either catecholamine excess or hypersensitivity. The existence of mixed type of both categories could be explained by a strong expression of catecholamine-induced micro vessel spasm. The two conditions can be separated by a high positive rate of results for myocardial ishcemia in ^{201}Tl exercise scintigram in the simple anoxia group and a high incidence of chest pain in the catecholamine-related group.

References

1. W. Likoff, B.L. Segal, and H. Kasparian, N. Engl. J. Med. 276 (1976) 1063.
2. D. Opherk, Zebe H, E. Weihe, G. Mall, C. Durr, B. Gravert, H.C. Mehmel,F.Schwarz, and W. Kubler, Circulation 63 (1981) 817.
3. R.O. Cannon, R.M. Watson, D.R. Rosing, S.E. Ebstein, J.Am. Coll. Cardiol. 1 (1983) 1359.
4. B. Strauer, J. Am. Coll. Cardiol. 15 (1990) 775.
5. R. Okada, M. Shimizu, S. Kawai et al., 1980 Report of Group Study on Cardio-myopathies Supported by Ministry of Health and Welfare in Japan (1981) 27.

COMPARISON OF THE DIAGNOSTIC INFORMATION OF EXERCISE 12–LEAD ECG AND BODY SURFACE MAP MEASUREMENTS

KOZMANN, GY.
Dept. for Biology, Research Institute for Material Science, Konkoly Thege u. 29–33, Budapest, Hungary

and

PREDA, I., BALOGH, I.
2nd Medical Clinic and Clinic for Radiology, Postgraduate Medical University, Szabolcs u. 33–35, Budapest, Hungary.

ABSTRACT

The diagnostic information of the 12 lead exercise ECG (XECG) measurements with respect to the exercise body surface mapping (XBSPM) was studied in a population of 32 coronary artery disease patients. Results show that approximately 80% of the maximal ST body surface depression can be detected by the XECG in average. The loss in XECG ST depression amplitudes was due to the significant mean distance between the location of the maximal body surface ST depression area and the nearest exploring XECG electrodes (average: 6.5 cm, maximal distance: 36 cm).

1. Introduction

Pioneer exercise body surface mapping (XBSPM) studies suggest that mapping methods significantly improve the sensitivity of coronary artery disease (CAD) detection, 5–24% according to the different authors, with respect of the standard 12–lead exercise ECG (XECG), without a loss in specificity[1]. Beyond this improved diagnostic performance, XBSPM may provide data for the estimation of the site and extension of the ischemic zones, number of vessels involved, etc. A comprehensive model study of the problem have been published by Selvester et al.[2], using a multidipolar heart model and a fine grid inhomogeneous, realistic shape volume conductor model of a male torso. The findings of the limited number small sample studies published in this field were summarized by Mirvis[1]. According to his conclusion the bulk of data available suggest only a limited role of XBSPM in localizing ischemic regions. However, larger studies using quantitative analytic methods may prove more successful than the simple approaches using pattern recognition methods.

In this study, the global and space dependent relative information loss of the 12 lead XECG measurements with respect to the XBSPM was analyzed statistically.

2. Methods

Thirty-two CAD patients were included into the study. Significant obstruction of one or more coronary arteries were validated by coronary arteriography and/or by T1-201 exercise scintigraphy. All or the patients with supine position underwent symptom or submaximal/maximal heart rate limited bicycle ergometer test. Seven seconds of BSPM data samples were taken by the Lux-type 32 electrode limited lead system[3] at rest, and at the end of each load increments. Data processing included cubic spline base-line adjustment[4] and high-frequency noise reduction by synchronized averaging. Subsequently, from the processed 32 measured ECGs 192 electrode XBSPMs were estimated, using the statistically derived transformation matrix valid for the whole population[3].

For the detailed analysis the following features were used: amplitude and location of the exercise induced maximal ST depression of the XBSPMs measured 60 msec after the J point. XBSPM data were also used for reconstructing 12 lead ECG signals where similar features were applied to characterize the maximal XECG ST response.

3. Results

The body surface scattering of maximal ST depressions found at the CAD patients are plotted in Fig.1.

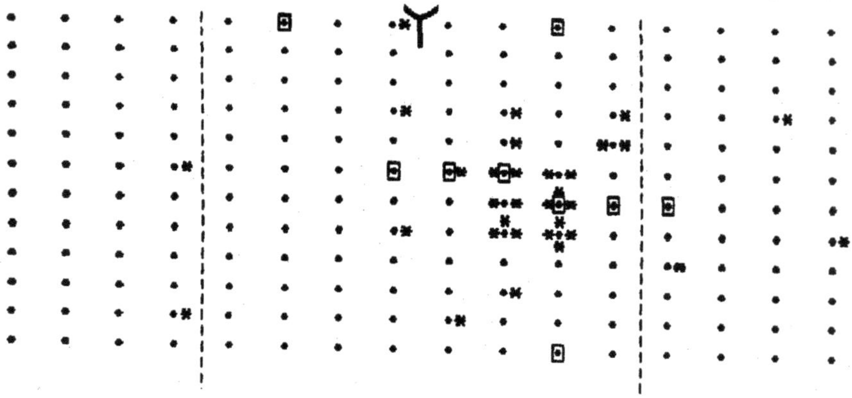

FIG.1. Scatter diagram of the maximal ST60 depressions. (Dots stand for the 192 electrode lead system[2], rectangles denote 12-lead ECG electrode positions, asterisks maximal ST60 depression locations.)

According to these data the maximal ST60 depressions in several cases are far from the location sampled by the 12 lead system (mean distance: 6.5 cm, maximal distance: 36 cm). Consequently, the maximal depression values observable by the 12–lead system are significantly lower in amplitudes than the values measured by BSPM (mean value: 80%). In a certain percentage of cases, this amplitude loss might result in false negative test interpretation, causing a deterioration in sensitivity.

The value of the maximal ST depression depends on the extension of the ischemic area. In this study we were interested in the relative performance of the two type of exercise tests, therefore the percentage of the depression recorded by the XECG was referred to the value measured in the BSPM.

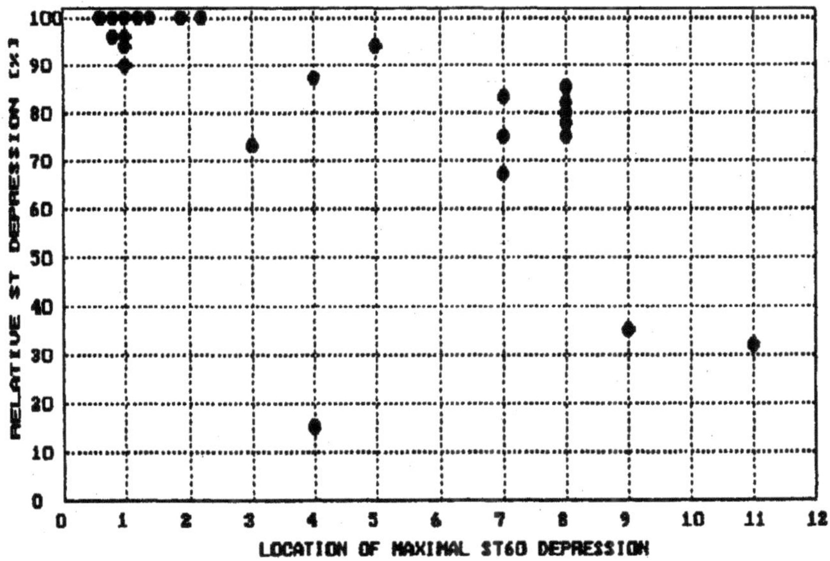

FIG.2. Relative depression of the 12–lead ECG with respect to the value measured in the BSPMs vs., the location of the maximal depression. Locations are coded according to Selvester et al.[2]

In Fig.2. the relative 12–lead ST60 depression amplitudes are plotted vs. the location of the max depressions in the BSPMs. More precisely, instead of the very exact locations, only the code of body surface areas are indicated based on the simulation results of Selvester et al.[2] In their study the latter authors assigned to each thoracic surface subregion an equivalent source location, based on a 12 element multidipolar model of the left ventricular sources and the chest as a volume conductor. In our notations subregions from 1 to 3 stand for the projection areas of antero–septal sources, lateral sources are projected into regions 4 to 6, postero–inferior sources into regions 10 to 12, and finally postero–septal sources into 7 to 9. In each source–triplet the lowest serial number always refers to an equivalent dipolar source near to the apex, while the increasing serial numbers refer to sources located in the midventricular region or at the basis of the heart. Obviously the antero–septal sources are recorded without a significant loss, but e.g. the infero–posterior location ST changes are seriously attenuated.

4. Conclusions

The loss in diagnostic information when using standard 12–lead XECG, steams from the inadequate exploration of the chest by electrodes. Single vessel CADs involving LAD usually are properly detected, but obstructions on the posterior heart surface can easily be overlooked, mostly because the main effect is projected in body surface regions not explored by electrodes.

The results suggests the need for location dependent diagnostic criteria, because alterations of the same size in different parts of the LV cause different amplitudes in the exercise induced ST response[2,5]. This conclusion seems to be strictly valid for one vessel disease. In multivessel CAD the contributions of the different ischemic regions may partly cancel each other, influencing the location of maximal ST depressions and its detectability by the 12 lead ECG, as well.

5. References

1. D.M. Mirvis, *Body Surface Electrocardiographic Mapping* (Kluwer Academic Publishers, Boston, 1988) p. 119.
2. R.H.S. Selvester, J.C., Solomon, G.D., Tolan, *Proc. 9th Annual Conf. of the EMBS* (IEEE Service Center, Piscataway, NJ, 1987) p. 507–508.
3. R.L. Lux, C.R. Smith, R.F. Wyatt, J.A. Abildskov, *IEEE Trans. BME–25* (1978) p. 270–276.
4. C.R. Meyer and H.N. Keiser, *Computers and Biomed. Research* **10** (1977) p. 459–470.
5. F. Kornreich, T.J. Montague, P.M. Rautaharju, (*In this volume*)

EXERCISE STRESS TEST vs DOBUTAMINE STRESS ECHOCARDIOGRAPHY IN THE DETECTION OF MYOCARDIAL ISCHEMIA

A. Pereirinha, M. Fiúza, P. Pedro, E. Dias, F. de Pádua and M. G. Lopes

Medicina IV - A (UCIM), Hospital de Santa Maria and LA 3 - CCUL, Faculdade de Medicina de Lisboa, Lisbon, Portugal

Since its introduction almost 50 years ago for the diagnosis of coronary artery disease (CAD), exercise testing has been the most widely used non invasive stress test [1]. In a metaanalysis study perfomed by Gianrosis et al [2] in 147 published reports, the exercise testing showed a sensitivity of 68%.

However this test has been shown to be unsatisfactory in certain patients, such as those presenting bundle branch block, Wolf-Parkinson-White, or left ventricular hypertrophy ECG patterns in which the electrocardiographic diagnosis of ischemia is impossible or very erroneous.

These and other limitations of the exercise stress testing determined the search for other stress modalities, namely the use of exercise echocardiography. Dobutamine stress echocardiography has been recently introduced in clinical practice with excelent sensitivity (85%) and specificity (87%) and without major complications [3].

Our objective was to compare the results of exercise stress test and Dobutamine Echocardiography test in patients with known or suspected CAD.

Population

The study population consisted of 35 patients (30 male, 5 female, mean age: 55± 11 years) with known or suspected CAD.

All patients (pts) performed treadmill exercise test and Dobutamine stress Echocardiography. (Dob ECHOCG).

Material and Methods

Exercise treadmill test was performed using Bruce or Naughton protocol.

Dob ECHOCG was performed according to UCIM protocol which includes Dobutamine infusion from 5 µg/Kg/min to 40 µg/Kg/min im 3 minute stages, until new wall motion abnormalities or 85% maximal predicted heart rate or any indication to stop the test. If none of the above occurs after maximal Dobutamine dose, Atropine (0,25 mg/min e.v. up to 1 mg) is administered.

Results

Treadmill exercise test performed either with Bruce or Naughton protocol was positive for myocardial ischemia in 19 pts (54%) and in the other 16 pts (46%) the test was considered negative. No major complications were observed.

The same pts performed a Dob ECHOCG a few days later. The test was positive in 14 pts (40%) and negative in the other 21 (60%) pts (Fig. 1). The concordance between the two tests was seen in 19 pts (54%).

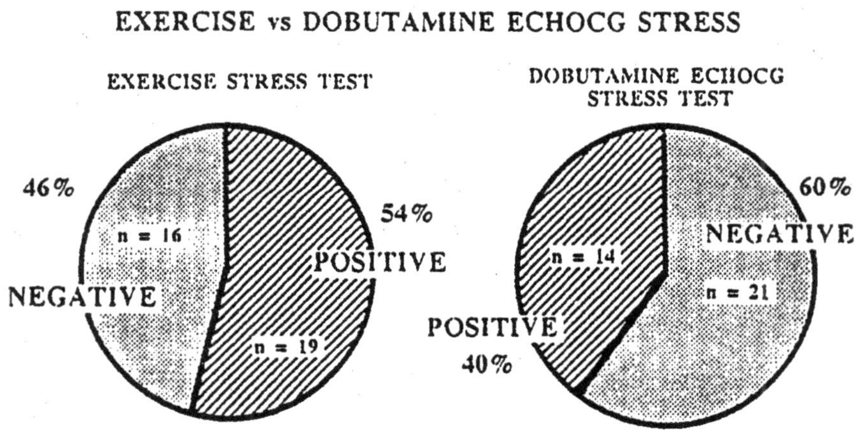

Figure 1. Positive and negative tests with exercise stress test and Dobutamine Echocardiography stress test.

In the 16 pts (46%) with discordant results, 9 pts had positive treadmill tests and negative Dob ECHOCG. Coronary angiography (CATH) was performed in 3 of these pts and no significant coronary artery lesions were identified.

In the other 7 pts, with discordance of the tests, exercise test was negative but Dob ECHOCG was considered positive. Four pts had coronary angiography which showed significant (> 50%) coronary lesions in all of the pts (Fig. 2).

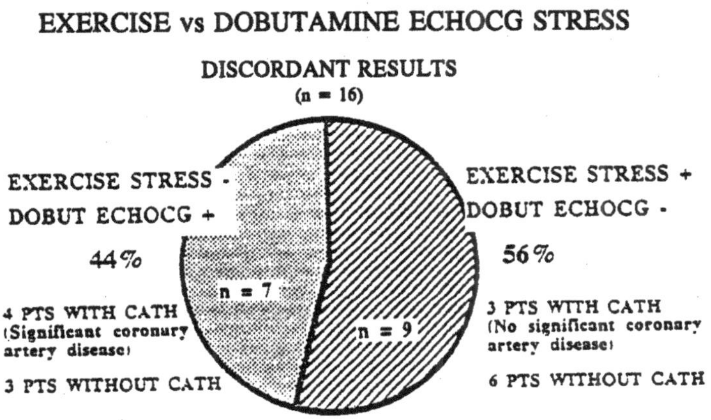

Figure 2 Coronary angiography in the patients with discordant tests.

Discussion

The classical treadmill stress test is a safe, non expensive test for the non invasive diagnosis of CAD, although with several limitations that can be a source of false positives and negatives for the diagnosis of ischemia. Stress echocardiography has emerged as an alternative to treadmill stress test to solve some of these limitations.

The logical for the use of stress ecocardiography lies in the fact that during the ischemic cascate, wall motion abnormalities occur before electrical (ST-T) abnormalities or pain. With pharmacological stress technical problems related with performing the echocardiographic study with the patient exercising are overcome. It is also a good alternative for pts who cannot exercise, and can be considered a safe and feasible diagnostic test for the non invasive diagnosis of CAD (3,4).

Beside to the diagnosis, stress echocardiography can be useful for the identification of the correct physiological significance of the coronary artery stenosis (5). It has also been shown to provide a method to identify viable myocardium after myocardial infarction (6).

Although training in stress echocardiography is important for the accuracy obtained with the test (7), good reproducibility can be achieved (8).
Stress echocardiography can be considered ready for routine clincal use (9).
Our results, with a concordance of 54% between treadmill stress test and Dobutamine ECHOCG are in agreement with their known sensitivity and specificity.
Not all our pts were submitted to coronary angiography. In those pts who had an angiography made, the results were in agreement with the Dobutamine ECHOCG.

Conclusions

In our population we found agreement between the results of treadmill exercise test and Dob ECHOCG stress test in 54% of the cases. Dob ECHOCG was superior to treadmill in the detection of myocardial ischemia and will probably have an increasing utilisation in the routine daily practice.

Bibliographic references

1. Master AM, Nuzie S, Brown Re et al: The electrocardiogram and the "two step" exercise: a test of cardiac function and coronary insufficiency. Am. J. Med.Sci. 1944, 207;435 - 450.

2. Gianrossi R, Detrano R, Mulvitill D et al: Exercise-induced ST depression in the diagnosis of coronary artery disease. Circulation 1989; 80:87-98.

3. Sawada SG, Segar DS, Ryant et al: Echocardiographic detection of coronary artery disease during Dobutamine infusion. Circulation 1991; 83:1605-1614.

4. A. Salustri, P.M. Fioretti, M.M. A. Pozzoli, A. J. McNeill and J. R. T. C. Roelandt: Dobutamine stress echocardiography: its role in the diagnosis of coronary artery disease. European Heart Journal 1992, 13: 70-77.

5. Byron F. Vandenberg, Steven R. Fleagle, David J. Skorton: Exercise Echocardiography and Quantitative Angiography: Improved Identification of Physiologically Significant Coronary Artery Stenoses. Editorial comment JACC, Vol. 15, Nº 5, April 1990, 1052 - 4.

6. Luc A. Piérard, Christian M. de Landsheere, Christian Berthe, Pierre Rigo, Henri E. Kulberus: Identification of Viable Myocardium by Echocardiography During Dobutamine Infusion in Patients with Myocardial Infarction after Thrombolytic Therapy: Comparison with Positron Emission Tomography.

7. Eugénio Picano, Fabio Lattanzi, Andrés Orlandini, Cecilia Marini, Antonio D'Abbate: Stress Echocardiography and the Human factor: The importance of Being Expert. J. Am. Cardiol. 1991, 17:666 - 9.

8. Albert Oberman, Po-Hoey Fan, Navin C. Nanda, Jeannette Y. Lee, William J. Huster, Julie A. Sulentic, Octavia F. Storey: Quantitative two-dimensional echocardiography immediately after exercise is highy reproducible providing a valuable tool for assessing serial changes in left ventricular function. J. Am. Cardiol. 1989; 14: 923 - 8.

9. S. Iliceto and P. Rizzon: Stress echocardiography: ready for routine clinical use? European Heart Journal. 1991; 12: 262 - 265.

PART VII

Diagnostic Criteria including Computer Applications

CONVENTIONAL ECG AS A NON-INVASIVE MARKER OF HEART REMODELLING IN RATS WITH ARTERIOVENOUS FISTULAS

LINO GONÇALVES
FÁTIMA PACHECO
CRISTINA SANTOS
LUÍS A. PROVIDÊNCIA
Department of Cardiology, University Hospital, Coimbra, Portugal

ABSTRACT

To assess the role of conventional ECG as a non-invasive marker of heart remodelling in rats with arteriovenous fistulas (AVF), we distributed 30 male Wistar rats in 3 groups: group A (control), group B (fistula) and group C (fistula+enalapril). An end to side (AVF) was produced in rats from groups B and C. A 12 lead ECG was recorded at the beginning and 8 weeks later in each rat, for QRS voltage analysis. Rats from group B developed structural remodelling of the heart. These changes were prevented in group C. There was an increase of QRS amplitude in group B, which achieved statistical significance in most of the leads studied. This increase was not seen in group A and C. In conclusion, in this particular model of volume overload, conventional ECG is a good non-invasive marker of structural remodelling of cardiac myocytes.

Introduction

After normal growth is completed, further cardiac growth can occur as an adaptation to pressure and/or volume loads, which usually develop in a precipitating stress pattern[1].

When an arteriovenous fistula (AVF) is produced in humans[2] and animals[3,4] the systemic blood pressure stays normal, the total peripheral resistance is reduced and there is an increase in cardiac output, stroke volume, and end-diastolic pressure. These changes induce an eccentric cardiac hypertrophy during the compensated phase, that is, chamber dilatation, and an increase in wall thickness. These changes, originated by volume overloading, are associated with an increase in myocyte length[5-7] rather than cross sectional area and can also be seen in hyperthyroidism[8], isotonic exercise[9], and excess growth hormone[10]. These changes in cell dimension and shape, seem to be an adaptive response that tends to minimise the effects of an increase in volume load on wall stress. The assessment of changes in myocyte length and cross sectional area is difficult because: a) true longitudinal sections are not easy to obtain due to the complex 3-dimension geometry of cardiac myocyte, b) a dramatic change in cell orientation occurs frequently c) distances between intercalated discs are different from cell to cell and within the same cell[7]. Isolated myocytes can be used in the study of cellular dimensions[11,12].

However, with this technique we have to sacrifice the animals, and 30% of cells are damaged during the procedure. With a non-invasive marker of these changes, one would be able to study the induction and regression of cardiac remodelling, without killing the animal. Despite the fact that ECG has lost his prominence in favour of echocardiography (ECHO), in assessing anatomic diagnosis[13], the latter is not practical in a rat model. In our study, we evaluate the role of ECG as a non-invasive marker of the structural remodelling of the cardiac myocytes in rats with (AVF)s.

Methods

Animal Model

Thirty male Wistar rats were distributed into 3 groups: Group A (control), group B (fistula) and group C (fistula+enalapril). They were anaesthetised using 0.2 ml/g of weight from a mixture of ketamine hydrochloride (75 mg) and chlorpromazine (50 mg). An ECG was then performed in each animal. The skin of the right thigh was incised and the right femoral artery and vein were isolated from the level of the inguinal ligament distal to the superficial epigastric artery and vein. An end to side anastomosis was performed between the femoral artery and vein. The rats were permitted to recover. Eight weeks later, the rats were again anaesthetised, and another ECG was performed in all groups. The patency of the fistula was visually confirmed. The rats were sacrificed with 2 ml of KCl (1 mEq per ml). The hearts were rapidly excised, weighed, and sent to macroscopic and microscopic study. The pathologist was blind as to which group the hearts belonged to.

Electrocardiography

All groups were submitted to a 12-lead ECG at the beginning of the study and 8 weeks later, for QRS voltage analysis. The ECG was performed with a Fukuda Denshi Cardiomax FK12 electrocardiograph using a sensitivity of 2mV and a paper velocity of 50 mm/s. Ten electrodes were placed on the four limbs and on the rat precordium.

Pathologic Measurements

The heart was sectioned just bellow the auriculoventricular valves, perpendicularly to the long axis. The septum and the right and left ventricle free wall thicknesses were measured. Sections 3 mm thick from these segments were examined histologically after fixation in 10% neutral buffered formalin. After processing through graded alcohols, clearing in xylene and embedding in paraffin, sections 5-μm thick were cut and stained with hematoxylin-eosin. Morphometric analysis was made using a point counting technique. A total of 30 fields were evaluated in each cardiac segment, using a square grid with 361 points of intersection. The morphometric sampling consisted on counting the total number of points of intersection that fit inside the myocyte nuclear/cytoplasm profiles in equal areas of tissue sections at ×400 magnification. Only those nuclei were measured in which the nuclear envelope was sharply defined at both ends. We used the following equation to determine the volume fraction of cytoplasm (Fc) [Eq. 1], in which n_c, are the number of points counted inside the cytoplasm:

$$F_c = \sum_{c=o}^{30} \frac{n_c}{30 \times 361} \qquad \text{[equation 1]}$$

Statistical analysis

Results are presented as mean ±SD computed from the average measurements obtained from each rat. Statistical evaluation of the results for comparisons between groups was performed with unpaired Student's t-test. Significance levels for comparisons between QRS voltage evolution within a group were calculated using the paired Student's t-test. Values of $p<0.05$ were regarded as significant.

Results and Discussion

In the present work an experimental model of cardiac volume overload by producing an (AVF) between the right femoral artery and vein is implemented. Others[14,15] have shown that a stabilized state of compensatory hyperfunction is achieved about 30 days after a load is placed on the heart. Gerdes et al[5] have also shown that after 10 weeks in rats with an (AVF) there was also cardiac hypertrophy in the absence of any signs of cardiac failure. In our study, a smaller period of time of 8 weeks was used. Body weight evolution was similar in all groups. Heart weight increased in group B (1.78±0.2 g) when compared to group A (1.55±0.11 g), ($p<0.01$), and was similar (p=n.s.) in groups A and C (1.58±0.13 g). When heart weight/body weight ratio was studied, there was also an increase of this ratio in group B (4.4±0.55 mg/g) when compared to group A (3.6±0.5 mg/g) ($p<0.01$), and was similar (p=n.s.) in groups A and C (3.66±0.4 mg/g). An increase in wall thickness was detected in group B in the right ventricle ($p<0.004$), septum ($p<0.05$) and left ventricle ($p<0.03$) when compared to groups A and C(Table I).

Table I

Wall Thickness

	Group A (mm)	Group B (mm)	Group C (mm)
Right Ventricle	1.3±0.15	1.5±0.16	1.21±0.3
Septum	3.2±0.3	3.6±0.2	3.2±0.4
Left Ventricle	3.2±0.3	3.6±0.25	3.0±0.7

Myocyte cytoplasm volume fraction was increased in group B (Table II), when compared with group A, in all segments studied (right ventricle p=0.011, septum p=0.025, and left ventricle p=0.031). Groups A and C were similar (p=n.s.).

Table II

Cytoplasm Volume Fraction

	Right Ventricle (%)	Septum (%)	Left ventricle (%)
Group A	97.2 ± 0.8	97.5 ± 0.5	97.3 ± 0.7
Group B	98.2 ± 0.8	98.1 ± 0.6	98.0 ± 0.7
Group C	96.9 ± 0.7	97.0 ± 0.8	97.0 ± 0.6

In humans beings, more accurate techniques, such as ECHO, are superior to and simpler than ECG in following the progression and regression of chamber enlargement[13]. However, ECHO has obvious technical difficulties in experimental rat models. Thus, despite the reported 73% sensitivity and 78% specificity of QRS voltage analysis in patients with cardiac hypertrophy[16], we tried to evaluate the role of ECG as a non-invasive marker of structural remodeling of cardiac myocytes in this cardiac volume overload model induced by an (AVF). The results are plotted in Table III.

Table III
QRS Voltage

Lead		DI	DII	DIII	aVR	aVL	aVF	V1	V2	V3	V4	V5	V6
Group A	0 w	2.7	4.2	3.5	2.9	2.2	3.7	5.4	7.9	5.2	3.5	2.6	2.0
(mm)	8 w	2.6	3.8	3.3	2.8	2.2	3.2	6.3	7.7	6.0	3.5	2.1	1.7
p=		n.s.	0.04	n.s.	n.s.	n.s.	n.s.	n.s.	n.s.	n.s.	n.s.	n.s.	n.s.
Group B	0 w	2.3	4.3	3.6	2.8	2.4	3.8	5.3	6.9	4.4	2.4	2.0	1.6
(mm)	8 w	3.4	4.7	4.5	3.6	2.8	4.3	7.1	10.6	8.8	5.4	3.3	2.2
p=		0.01	n.s.	0.04	0.006	n.s.	n.s.	0.04	0.005	0.01	0.01	0.01	n.s.
Group C	0 w	3.5	5.4	5.1	4.1	3.0	5.1	6.2	8.1	6.1	4.0	2.8	2.1
(mm)	8 w	2.8	5.6	4.5	4.2	2.3	5.1	6.7	9.5	8.0	4.4	3.5	2.1
p=		n.s.	n.s.	n.s.	n.s.	n.s.	n.s.	n.s.	n.s.	n.s.	n.s.	n.s.	n.s.

There is an increase in QRS voltage in all leads in group B, achieving in most of them statistical significance. No increase in QRS voltage was found in groups A and C.

Conclusion

Heart remodelling was produced by a volume overload model, in which a shunt between the right femoral artery and vein was induced. Enalapril prevented the cardiac remodeling as assessed by gross anatomical and microscopic studies. ECG proved to be a non-invasive marker of the structural remodelling of cardiac myocytes in this model.

References

1. W. Grossman , B. A. Carabello, S. Gunther, M. A. Fifer, in *Perspectives in Cardiovascular Research, Myocardial Hypertrophy and Failure*, ed. N. R. Alpert, (Raven Press, New York, 1983) 7, p 1.
2. F.H. Epstein, O. W. Shadle, T. B. Fergusson and M. E. McDowell, *J. Clin. Invest.* **32** (1953) 543.
3. S. F. Flaim, W. J. Minteer and S. H. Nellis, *Am. J. Physiol.* **236** (1979) H698.
4. A. V. Loo and E. C. Heringman, *Am. J. Physiol.* **158** (1949) 103.
5. *A. M.* Gerdes, S. E. Campbell and D. R. Hilbelink, *Lab. Invest.* **59** (1988) 857.
6. W. Grossman, D. Jones and L. P. McLaurin, *J. Clin. Invest.* **56** (1975) 56.
7. P. Y. Hatt, K. Rakusan, P Gastineau and M. Laplace, *J. Mol. Cell. Cardiol.* **11** (1979) 989.
8. A. M. Gerdes, J. A. Moore and J. M. Hines, *Lab. Invest.* **57** (1987) 708.
9. I. P. Panidis, M. N. Kotler, J. F. Ren, G. S. Mintz, J. Ross and P. Kalman, *J. Am. Coll. Cardiol.* **3** (1984) 1309.
10. L. Q. Lei, S. A. Rubin and M. C. Fishbein, *Lab. Invest.* **59** (1988) 357.
11. *S. P.* Bishop and J. L. Drummond, *J. Mol. Cell. Cardiol.* **11** (1979) 423.
12. A. M. Gerdes, J. A. Moore, J. M. Hines, P.A. Kirkliand and S. P. Bishop, *Anat Rec* **215** (1986) 420.
13. B. Surawicz B, *J. Am. Coll. Cardiol.* **8** (1986) 711.
14. E. A. Breisch, C. W. Francis and C. M. Bloor, *Lab. Invest.* **51** (1984) 333.
15. D. B. McCallister and A. L. Brown, *Lab. Invest.* **14** (1965) 692.
16. *D. L.* Vine, R. N. Finchum, H. T. Dodge, W. H. Jr. Bancroft and D. C. Hurst, *Circulation* **43** (1971) 547.

THE U WAVE AND ITS ECHOCARDIOGRAPHIC IMAGE

BORISLAV G. GEORGIEV
National Centre of Cardio-Vascular Disease
1309 Sofia, Bulgaria

ILIA TZENOV
National Centre of Cardio-Vascular Disease
1309 Sofia, Bulgaria

The U wave is an ECG event with unknown genesis. The contradictory data for its appearence, morphology and relations with pathological states made us to discuss its relations to cardiac cycles. We studied 180 persons (124 men and 56 women) of average 48 years of age -100 of them were healthy and 80 - with cardio-vascular diseases. We found that the positive U wave in ECG precordial leads V_2, V_3, (V_4) coincided with the contact between Ep of Anterior Mitral valve (AMV) and systolic septal thickness in M-mode echocardiogram. The positive U wave in (V_4), V_5, V_6 also coincided with contact between E'p of Posterior Mitral valve(PMV) and posterior left ventricular wall, and the positive U wave in ECG leads (V_1), V_2-V_6 - with a contact between Ep of AMV, E'p of PMV and the left ventricular endocardium. In cases with severe calcified changes of mitral valves and after inplantation of mitral valve prosthesis the appearence of U wave coincided with an increased echogenesity of a zone of interventricular septum, most probably due to previous contact between Ep of AMV and interventricular septum. The appearence of U wave in cases of intermitent U wave coincided with the contact of mitral valve with left ventricular endocardium.We suggested, that the U wave was a left ventricular diastolic phenomenon due to an impulse provoked by the mechanical stimulation of the left ventricular endocardium by the mitral valve.

It has been suggested that the U wave was diastolic phenomenon with unclear genesis. In a polycardiographic recording, its peak appeared 0,03 sec. after the second heart sound and it was synchronous with the pulse of jugularis vein. It has been suppoused that the U wave represented a surface reflection of negative afterpotential [1,2]. The two prevailing concepts about its mechanism included repolarization of Purkinje fibers [3,4,5] or a mechanical event, probably diastolic relaxation of the myocardium [6,7]. The U wave is upright with an amplitude 5-25 (50) per cent of that of T wave [8] and the highest one is recorded in ECG precordial leads V_2 and V_3. Generaly the U wave is clearly separated from the T wave, but it may appears earlier in conditions such as states with foreshortened ventricular filling and ejection or when the Q-T interval is prolonged. On the other hand the U wave can be easely identified when the Q-T interval is foreshortened [9]. The aim of this study was to understand more about the genesis of the U wave, its relation with the cardiac cycles and its echocardiographic image equivalent.

Patients and Methods

Hundred and eighty persons with ECG data for U wave were studied in the National Centre of Cardio-Vascular Disease. Hundred and twenty four of them were men and fifty six - women, aged from 20 to 75 years (of average 48 years of age). Hundred of the studied people were with normal ECG and Echocardiograms (EchoCGs) and eighty had pathological changes. All persons had upright U wave in the standart and precordial ECG leads. Constant U wave was found in ninty three of healthy people and intermitent U wave was registrated in seven of them after physical activity. All eighty patients with cardio-vascular diseases were as follows : mitral valve disease - 34, after mitral valve replacement surgery - 12, arterial hypertension and left ventricular hypertrophy- 24, hypertrophic cardiomyopathy - 10. All persons from the studied group have had a good echocardiographic window, that allowed us to obtain good echocardiographic image in different positions and sections.

Results

In a previous study[10] we found several cases of a short E point septal separation (EPSS) during our studies on the kinetics of the mitral valve. In a group of persons we saw that E point (Ep) of Anterior Mitral valve (AMV) have touching left ventricular septal endocardium, and we found that the contact between Ep of AMV and interventricular septum coicided with the U wave, that could be also seen in transversal section on the level of mitral valve. Seventy five of hundred healthy persons have had an upright U wave in leads V_2,V_3,(V_4) and we found that it coincided with the contact between Ep of AMV and interventricular septal endocardium. The second systolic thickness of interventricular septum below the mitral valve seen on the EchoCG of these people also coincided with U wave. In 12 of 100 persons we found U wave only in V_5 and V_6 and in parasternal echocardiographic section we saw a contact between E'p of Posterior Mitral valve (PMV) and posterior left ventricular wall. We did not registrate a second systolic thickness of posterior wall below mitral valve. Six of hundred patients had U wave in precordial leads (V_1),V_2-V_6.Their EchoCGs showed a contact between Ep of AMV and interventricular septum and E'p of PMV and posterior wall. In seven cases we did not find U wave in the last ECG recording, but we found it in previous ECG. During the first echocardiographic examination we did not see any contact between mitral valve and left ventricular endocardium, but we measured only a short EPSS. After physical efforts we saw contact between Ep of AMV and interventricular septal endocardium and an U wave appeared in ECG precordial leads V_2,V_3,(V_4) in all of them.

The problem about the U wave and its relations with the cardiac cycles in cases of cardiac damages is not so clear. All of the patients with mitral valve lesions had a hystory of rheumatic disease with mean mitral stenotic orificial area 1,47 cm^2 with fibrous changes or calcifications.In 22 of 34 patients with mitral valve disease we found a contact between mitral valve and left ventricular endocardium with the characterisation of the healthy people. In the group of patients with mitral valve prosthesis and in 13 of 34 mitral stenotic patients we could not see contact between left ventricular endocardium and mitral valve,valve prosthesis or remained part of papillary muscles but in their ECGs an U wave in leads (V_2),V_3 was registrated. In those patients we have seen in the upper third of interventricular septal endocardium a zone more echogenic than the surrounding myocardium, most probably due to a previous contact between Ep of AMV and interventricular septum. M-mode parasternal EchoCG visualized second systolic thickness like in healthy persons. We supposed that there was a difference between the electrical potentials of fibrouse tissue and surrounding myocardium and it could potentiate impulses with the image of U wave. The mechanical event was most probably due to the whirle of blood stream trough mitral valve during left ventricular diastole.

In the groups of patients with arterial hypertension and left ventricular hyprtrophy and with hypertrophic cardiomyopaty we have seen a contact between mitral valve and left ventricular endocardium. In some cases we saw U wave with a highest amplitude which coincided with a continued contact between Ep of AMV and the septum. In cases of hypocalemia we did not visualized any changes in the contact areas seen before,after and during hypocalemia, and we supposed that the augmentation of vulnerability of myocardial cells reflects on a potenciation of a tallest U wave. It was not easy to differenciate the U wave in case of atrial flutter, but if there was a contact between mitral valve and endocardial surface the careful analysis could differenciate some F waves with abnormal morphology.

Conclusions

From the presanted data we could suggest that the U wave was a diastolic phenomenon caused by mechanical stimulation of the left ventricular endocardium by mitral valve. When there was a contact between Ep of AMV and interventricular septum the U wave appeared in ECG precordial leads V_2,V_3,(V_4) and on the septal M-mode EchoCG was seen a second systolic thickness. When the contact was between E'p of PMV and posterior left ventricular wall the U wave was in leads V_5,V_6 and it was with a lower amplitude than the T wave amplitude. We suppose that states with an incresed myocardial vulnerability could be presented with an augmentation of the amplitude of U wave due to an increased electrical impulse generation. In some young healthy people the U wave could be intermitent and it appeared when the contact between mitral valve and left ventricular endocardium was effected. In mitral stenotic patients the U wave could be generated without contact between mitral valve and endocardial surface, but in the zone of previouse contact of Ep of AMV and the septum the whirle of blood stream trought mitral orifice could generate the U wave.

Acknowledgement

We are kindly acknowledged Hellige PPG who gave us the possibility to present this trial at the XIX International Congress on Electrcardiology and M. Bogdan Stoyanov who helped us in the preparing of this article.

References

1.E.Lepeschkin: Arch Intern Med,**96** (1955)600

2.E.Lepeshkin et al: Ann NY Acad Sci; **65**(1957)942

3.B F Hoffman, P E Cranfield(Electrophysilogy of the heart, Mc Grew -Hill, New York 1960) p 180

4.I Watanabe: Circulation;**51**(1975)1030

5.I Watanabe, H Toda : Am J Cardiol **41**(1978)23

6.E.Lepeschkin E (Advences in Electrocardiography; Grune and Stratton; New York 1972) p 431

7.H .Kishida , J S Cool B Surawicz : Am J. Cardiol ;**49**(1982)2030

8.C Fisch (Heart Disease,Philadelphia ,W.B.Saunders Co,1992) p 140

9.E Lepeschkin Mod Concepts Cardiovasc Dis;**38**(1969)39

10.B.Georgiev,I.Tzenov(IV National Congress on Cardiology, Abstract book, Plovdiv-Bulgaria,1992) p.29

Artificial Neural Networks for the Diagnosis of Atrial Fibrillation

T.F. Yang, B. Devine, P.W. Macfarlane.
University Department of Medical Cardiology,
Royal Infirmary, Glasgow , Scotland.

ABSTRACT

The purpose of the present study was to compare software based neural networks versus deterministic logic for separating sinus rhythm with supraventricular extrasystoles and/or ventricular extrasystoles from atrial fibrillation at a particular point in the diagnostic logic of the Glasgow Program. 460 ECGs were selected for a training set., 263 had atrial fibrillation and 197 had sinus rhythm accompanied by supraventricular extrasystoles and/or ventricular extrasystoles. The training set ECGs were fed into various neural networks containing different input variables and a different number of neurons in the hidden layers but all with only one output layer. The configuration of the neural network with the best result for the test set contained 9 input variables and 2 hidden layers each with 30 neurons. A separate test set containing 470 cases with the same mixture as for the training set was then studied. For the artificial neural networks, the sensitivity was 95.2% (vs 94.6% by the Glasgow Program) and the specificity was 96.5% (vs 98.6% by Glasgow program). The use of neural networks seemed not to lead to any noticeable improvement. Further investigation is mandatory to improve the performance of the neural network by incorporation into the deterministic logic.

Introduction

Atrial fibrillation is a common arrhythmia, with a prevalence of approximately 2% in the general population[1]. It is more common in the elderly, affecting about 5% of persons over 60 years of age[2]. The importance of atrial fibrillation is emphasized by its association with between 6% and 24% of ischemic strokes and with about 50% of cardioembolic strokes[3,4]. The diagnosis of atrial fibrillation is usually made by electrocardiograms showing an absence of discrete atrial activity, an irregular undulating baseline and a variable RR interval. Before the use of computers for ECG interpretation, each ECG had to undergo visual classification by cardiologists. The demand for ECG recordings has increased in recent years resulting in additional work for cardiologists. For this reason it was hoped that the utilization of computers for ECG analysis could not only save time but perhaps improve the accuracy of ECG interpretation. Because artificial neural networks are not rule-based and can be applied in areas where rules are difficult to formalize or are ill-defined, they are theoretically particularly suitable for application to visual pattern recognition problems. Deterministic logic is currently applied to rhythm analysis in computer-assisted ECG interpretation methods developed in Glasgow Royal Infirmary[5]. This is an area requiring further investigation. For this reason, the aim of the present study was to compare an artificial neural network versus deterministic logic for separating sinus rhythm with supraventricular extrasystoles and/or ventricular extrasystoles from atrial fibrillation at a particular point in the diagnostic logic of the Glasgow Program.

Materials and Methods

The Glasgow program for ECG analysis uses 3 leads selected from the 12-lead ECG for interpretation of cardiac rhythm. These 3 leads are selected from a study of the average beats which have been calculated by the main wave measurement logic. From these 3 selected leads, measurements on PR interval variability, RR interval regularity, presence or absence of discrete P waves, presence or absence of multiple P waves and so on are determined. In the presence of atrial fibrillation, it is likely that fibrillatory waves may for the purposes of rhythm analysis be detected as P waves and hence the concepts of multiple P waves and PR regularity etc still apply[5].

930 ECGs with irregular rhythm (including atrial fibrillation, sinus rhythm with supraventricular extrasystoles or ventricular extrasystoles) were selected from the data bank in the department of Medical Cardiology, Glasgow Royal Infirmary. These ECGs were recorded from the patients attending the outpatient clinics and admitting to the wards of Royal Infirmary from 1981 to 1992. The interpretation of the ECGs was performed both by the deterministic logic in the Glasgow Program and by two cardiologists. The 930 ECGs were divided equally into a training set and a test set which were randomly separated. They contained both atrial fibrillation and sinus rhythm with supraventricular extrasystoles or ventricular extrasystoles. The training set consisted of 460 ECGs. 263 of them were Atrial fibrillation and 197 were sinus rhythm always accompanied by either supraventricular extrasystoles and/or ventricular extrasystoles. These ECGs with appropriate classifications were fed for training purposes to a variety of artificial neural networks containing a different number of input and hidden layers but all with a single output layer. Artificial neural networks with 7, 9, and 10 neurons in the input layer and various numbers of neurons in the hidden layer(s) were trained. The training process was performed through the mechanism of back-propagation[6]. After the training processes were completed, a separate test set containing 186 ECGs of atrial fibrillation and 284 ECGs of sinus rhythm with supraventricular extrasystoles or ventricular extrasystoles was then studied using the trained neural network.

Results

The results from the test set applied to networks with 7,10 and 9 input variables are shown in Table1-3 respectively. The artificial neural network with 9 input variables was found to be the best performing network. The 9 input variables for the optimal performance of the artificial neural network were as follows:

(1) PR interval variability;
(2) RR interval regularity;
(3) presence or absence of discrete P waves in the precordial leads;
(4) presence or absence of discrete P waves in the limb leads;

(5) presence or absence of multiple P waves;
(6) percentage regularity of RR interval;
(7) number of leads with definite P waves;
(8) Maximum PR interval;
(9) Minimum PR interval.

The effect of the varying design of the hidden layer(s) on the network with 9 input variables shown in Table 3. The artificial neural network with the best performance was found to be the network with 2 hidden layers each with 30 neurons. For the Glasgow program, sensitivity was 94.6% (176/186) and specificity was 98.6% (280/284); while for the artificial neural networks, sensitivity was 95.2% (177/186) and specificity was 96.5% (274/284).

Table 1. The effect of varying design of the hidden layers on the neural network with 7 input variables.

Input layers	Number of neurons in hidden layers	Output layers	Sensitivity %	Specificity %
7	20	1	86.0	98.3
7	30	1	89.2	96.5
7	40	1	88.7	97.6
7	20-20	1	82.3	98.3
7	30-30	1	88.2	97.9
7	30-30v2	1	90.3	98.3
7	40-40	1	86.6	98.6

Table 2. The effect of varying design of the hidden layers on the neural network with 10 input variables.

Input layers	Number of neurons in hidden layers	Output layers	Sensitivity %	Specficity %
10	20	1	86.6	98.3
10	30	1	87.1	95.8
10	40	1	85.5	95.8
10	20-20	1	87.6	98.6
10	30-30	1	84.9	97.6
10	30-30v2	1	83.9	99.3
10	40-40	1	87.1	98.3

Table 3. The effect of varying design of the hidden layers on the neural network with 9 input variables.

Input layers	Number of neurons in hidden layers	Output layers	Sensitivity %	Specificity %
9	5	1	96.8	94.4
9	10	1	97.3	94.0
9	15	1	93.5	94.4
9	20	1	96.2	94.4
9	30	1	97.3	94.7
9	40	1	97.3	91.9
9	5-5	1	96.2	94.7
9	10-10	1	94.6	96.1
9	15-15	1	95.2	94.7
9	20-20	1	94.6	94.0
9	20-20v2	1	93.0	95.8
9	30-30	1	95.2	96.5
9	30-30v2	1	95.2	96.1
9	40-40	1	93.0	95.4

Conclusion

The use of artificial neural networks seemed not to produce any noticeable improvement for the diagnosis of atrial fibrillation. It remains to determine whether application of artificial neural networks at a more specific point in the logic, or whether a combination of artificial neural networks with the original deterministic logic would bring enhanced benefit. This study is currently in progress.

References

1. M. Dunn, J. Alexander, R. de Silva, and F. Hildner,
Chest, **95** (1989) 118S- 127S.
2. W. B. Kannel, R. D. Abbott , D. D. Savage,and P. M. McNamara,
New England Journal of Medicine, **306** (1982) 1018-1022.
3. Cerebral Embolism Task Force.*Archive of Neurology*, **43** (1986) 71-84.
4. Cerebral Embolism Task Force.*Archive of Neurology*, **46** (1989) 727-743.
5. P. W. Macfarlane, B. Devine, S. Latif, S. McLaughlin, D. B. Shoat, and
M. P. Watts ,*Methods of Information in Medicine*,**29** (1990) 354 - 361.
6. B. Devine,*Neural Networks in Electrocardiography*
MSc thesis,University of Glasgow,1990.

A METHOD FOR IMPROVING THE REPEATABILITY OF AUTOMATED ECG ANALYSIS

STEPHANIE C. McLAUGHLIN
University Department of Medical Cardiology, Royal Infirmary, Glasgow, Scotland.

THOMAS C. AITCHISON
Department of Statistics, University of Glasgow, Glasgow, Scotland.

PETER W. MACFARLANE
University Department of Medical Cardiology, Royal Infirmary, Glasgow, Scotland.

ABSTRACT

This paper describes a method for improving the repeatability of the computer-assisted diagnosis of Left Ventricular Hypertrophy (using the Glasgow program) by the use of statistical smoothing techniques.

Computer-assisted interpretation of the ECG is a long established technique initiated by Caceres[1] in the early 1960s. The Glasgow program[2] has been developed continually since its inception in the early 1970s. However, one of the main drawbacks to the automated interpretation of the ECG is a lack of repeatability which can arise from day to day and even from minute to minute. In fact, Bailey et. al.[3] demonstrated that when the same digitised ECG tracing is split into two, one composed of the odd samples and the other the even samples, variation in interpretations can still be found.

The impetus behind the current study was therefore to attempt to improve the agreement in the computer diagnoses of Left Ventricular Hypertrophy from day to day using the Glasgow program applied to the same patients.

Consider the following two ECGs recorded on consecutive days from a 51 year old male being investigated for suspected valvular heart disease (Figure 1).

It can be seen that the diagnoses produced by the Glasgow program are inconsistent with no indication of LVH being reported on day 1 and probable LVH being diagnosed on day 2. Clearly this is an undesirable occurrence since the patient was in a stable condition. Methods which removed such discrepancies would therefore augment the technique.

The Glasgow program uses a point-scoring system to make a diagnosis of LVH. Various criteria are examined, with points being scored depending on whether an ECG measurement exceeds a specified threshold value or not. These points are then totalled to give an overall LVH score for diagnostic decision making. If this overall score ≥ 4 then LVH of some form or another is reported, i.e.

LVH Score ≤ 3 then No LVH
LVH Score $= 4$ then Possible LVH
LVH Score $= 5$ then Probable LVH
LVH Score ≥ 6 then Definite LVH

DAY 1 **DAY 2**

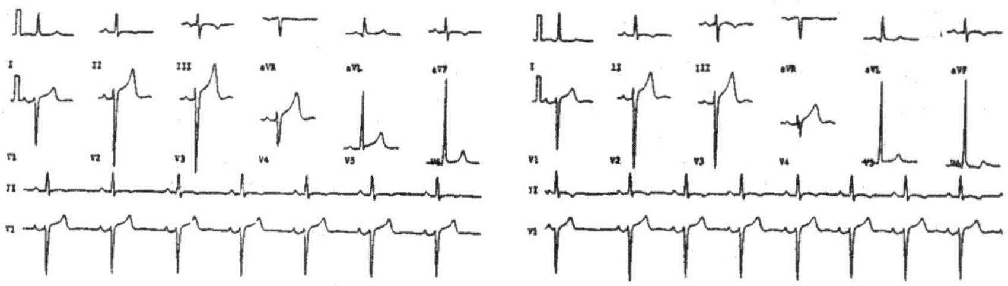

DAY 1

Anterolateral ST Elevation
MARKED ST ELEVATION - NON SPECIFIC
T wave changes in the inferior leads
APPEARANCES ARE BORDERLINE ABNORMAL AND
ARE POSSIBLY DUE TO MYOCARDIAL ISCHAEMIA

DAY 2

Broad P waves
CONSIDER LEFT ATRIAL ABNORMALITY
High praecordial voltages
Abnormally high SV1+RV5
PROBABLE LEFT VENTRICULAR HYPERTROPHY
T wave changes in the inferior leads
APPEARANCES ARE BORDERLINE ABNORMAL AND
ARE POSSIBLY DUE TO MYOCARDIAL ISCHAEMIA

Figure 1 Day 1 and Day 2 ECG recordings from a 51 year old male.

Many of the upper limits of normal for the ECG voltage measurements are categorised according to age and are in the form of step-functions with different limits applying to each age category. The nature of these limits may contribute to a lack of repeatability if, for example, a patient's age category alters from one recording to another but the ECG measurement under consideration does not change significantly. Replacing these discrete limits with equations which change smoothly and continuously throughout the age range will help alleviate the problem of inconsistent diagnoses arising as a direct result of this situation.

A further contributory factor to a lack of repeatability is the situation whereby measurements lying close to, but below, a threshold value will contribute 0 points to a final diagnosis of LVH whereas measurements lying close to, but above will score K points (in the general case), i.e.

$$S(x) = \begin{cases} K & \text{if } x \geq b \\ 0 & \text{if } x < b \end{cases}$$

Again, it is easy to see that conflicting scores may be recorded by ECG measurements x which are not significantly different from each other but still cause the threshold value b to be crossed.

An appealing solution to this problem is to replace this discrete form of score function with a smoothed version which will gradually increase from 0 to K. This new score function $S_m^*(x)$ was developed using the logistic cumulative distribution function as a basis, and knowledge of the amount of day-to-day variation in the relevant ECG measurements provided a guide to the rate of increase of the function. Both score functions can be seen in Figure 2.

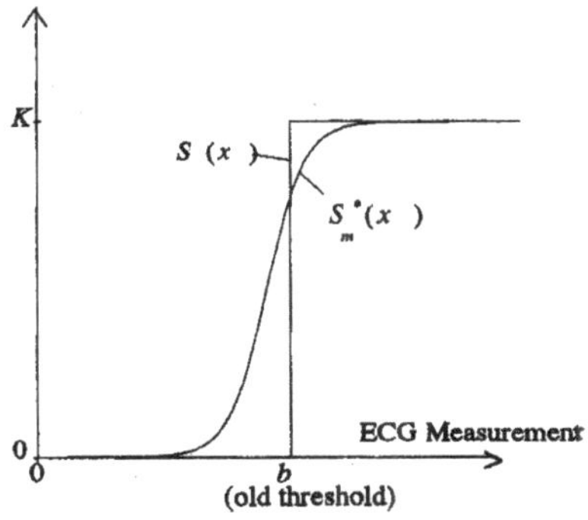

Figure 2 Comparison of the new and the old score functions

The new function has essentially smoothed out the sharp corners of the discrete step function and ensures that similar measurements receive comparable scores, even when close to the boundary value.

An algebra of score construction was then developed which allowed various combinations of criteria to be catered for, involving union, intersection, maxima, etc. For example, making use of some basic algebraic rules, it was possible to calculate a new smooth score function for the identification of an abnormal P terminal force which, in the Glasgow program, relies on the amplitude of the P wave in lead V1 being more negative than -110μV and the duration being longer than 40msecs.

Smooth scores were calculated for each of the six criteria involved in the point-scoring system for the identification of LVH. These were in turn totalled to provide an overall LVH score. A cutpoint was required in order to separate those who will be diagnosed as having LVH from those who will not. A receiver operating characteristic curve (ROC curve) was constructed using a database of 84 clinically documented LVH cases and 136 non-LVH cases where a diagnosis of LVH was made on the basis of an M-mode echocardiogram, comparing the indexed left ventricular mass to critical values for males and females.

The optimal point on the ROC curve is that point which lies closest to the origin, minimising the percentage of false positives and the percentage of false negatives simultaneously. In this case, a score of 3.5 appears to be the best separating point.

A comparison of both sensitivity and specificity using McNemar's test revealed that there were no significant differences between the old and the new versions of the Glasgow program so that it was now possible to proceed and compare the repeatability of the computer diagnosis of LVH from day to day.

The repeatability of each method was assessed using a database of 250 day 1 and day 2 ECGs which were recorded at least 24 hours apart using no standardising procedures. The patients were being investigated for suspected ischæmic or valvular heart disease and were considered to be stable.

Table 1 illustrates that when the conventional Glasgow program was used there were 13 individuals who were diagnosed as having no LVH on one occasion and LVH of some form or another on another day. However, using the smoothing techniques produces only 5 inconsistent diagnoses from day to day (see Table 2).

Table 1 Repeatability of conventional program

		DAY1	
		NO	YES
DAY2	NO	207	13
	YES		30

Table 2 Repeatability of modified program

		DAY1	
		NO	YES
DAY2	NO	212	5
	YES		33

It was also of interest to establish the relative seriousness of the discrepancies from day to day given that a day 1 diagnosis of no LVH followed by one of possible LVH might be more acceptable than no LVH followed by definite LVH.

A simple index of repeatability was calculated for each method, assigning weights of 0 for those individuals whose day 1 and day 2 diagnoses were completely in agreement, weights of 3 for all those exhibiting a discrepancy of 3 categories (i.e. No LVH followed by definite LVH) and intermediate weights of 1 and 2 to each pair demonstrating discrepancies of 1 and 2 categories respectively. The lower this index, the more repeatable is the method of diagnosis. The conventional method produces a 'Repeatability Index' of 41, which falls to 15 when the modified version is used.

In conclusion smoothing techniques have been implemented successfully with the effect of improving the repeatability of the LVH diagnosis in the Glasgow program by 63%.

References

1. C. A. Caceres, *Archives of Internal Medicine* **111** (1963) 114.
2. P. W. Macfarlane, *Cardiovascular Research* **5** (1971) 141.
3. J. J. Bailey, S. B. Iscoitz, J. W. Hirshfield, L. E. Grauer and M. Horton, *Circulation* **50** (1974) 73.

A Study of Right Ventricular Hypertrophy in the Patients with Chronic Obstructive Lung Disease Compared with Electrocardiogram and Ultrafast Computed Tomography

Fumitake Inomata
The Department of Cardiology
Kikuna Memorial Hospital
4 – 4 – 27, Kikuna, Kohoku – ku, Yokohama – shi,
Kanagawa – ken, 222, JAPAN

Abstract

I evaluated diastolic volume and weights of right and left ventricule using ultrafast computed tomography (UFCT), and compared with electrocardiographic (ECG) diagnostic criteria of cor pulmonale (CP) and right ventricular hypertrophy (RVH)in the patients (pts) with chronic obstructive lung disease (COLD) and healthy adults.

28 persons were performed ECG – triggered and enhanced UFCT;13 healthy adults and 15 COLD pts without organic heart disease and hypertensive heart disease.

Results: The ratio of the left ventricular to the right ventricular weight (LVW/RVW) in healthy adults and pts with COLD were as follows;(5.1 ± 1.5 vs 3.8 ± 1.3, respectively, $p<0.05$). There were no satisfaction of ECG diagnostic criteria of CP and RVH in neither group, but there were smaller value in sv5 and sv6, and larger volume R/Sv6 in COLD group respectively.

Conclusion: 1) Pts with COLD have lower value of ratio of LVW/RVW significantly before satisfactin of ECG criteria of CP and RVH. 2) It is useful to consider latent CP using above lowere ratio as a parameter. 3) ECG criteria emphasize in alteration in R/S ratio and S amplitude than axis that may be obscured in pts with possibility of reflection of early treatment with right ventricular hypertrophy in the pts with COLD by UFCT than ECG.

The WHO definition of cor pulmonale:"right ventricular hypertrophy as a result of disease which affect the structure or function of the lung" is a pathological definition that has not found favor clinically, since measurement of right ventricular hypertrophy in life is difficult. Ultrafast computed tomography (UFCT) is suitable for to take photography to the heart because of multi – tomographic computed graphics by 50 msec. And it is capable to calculate cardiac volume and weight to use UFCT.

I evaluated diastolic volume and weight of right and left ventricule using UFCT. The purpose of this study is the comparison of these volume and weight and electrocardiographic criteria of cor polumonale (CP) between healthy adults and the patients with Chronic Obstructive lung disease (COLD).

Patient selection

13 healthy adults and 15 COLD pts without organic heart disease and hypertensive heart disease were examined. The pts with COLD were diagnosed clinically and have $FEV_{1.0}\%$ below 70%. In healthy adults, 8 male and 5 female, age was from 26 to 76 years old, mean age: 58.0 years old. In the pts with COLD, 11 male and 4 female, age was from 41 to 88 years old, mean age :69.3 years old.

Method

UFCT(Imatrou C – 100) was used to the pts at supine position putted on ECG. ECG – triggered acanning enhanced film, at the time of diastolic phase, was took and coverd with overall the whole heart by 100msec photographic time on each 1 to 2 beat by using non – inonic contrast medium from 1 to 2 ml per second intravenously. I traced 8 to 20 left and right ventricular silhoettes manually. Left and right ventriular volume were calculated from sum of these traced data. And left and right ventricular weight were calculated from sum of left and right ventricular free wall data as same method of ventricular volume. I calculated the ratio of Left ventricular weght/right ventricular weight. And calculated P_{max}, R/S_{v5}, R/S_{v6}, S_{v5}, S_{v6} and axis from 12 lead ECG.

Results: Table

Conclusion

1) Pts with COLD have lower value of ratio of LVW/RVW significantly before satisfaction of ECG criteria of CP

and RVH.
2) It is useful to carsider latent CP using above lower ratio as a parameter.
3) ECG criteria emphasize in alteration in R/S ratio and S amplitude than axis that may be obscured in pts with possibility of reflection of early treatment with RVH in the pts with COLD by UFCT than ECG.

Table

Results

	Healthy	COLD	
LV volume	113.6 ± 28.9	98.7 ± 24.7	
LV weight	92.2 ± 19.3	85.6 ± 24.4	
RV volume	111.9 ± 21.3	108.0 ± 24.0	
RV weight	19.0 ± 6.0	25.5 ± 14.6	
LVW/RVW	5.1 ± 1.5	3.8 ± 1.3	*4
Pmax	1.3 ± 0.5	1.5 ± 0.9	
R/S_{V5}	4.6 ± 5.2	5.4 ± 3.6	
R/S_{V6}	3.4 ± 2.0	10.5 ± 5.8	*1
S_{V5}	6.3 ± 4.0	3.7 ± 1.9	*2
S_{V6}	2.7 ± 0.9	1.3 ± 0.4	*3
Axis	37.7 ± 67.0	50.2 ± 35.0	

*1 $P<0.02$ *2 $P<0.01$

*3 $P<0.001$ *4 $P<0.05$

Reference
1) WHO: Chronic cor pulumonale. A report of the expert committee. Circulation 27:594, 1933.
2) Reiter S. J. et al: Circulation 74:890, 1986
3) Furray S.A. et al: Am. Heart J. 107:404, 1984.

SIGNIFICANCE OF ELECTROCARDIOGRAPHICAL ASPECTS DURING CHEST COMPRESSION IN PATIENTS WITH CARDIAC ARREST.
THE MECHANOELECTRICAL FEEDBACK DURING CARDIOPULMONARY RESUSCITATION

C.Carp, Carmen Ginghina, Doina Rogozea, Ioana Stoian,
Romanian Institute of Cardiology, Fundeni Hospital, Fundeni-Way,258, Bucharest, Romania.

ABSTRACT

The electrocardiographical aspect induced by mechanoelectrical feedback activity during chest compression was studied in 56 patients (pts). The affections were: coronary heart disease with old or new myocardial infarction in 36 pts, valvular heart disease in 8 pts, dilated cardiomyopathy in 3 pts and congenital heart disease in 2 pts. Chest compression was applied during cardiac arrest or slow ventricular rhythm. The electrical activity of the heart was monitored during cardiopulmonary resuscitation with chest compression. We noticed of the beginning of the chest compre -sion two types of electrical aspects :

1) distinct QRS complex, nearrow or wide in 8 pts.
2) wide wave without distinct QRS complex wave and T wave.

Both electrical aspects were isolated or associated with slow idioventricular activity. The presence of type one coresponded to an early cardiopulmonary resuscitation to a better anterior cardiac function and a more favourable response with cardiac recovery. The presence of type two showed a poor response to cardiopulmonary resuscitation. Type two with large wave slowely decrease in amplitude with increasing in wide and finaly absence of electrical activity in pts. with not favourable response.
In conclusion, we noticed two types of electrical activity of the heart during chest compression by mechanoelectrical feedback with different prognosis.

Acute coronary occlusion clinicaly and experimentaly is accompanied by ST segment elevation and acute local ventricular bulging. The question was that this association is coincidental or causal (1). Using an experimental model we demonstrated a relationship between systolic expansion during myocardial injury and increase of ST segment elevation (2,3). The notion that mechanical dilatation influence the electrical activity by mechanoelectrical feedback was established experimentaly (Lab.). The existence of stretch-activated ion channels was reported in neonatal rat myocytes. (4) and was demonstrated that diastolic stretch induces arrhythmias (5). We consider that chest compression during cardiopulmonary resuscitation induce not only an mechanical vitae organ perfusion but also an electrical heart activity by a mechanoelectrical feedback acti--vity. The aim of the present study was to investigate the significan -ce of the electrocardiographical aspect during chest compression in patients with cardiac arrest. We have evaluated specific effects :

1. The morphology of the electrical heart activity induced by the chest compression during cardiopulmonary resuscitation.
2. The principal electrocardiographical aspect of the QRS complex induced by mechaelectrical mechanism.
3. The evolution of the morphology of QRS complex aspects during car -diopulmonary resuscitation .
4. The relation between QRS complex wave aspects, the evolution of the morphology of QRS complex and prognosis.

Patients and Methods.

We have studied 56 patients, 36 male and 17 females. The affections present was :

old or new myocardial infarction	36 pts.
valvular heart disease	8 pts
complete A-V block	7 pts
Dilated cardiomyopathy	3 pts
Congenital heart disease	2 pts

Cardiac arrest was present in all patients. The chest compression was applied during cardiopulmonary resuscitation for cardiac arrest following events: electrical shock for ventricular fibrillation, asystole or very slow rhythm in complete A-V block, primary asystole or the descendent arrest of sinus and A-V node and finale cardiac asystole. The electrical heart activity during cardiopulmonary resuscitation and chest compression was monitored and registered.

RESULTS.

A. We noticed of the beginning of the chest compression the principal types of electrical QRS wave morphology :

1. Distinct, narrow or wide QRS complex in 8 pts. (Fig. 1, Fig. 2).

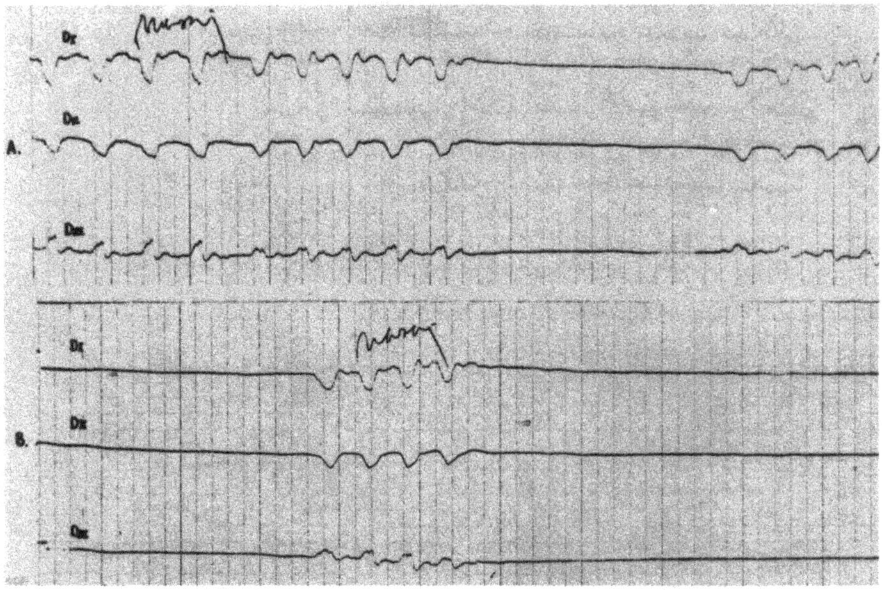

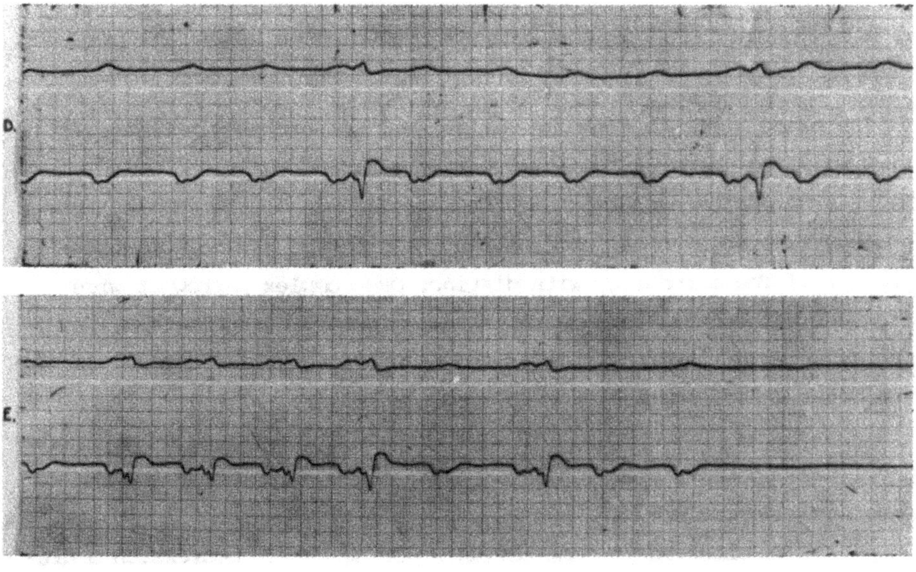

2. Wide wave without distinct QRS complex and T wave in 33 pts.(Fig 3

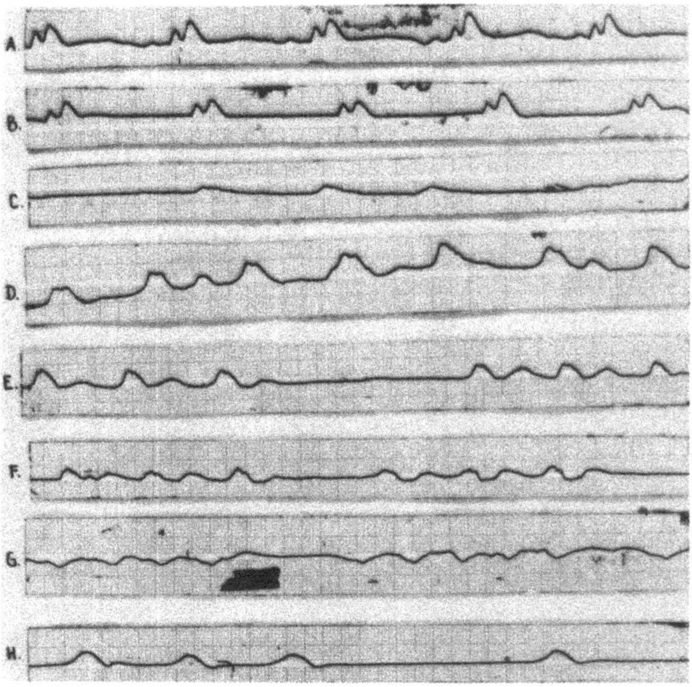

3. Both distinct QRS complex and wide indistinctly wave in 8 pts.(Fig. 4).

4. The association in the same patients of the mechanoelectrical activity with the proper idioventricular rhythm.

B. We studied the evolution and the significance of the QRS wave morphology induced by chest compression. We observed the following aspects : 1) The morphology with distinct QRS complex narrow or wide frequent coresponded to an early cardiopulmonary resuscitation, to a better anterior cardiac function and a more favourable response during and after chest compression with cardiac recovery.

2) The presence of wide wave without distinct QRS complex wave and T wave showed a poor response to the chest compression and the resuscitation procedure.

3) We observed in some patients during chest compression a gra-

dually decrease of amplitude and increase in width of QRS complex. These patients also have an unfourable evolution.

Fig. 4. Patient SP: Wide waves without distinct QRS complex wave and T wave intermitent idioventricular rhythm induced by the chest compression

A.

B.

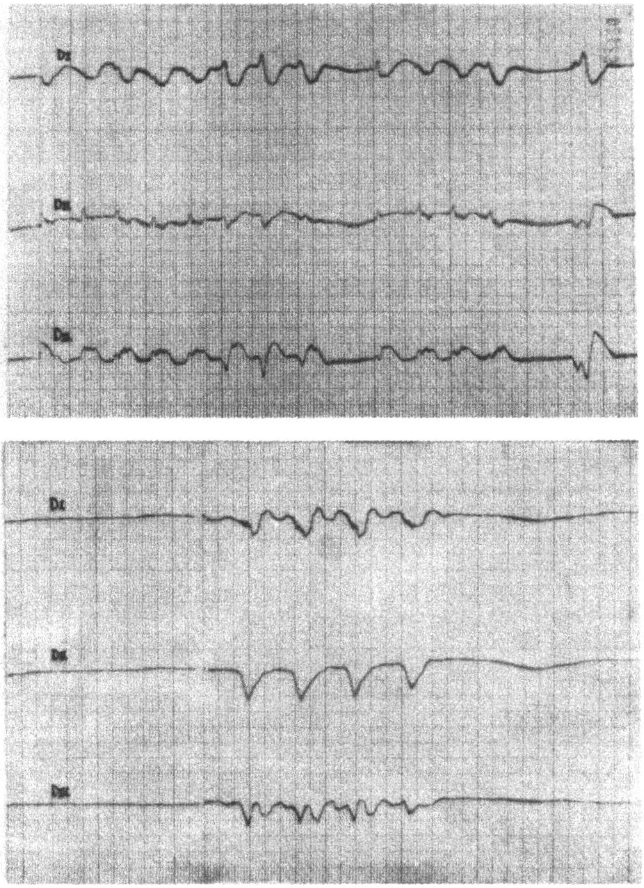

DISCUSSION

The influence of myocardial contractility on electrical heart activity was studied before in different way.
Using an experimental model was establiseh a cause to effect realationship between systolic expandion during myocardial injury and increase of ST segment elevation (2).
The hypothesis that diastolic strech induces arrhythmias was proved (Hansen) and also that the mechanical dilatation can influence the electrical activity of the heart by mechanoelectrical feedback(5).
The demonstration recently of the existance of stretch-activated channe-ls (4) offered the mechanism of the electrical activity induced by chest compression during cardiopulmonary resuscitation. In our study we observed during chest compression different aspects of electrical activity. We described two principal types of QRS complex. The first type coredpond to an distinct QRS complex narrow or with wide aspect. This aspect was observed at beginning of the cardiac arrest or in the patients with some response to the cardiopulmonary resuscitation.
We consider this type of the electrical response because proved the posibility of recovery.
The second type with very large and indistinctly QRS complex corespond to the late cardiopulmonary resuscitation with poor prognosis. The situation appear during the chest compression the QRS complex gradually become small or increase in width. We consider the patient have an identical poor prognosis.
During the chest compression with mechanoelectrical activity in some patients appear a spontaneously ventricular rhythm and then sinus rhythm is established. It is demonstrated in this situation that myocar-dial stretch can induced ectopic beats (5), idioventricular rhythm and probably by keeping the mechanical cardiac activity appear sinus rhythm.
We conclude from this study :

1. The chest compression during cardiopulmonary resuscitation induced two principal types of QRS complex.
2. The mechanoelectrical activity can be correlated with the evolution and prognosis of the patients.
3. The presence of wide and not distinct QRS complex showed a poor response to the resuscitation procedure.
4. The unfavourable evolution is observed with wide and decreased amplitude of QRS complex during chest compression.

References

Braunwald E., Maroko P.P., Causes of the ST-segment (the authors' repy).Circulation 1977, 56, 499.

Carp C., The Relationship between Electrical Activity and Myocardial Contractility Following Acute Coronary Occlusion., Rev.Roum Med. 1979,17,3,245.

Carp C.I., Causes of the ST segment elevation ,Circulation 1977, 56, 498.
Lab M.J.Contraction-excitation feedback in myocardium,Circ.Res.1982 5o,756.

Craelius W.,Chen V., El-Sherif N., Stretch activated ion channels in ventricular myocytes. Biosci.Rep.1988, 8, 4o7.

Hansen D.E., Craig S.C., Handeghem L.M., Stretch-Induced Arrhythmias in the isolated canine Ventricle. Evidence for the Importance of Mechanoelectrical Feedback. Circulation 199o, 81,3,1o94.

VECTORCARDIOGRAPHIC AND ECHOCARDIOGRAPHIC STUDY IN PATIENTS WITH THALASSEMIA MAJOR

Tedesco MA, MD, Ratti G, MD, Iarussi D, MD, Gualtieri S, MD, Irace L, MD, Romano A, MD, Guadagno I, MD, Coppolino P, MD, Iacono A, MD

Cardiology, Ist Medical School, University of Naples, Italy

Abstract

This work try to assess the correlation between the presence of VCG bites and echocardiographic parameters of left ventricular morphology and function in patients with thalassemia major. 30 patients with thalassemia major were studied. The patients with VCG bites (20%) showed also a significant alteration of echocardiographic parameters. No echocardiographic modifications were present in patients without bites. Therefore VCG could be an useful method to assess the presence of myocardial involvment in thalassemic patients.

Introduction

Cardiac haemosiderosis is still a complication of repeated transfusions used in the therapy of anemia secondary to thalassemia major (TM). Although iron chelation therapy with deferoxamine has been introduced to prevent myocardial fibrosis, this aspect is very frequent in thalassemic patients. Vectorcardiography (VCG) could be used to detect the myocardial fibrosis through the presence of VCG-bites, as already proved in diabetes and myocardial infarction (1-4). Aim of this study was to asses the correlation between the VCG bites and left ventricular morphology obtained through M-mode and 2-D echocardiographic technique in patients (pts) with homozigous TM.

Methods

Selection of patients

30 pts (mean age 12.8 yrs) with TM, in absence of cardiac symptoms or clinically apparent heart disease using standard transfusional therapy (every 4 weeks, with mean haemoglobin level between 10.5 and 13.5 g/dl) and iron chelation therapy (deferoxamine dosages ranged at 25-40

mg/kg body wt/day subcutaneously) were studied (group A). 33 normal subjects, age-matched (mean age 13.6 yrs) were used as a control group (group B).

Vectorcardiography
All the subjects were examinated by VCG (Mx 1000 r3.2 Peretti) according to Frank's method and the following parameters were considered: morphology, lenght, direction of the QRS-loop on the three classic planes (orizzontal, saggittal and frontal plane). Moreover the bite was identified as an indentation of QRS-loop with an amplitude more than 0.15 mV and a duration egual or more than 10 msec on at least two of the three planes considered (5).

Echocardiography
The pts with TM and normal controls underwent to echocardiographic examination with an Acuson MPX/3 device equipped with 3.5 Mhz transducer while patient recumbent in left lateral position.M-mode echocardiograms were derived from the 2-D images and the following parameters were considered: left ventricular end diastolic diameter (LVEDD), left ventricular end systolic diameter (LVESD), interventricular septum thickness (IVST), left ventricular posterior wall thickness (LVPWT), fractional shortening (FS) according to the reccomendation of the American Society of Echocardiography (6). Left ventricular mass was calculated with the formula of Devereux (7)

Statistical analysis
Data are expressed as mean values ± SD; mean differences were analyzed by using the unpaired Student's T test. Echocardiographic data exceeding the 95% were considered as abnormal values on a confidence interval basis taken out of the control group.

Results
The clinical characteristics of the groups are shown in table I: no statistically significant difference was found in age, sex distribution and body mass index.

Table I

	A1	A2	B	p
Age (yrs)	16 ± 6	13 ± 6	13 ± 5	ns
Sex	4M/2F	14M/10F	20M/13F	
BMI (m^2)	1.2±0.4	1.4±0.6	1.3±0.5	ns

The group A1, with VCG bites, was consisted of 6 (20%) pts, the group A2, without VCG bites, was formed by 24 pts (80%). Left ventricular hypertrophy occurred in 4 pts of the group A1. No other modification of VCG loop was found in the group A2.
The 6 pts of group A1 showed also a significant increase of the following echocardiographic parameters: IVST in 4 pts, LVEDD in 3 pts, LVESD in 2 pts, LVPWT and cardiac mass in all. Further on, the %FS was normal in every one.
The control group did not show any VCG modification or echocardiogrphic parameters.

Discussion

Thalassemia major is an inborn errorr of haemoglobin synthesis which results in an absence of ß-chain. Clinical manifestations are severe anemia and very active, however inefficacious, haerythropoiesis. Therefore repeated transfusions are needed to maintain life. This therapeutic approach, in addition to increased gastrointestinal absorption causes a cardiac haemosiderosis that appear after few years of therapy (3-4 yrs) (8).
Cardiac complications (as congestive heart failure and arrhytmias) develop during second or third decade of life; the time of developing these cardiac complications is slightly longer in the pts subject to a complete transfusional-chelation therapy with deferoxamine.
At anatomopathological observation the heart shows atrial and ventricular dilatation, ventricular wall thickening, cardiac mass increase, heavy fibrosis of the myocardium and of the conduction system (8).
VCG could be used to detect loop modifications in these patients and could also improve sensibility to detect the presence of fibrosis with the checking of VCG-bites, that are indentations of QRS-Loop with an amplitude more than 0.15 mV and a duration equal or more than 10 msec. To be more specific we included only bites that are present on at least two planes of VCG examination and we found echocardiographicc alterations in all patients with VCG-bites and no modifications in those without. Therefore we can suppose that in patients with cardiac mass increase also a variable degree of fibrosis could be present and this could be of bad prognostic significance for the developing of congestive heart failure.
Although prospective studies are needed to verify this hypothesis from our data it can be desumed that:
- myocardial damage is still a complication in pts with TM, even iron chelation therapy;
- VCG could be an useful and an unexpensive method to assess the presence of myocardial involvment in these patients.

References

1. Selvester RH, Rubin HB, Hamlin JA, Pote WW: New quantitative

vectorcardiographic criteria for the detection of unsuspected myocardial infarction in diabetics. Am Heart J 75, 1968, 335

2. RIff ER, Riff KM: Abnormalities of myocardial depolarization in overt, subclinical and prediabetes: a vectorcardiographic study. Diabetes 23, 1974, 572

3. Zoneraich O, Zoneraich S: A vectorcardiographic study of spatial P, QRS and T loops in diabetic patients without clinically apparent heart disease. J Electrocardiol 10, 1977, 207

4. Tedesco MA, Irace L, Iarussi D, Langella S, Elettrico C, Coppolino P, Russo R, Iacono A: Correlazione tra bites vettorcardiografici e funzione miocardica regionale in pazienti con diabete mellito tipo I. Cardiologia, 36, 1991, 120

5. Ebenbrandt L, Ek A, Lundh B, Pahlm O: Vectorcardiographic bites. J Electrocardiol 22, 1989, 325

6. Sahn DJ, De Maria A, Kisslo J, Weyman A: The Committee on M-Mode standardization of the American society of echocardiography: reccomendations regarding quantitation in M-Mode echocardiography:results of a survey of echocardiographic measurements. Circulation 58, 1978, 1072

7. Devereux RB, Alonso DR, Lutas EM: Echocardiographic assessment of left ventricular hypertrophy: comparation with necropsy findings. Am J Cardiol 57, 1986, 450

8. Engle MA: Cardiac involvement in Cooley's anemia. Ann NY Acad Sci 119, 1969, 694

DOXORUBICIN CARDIOTOXICITY ASSESSED WITH VECTORCARDIOGRAPHIC AND ECHOCARDIOGRAPHIC TECHNIQUES

Tedesco MA, MD, Iarussi D, MD, Ratti G, MD, Gualtieri S, MD, Irace L, MD, Romano A, MD, Guadagno I, MD, Coppolino P, MD, Iacono A, MD

Cardiology, Ist Medical School, University of Naples, Italy

Abstract

This work studied the correlation through VCG-bites and left ventricular morphology and function in patients long after the ending of doxorubicin treatment. 24 patients (mean age 13 yrs) underwent to echocardiographic and vectorcardiographic examination. The patients with VCG-bites (25%) showed increase of LVEDD and LVESD and a decrease of %FS respect to a control group. VCG bites were detected only in patients receiving a high dosage of doxorubicin (>300 mg/m²). Therefore the presence of VCG bites is related to functional and morphological myocardial alterations detected by echocardiography.

Introduction

Doxorubicin (DXR) is a highly effective antineoplastic agent, but its use is limited by a cumulative dose-related cardiomyopathy (1-2). It can cause histomorphological changes: diffuse myocyte damage with marked cellular changes and frank necrosis, evolving to fibrosis. The vectorcardiogram (VCG) could be used to detect the myocardial fibrosis through the presence of VCG-bites, as already proved in diabetes, myocardial infarction and also in patients treated with adriamycin (3-7).

Aim of this study was to asssess the correlation between the VCG bites and left ventricular morphology and function with Echocardiography (ECHO) in patients (pts) long after the ending of anthracycline therapy.

Methods

Selection of patients

24 pts (mean age 13 yrs) with malignancies, 68±24 months after the ending of chemiotherapy (ET) were studied (group A), in absence of

cardiac symptoms or clinically apparent heart disease. 8 pts (33.7%) received a cumulative dose <300 mg/m² of DXR, 16 pts (66.3%) received a cumulative dose >300 mg/m² of DXR. 28 normal subjects age-matched (mean age 13.5 yrs) were studied as control group (group B).

Vectorcardiography
All the subjects were examinated by VCG (Mx 1000 r3.2 Peretti) according to Frank's method and the following parameters were considered: morphology, lenght, direction of the QRS-loop on the three classic planes (orizzontal, saggittal and frontal plane). Moreover the bite was identified as an indentation of QRS-loop with an amplitude more than 0.15 mV and a duration egual or more than 10 msec on at least two of the three planes considered (8).

Echocardiography
The pts with TM and normal controls underwent to echocardiographic examination with an Acuson MPX/3 device equipped with 3.5 Mhz transducer while patient recumbent in left lateral position. M-mode echocardiograms were derived from the 2-D images and the following parameters were considered: left ventricular end diastolic diameter (LVEDD), left ventricular end systolic diameter (LVESD), interventricular septum thickness (IVST), left ventricular posterior wall thickness (LVPWT), fractional shortening (FS) according to the reccomendation of the American Society of Echocardiography (9). Left ventricular mass was calculated with the formula of Devereux (10).

Statistical analysis
Data are expressed as mean values ± SD; mean differences were analyzed by using the unpaired Student's T test. Echocardiographic data exceeding the 95% were considered as abnormal values on a confidence interval basis taken out of the control group.

Results
The clinical characteristics of the groups are shown in table I: no statistically significant difference was found in age, sex distribution and body mass index.

	A1	A2	B	p
Age (yrs)	14 ± 3	13 ± 4	13 ± 5	ns
Sex	5M/1F	12M/6F	18M/10F	
BMI (m²)	1.1 ± 0.3	1.3 ± 0.5	1.3 ± 0.5	ns
ET (months)	67 ± 11	69 ± 14	--	ns

The group A1, with VCG bites, was consisted of 6 (25%) pts, the group A2, without VCG bites, was formed by 18 pts (75%). No other modification of VCG loop was found in the group A2.
The 6 pts of group A1 showed the increase of the following echocardiographic parameters: LVEDD in 2 pts, LVESD in 4 pts. There was a decrease in %FS (<28%) in 3 pts, while IVST, LVPWT and cardiac mass were normal in every one. The VCG bites presence was found only in pts using high dose of DXR (>300 mg/m²). The group B did not show any VCG or ECHO alteration.

Discussion

Our study demonstrate the presence of the VCG bites in 6 pts with high dose of DXR treatment. Further on, ECHO shows an increase of LVEDD and/or LVESD, expression of ventricular dilatation in the same pts. The systolic function was reduced in 3 of them, as demonstrated by the decrease in %FS.
In conclusion:
- myocardial damage is a complication of the high dose DXR treatment;
- VCG could be an useful method to assess the presence of myocardial fibrosis;
- VCG bites are correlated to morphological and functional alterations detected by ECHO.

References

1. Bristow MR, Mason JW, Billingham ME, Daniels JR: Dose effect and structure-function relationship in doxorubicin cardiomyopathy. Am Heart J 102, 1981, 709

2. Pisacane C, Iarussi D, Buono S, Gualtieri S, Coppolino P, Iacono A: Utilità clinica dell'analisi ecocardiografica bidimensionale quantitativa della cinesi segmentaria del ventricolo sinistro nel monitoraggio dei pazienti neoplastici trattati con antracicline. G Ital Cardiol 21, 1991, 1259

3. Selvester RH, Rubin HB, Hamlin JA, Pote WW: New quantitative vectorcardiographic criteria for the detection of unsuspected myocardial infarction in diabetics. Am Heart J 75, 1968, 335

4. RIff ER, Riff KM: Abnormalities of myocardial depolarization in overt, subclinical and prediabetes: a vectorcardiographic study. Diabetes 23, 1974, 572

5. Zoneraich O, Zoneraich S: A vectorcardiographic study of spatial P, QRS and T loops in diabetic patients without clinically apparent heart disease. J Electrocardiol 10, 1977, 207

6. Tedesco MA, Irace L, Iarussi D, Langella S, Elettrico C, Coppolino

P, Russo R, Iacono A: Correlazione tra bites vettorcardiografici e funzione miocardica regionale in pazienti con diabete mellito tipo I. Cardiologia 36, 1991, 120

7. Vitolo E, Madoi S, Colli AM: The meaning of bites on the vectorcardiogram: study in adriamycin cardiomyopathy. J Electrocardiol 15, 1982, 265

8. Ebenbrandt L, Ek A, Lundh B, Pahlm O: Vectorcardiographic bites. J Electrocardiol 22, 1989, 325

9. Sahn DJ, De Maria A, Kisslo J, Weyman A: The Committee on M-Mode standardization of the American society of echocardiography: reccomendations regarding quantitation in M-Mode echocardiography:results of a survey of echocardiographic measurements. Circulation 58, 1978, 1072

10. Devereux RB, Alonso DR, Lutas EM: Echocardiographic assessment of left ventricular hypertrophy: comparation with necropsy findings. Am J Cardiol 57, 1986, 450

A NEW ELECTROCARDIOGRAPHIC SIGN TO DETECT LATERAL MYOCARDIAL INFARCTION. ECHOCARDIOGRAPHIC CORRELATION

CABRERA-SOLE R; DOMINGUEZ P; AGUILERA M; SIQUIER J; PURAS A.
Department of Cardiology.General Hospital of Albacete.Albacete. Spain.

ABSTRACT

To evalue the electrocardiographic characteristics of the anterior myocardial infarction (anMI) and to compare them with those of anterolateral myocardial infarction (alMI),we prospectively studied 110 patients (P),who were admitted in the hospital with proved diagnosis of acute myocardial infarction.All of them underwent to an echocardiographic study in order to evalue the left ventricular segmentary contrac tion and according to it,the P were divided in two groups: 64 P with anMI and 46 P with alMI.After this,we analyzed a standard electrocardiogram which was done at 7.3 ∓ 3 days following the infarction.The results showed that Q-QS waves in V1 to V4 leads were present in 62 P with anMI and in 41 P with alMI (not significant),but,Q wave in V5-V6 were in 2 P with anMI and in 20 P with alMI ($p < 0.001$), Q waves in lead I were present in 5 P with anMI and in 17 P with alMI ($p < 0.001$) and Q in aVL were in 3 P with anMI and in 8 P with alMI ($p < 0.05$).With respect to T wave,we found negative T wave in lead I in 9 P with anMI and in 26 P with alMI ($p < 0.01$),in aVL were in 7 P with anMI and in 27 P with alMI ($p < 0.001$),and in leads V5-V6 in 17 P with anMI and in 22 P with alMI ($p < 0.05$).Finally,positive T wave in aVR we found in 43 P with alMI and not one in anMI group.We can conclude that presence of positive T wave in the context of myocardial infarction is a useful signs,without previous description,to detect lateral affectation of left ventricle and joined to another classical signs for alMI,improve the possibility to identify this localization of infarction.

INTRODUCTION

Some times,lateral myocardial infarction is very difficult to detect,overall if it is accompaning an anterior myocardial infarction,because the classical signs of anterolateral myocardial infarction (alMI)[1] are overlaped by those of anterior myocardial infarction (anMI)[2].
At first hours of anMI which has lateral extention it is possible to see an elevation of ST segment in I,aVL,V5 and V6 leads,accompaning the classical signs of the anMI,but,after some days of infarction,ST return to baseline situation,then,there are difficulties to see,examining the electrocardiogram,if there really was an lateral extention.In these cases an echocardiogram can solve the problem.Herein we present a study in which we compared the electrocardiogram of patients with anMI and those with alMI in order to find the differences,if there are,between them.

OBJECTIVE OF THE STUDY

To evalue the electrocardiographic differences between anMI and alMI.

MATERIAL AND METHODS

We have prospectively studied,110 patients (P),who were admitted in the hospital with proved diagnosis of acute myocardial infarction (MI).We excluded those patients who previously suffered another MI or P who died before complete their study.All of them submited to an intrahospital echocardiographic study,in order to evalue segmentary affectation of left ventricle,following the American Society of Echocardiography recommendations[3],and according to it,patients were divided in two groups:64 P with asynesia or severe hypokinesis of anterior and septal segments and 46 P with anterior,septal and lateral affectation.After this,we analyzed the standard electrocardiogram of each patients which were done at 7.3 ∓ 3 days after the infarction.Results are shown in the following table:

Data of ECG	anMI	alMI	p value
total patients	64	46	
- QS or Q V1-V4	62	41	NS
- Q in V5-V6	2	20	<0.001
- Q in I	5	17	<0.001
- Q in aVL	3	8	<0.05
- without Q	2	5	NS
- T (-) in I	9	26	<0.01
- T (-) in aVL	7	27	<0.001
- T (-) in V5-V6	17	22	<0.05
- T (+) in aVR	-	43	<0.001

DISCUSSION

One of the most valuable contributions of the ECG is in the diagnosis of myocardial infarction[6-7],and usually it is the first test performed in a patient with supicion of acute myocardial infarction.The technique is reliable,reproductible and can be used serially,being,properly interpreted,the cornestone of the diagnosis of myocardial infarction.The initial ECG is diagnostic of acute infarction in approximately 60% of the patients,abnormal but not diagnostic in 25% and normal in about 15%.Serial tracings increase the sensitivity to near 95%.The ECG changes of myocardial infarction are those of ischemia,injury and death and are,within certain limits,reflected by T-waves changes,ST segment displacement and the appearence of Q waves respectively[8].Such a clear-cut differentiation,although clinically useful,may be overly simplistic and some time artificial,because for example,T wave changes,may be due to ischemia,injury or death of muscle.Similarly, a Q wave may be due to another causes and not necessarily cellular death.However we must considerer that the diagnostic feature of myocardial infarction is the Q wave.

The classic evolution of acute myocardial infarction is documented in approximately two thirds of the patients,while in those remainig the infarct is manifested by ST segment,T wave,and non Q wave changes[9-10].

A precise anatomical location of anMI,based on ECG,is not always possible.Accuracy of such localization is influenced by different factors such as diameter of the chest,distance of the electrodes from the heart,between other,which varies considerably among individuals.So,on the basis of the presence of Q waves,an infarct is consedered septal when a Q wave is present in leads V1 and V2,anteroseptal when they are present in V1 to V4,inferior when present in leads II-III and aVF,high lateral when present in leads I-aVL,low lateral if there are Q waves in V5-V6 and anterolateral when present in leads I,aVL and V3 to V6[11].However,lateral infarction, some times is very difficult to detect because is overlap by anMI signs.In this study,we found that Q wave in V5-V6 leads were present in 2 P with anMI and in 20 P with alMI with a significant p value,but,Q waves in aVL,were present in 3 P of the first group and in 8 P of second group.This data is very important,because they say that Q waves in aVL,not always represent lateral myocardial infarction.On another hand,isolated lateral infarction is very difficult to find,and frecuently it is accompaning to an anterior infarction.In our study,QS waves in V1 to V4 were present in 62 of 64 P with anMI and in 41 of 46 P with alMI without significant differences between them.

When we analyzed T waves (see TABLE),we detected in aVR,a lead frecuently ignored,a curious sign:positive T waves were present in 43 patients with alMI and in not one of the anMI group.Normally, T waves are upright in all unipolar leads except in aVR in which are negative,for that,this sign could be useful,joined to another classical signs to identify lateral infarction.However,we must considerer that alterations in T waves do not have the same meanings of those of Q waves to detect infarction.

LIMITATIONS OF THIS STUDY

From our point of view,the patients included in this study could be not sufficient to fulfil the purpose of this study,and could be necessary more information about this subject.On another hand,we do not know if positive t wave in aVR is possible to find in another cardiac diseases different to those exposed here,because we did not considerer diseases like as hypertension,bundle branch blocks or valvular disease[3] in which there are some electrocardiographic alterations which can influence on T waves changes.Finally we saw this sign 7 days after infarction,being difficult to assign it some role in the acute phase of infarction.However,in the context of anterolateral myocardial infarction,this sign described before, and without previous reference in the literature,is useful to detect lateral infarction.

CONCLUSIONS

Lateral myocardial infarction is difficult to diagnosis and there are several signs to detect this infarction.We think that,to find positive T wave in aVR in the context of myocardial infarction can be useful to identify lateral affectation.

REFERENCES

1- W.J.Dunn;J.E.Edwards;R.D.Pruitt: The electrocardiogram in Infarction of Lateral Wall of the Left Ventricle. Circulation 14;1956.540.

2- J.A.Tullogh: The Electrocardiographic Features of High Posterolateral Myocardial Infarction. Brit Heart J 14;1952.379.

3- C.E.Cabrera and J.R.Monroy: Systolic and Diastolic loading of the Heart.Am Heart J 43;1952.661.

4- Report of the American Society Commitee on Nomenclature and Standards: Identification of Myocardial Wall Segments. November 1982.

5- W.D.Edwards;A.J.Tajik;J.B.Seward: Standardized Nomenclature and Anatomic Basis for Regional Tomographic Analysis of the Heart. Mayo Clinic Proc 56;1981.497.

6- F.N.Wilson;A.G.Mac Leod;P.S.Barker et al: The Electrocardiogram in Myocardial Infarction with Particular Reference to the Initial Deflection of the ventricular Complex. Heart 16;1933.155.

7- L.W.Klein;R.H.Helfant: The Q Wave and non Q Wave Myocardial Infarction: Difference and Similarities. Prog Cardiovasc Dis 29;1986.205.

8- R.Cabrera-Sole and J.Almendral in Semiologia Basica del Electrocardiograma,ed CEA.Madrid 1987.

9- H.Blanke;M.Cohen;G.V.Slueter et al: Electrocardiographic and Coronary Arteriographic Correlation during Acute Myocardial Infarction. Am J Cardiol 54;1984.249.

10- C.K. Friedberg and A.Zager: "Nonspecific" ST and T-wave changes.Circulation 23;1961.655.

11- B.Surawicz;H.Uhley;K.Borum et al:Tenth Bethesda Conference: Optimal Electrocardio graphy. Am J Cardiol 41;1978.130.

IS THE CENTRAL NERVOUS SYSTEM RESPONSIBLE FOR ST-T WAVE ABNORMALITIES IN THE ELECTROCARDIOGRAM OF ASYMPTOMATIC SUBJECTS?

ANGELOS G. ECONOMOU, ANDREAS N. FORTOS, LUIS I. CONSTANTINOU
Department of Cardiology, 4th Hospital of Social Security Foundation, Athens, Greece

ABSTRACT

To test the hypothesis that the central nervous system contributes to ST segment and T wave abnormalities in routine ECG of asymptomatic subjects two groups of cases were prospectively compared: Group A consisted of 35 consecutive asymptomatic subjects (10 men and 25 women, aged 51 ± 8 years) with ST-T changes without any evidence of organic or nervous system disease and group B consisted of 35 healthy subjects, serving as control, matched to A for age and sex with normal rest ECG. All studied cases conserned right-handed persons. Both groups underwent complete electroencephalographic study. The only discriminating parameter was found to be the relative lack of expected asymmetry of alpha rhythm in cases with ST-T changes (symmetry 65.7% in group A vs 34.3 in group B, $p<0.01$ and right dominance 25.7% in group A vs 65.4% in group B, $p<0.001$). It is concluded that asymptomatic subjects with ST-T changes in the resting ECG without organic heart or nervous system disease have a variant electroencephalographic pattern of alpha rhythm, probably a marker of a not explicitely defined influence of the central nervous system to the heart.

Introduction

The finding of ST segment and T wave repolarization abnormalities identical with myocardial ischaemic changes in routine electrocardiogram (ECG) of asymptomatic and apparently healthy people presents a difficult and socioeconomic problem, since their prevalence in general population is not so rare[1].

Also, ST-T wave changes, in association with various neurologic lesions have been known for more than three decades[2].

The aim of this study was to test the hypothesis that the central nervous system (CNS) contributes to the repolarization abnormalities in the resting ECG of asymptomatic subjects.

Subjects and Methods

In a prospective study two groups of right-handed asymptomatic subjects were compared: Group A consisted of 35 subjects (10 men and 25 women), aged 51±8 years with ST segment and T wave changes in resting ECG. Group B consisted of 35 healthy subjects, serving as controls, matched to A for age and sex, with normal rest ECG.

Organic cardiac or nervous system disease in both groups was ruled out by history, normal physical examination, X-rays, echo-studies and exercise electrocardiography (Bruce's protocol). Only cases with reversion of repolarization to normal and no pain after exercise were selected for group A.

Both groups underwent complete electroencephalographic (EEG) study including the measurements of frequency (cycles/sec), amplitude (μV), quantity (abudance), distribution as well as the symmetry over the two hemispheres of the alpha, beta, theta and rapid rhythms.

Results

The only discriminating parameter in the EEG study was found to be the relative lack of expected asymmetry of alpha rhythm, confined in cases with ST-T changes (Table 1).

On the other hand there was no difference concerning the various parameters of the other EEG-phic rhythms.

Table 1. Electroencephalographic characteristics of alpha rhythm.

	Group A (with ST-T changes)		Group B (with normal ECG)		P value
Frequency (cycles/sec)	10.84± 1.29		10.38± 1.15		NS
Amplitude (μV)	45.42±27.47		38.75±19.09		NS
Distribution	all cases posterior		all cases posterior		NS
Abudance	%	N	%	N	
high proportion	11.4	(4)	18.1	(6)	
average proportion	57.7	(20)	45.7	(16)	NS
small proportion	31.0	(11)	37.1	(13)	
Symmetry (concerning amplitude and distribution over the two hemispheres)	%	N	%	N	
symmetrical	65.7	(23)	34.3	(12)	<0.01
left dominance	8.5	(3)	0		NS
right dominance	25.7	(9)	65.7	(23)	<0.001

Discussion

The incidence of ST-T changes in the resting ECG of asymptomatic subjects has been variously reported. The prevalence of these changes in epidemiological studies ranges betwen 0.5% and 4%[1] and it is higher in athletes and negroes[3]. With regard to selected highly-trained groups the prevalence ranges between 4.1% and 18%[3].

The autonomic nature of these RA has been suggested by many workers[3,4]. Also, ST segment and T wave changes may be produced by CNS disease[2] and has been experimentally induced either by unilateral stimulation or by removal of stellate ganglia[5,6] or by brief or prolonged cardiac nerve stimulation[7] or catecholamine infusion[4]. Neurogenic ST segment and T wave changes have been attributed to localized changes in the duration of individual ventricular action potential[5].

EEGphic studies in asymptomatic subjects with ST-Twave changes have not been previously reported.

In the cases studied here the probability of coronary artery disease in the two groups was the same and very low because of the absence of history of angina and of the entirely negative maximal exercise testing[8]. Thus ST and T wave changes in group A could not be attributed to ischaemia.

The only discriminating parameter in the EEG study between the two groups was found to be the relative lack of the expected asymmetry (increase proportion of symmetry and diminished proportion of right hemisphere dominance) of alpha EEG rhythm, confined in cases with ST-T wave changes, though all studied cases concerned righ-handed persons. Usually in right-handed subjects alpha rhythm is of higher mean voltage and of wider distribution over the right hemisphere (smaller over the dominant hemisphere). It is believed that the characteristics of the alpha rhythm are genetically determined[7]. Thus cases with ST-T wave changes studied here may be associated to a CNS influence to the heart not explicitely defined. ST-T wave changes in rest ECG presumably are consequent to the inhomogeneity of ventricular repolarization due to the regionally altered autonomic tone in the myocardium, centrally-mediated. The variant pattern of alpha rhythm may be a marker or closely related to altered autonomic tone in the myocardium.

References

1. J. H. Atterhög, L. C. Ekelound, G. Ericsson and B. Ahlborg, *Upsal. J. Med.* **85** (1980) 125.
2. G. E. Burch, R. Meyers and J.A. Abildskov, *Circulation* **9** (1954) 719.
3. P. Zeppili, M.M. Pirrami, M. Sassara and R. Fenici, *Am. Heart. J.* **100** (1980) 213.
4. P. Taggart, M. Carruthers, E. Joseph, et al, *Br. Heart J.* **41** (1979) 214.
5. P. J. Shwartz, P. L. Verrier and B. Lown, *Cir. Res.* **40** (1977) 536.
6. F. Yanowitz, J.B. Preston and J. A. Abildskov, *Cir. Res.* **18** (1966) 416.
7. A. Abildskov, *Am. Heart J.* **92** (1976) 210.

8. G.A. Diamond and J. S. Forrester, *N. Engl. J. Med.* **300** (1979) 1350.
9. F.Vogl, *Electroenceph. Clin. Neurophysiol.* **19** (1965) 196.

IS THE HYPERADRENERGIC ACTIVITY RESPONSIBLE FOR REPOLARIZATION IN THE ELECTROCARDIOGRAM OF ASYMPTOMATIC SUBJECTS?

A.G.ECONOMOU, Th.KALFOGLOU, L.GEORGACOPOULOS, H.MANTZOURATOS

Department of Cardiology, 4th Hospital of Social Security Foundation, Athens, Greece

ABSTRACT

To test the hypothesis that hyperadrenergic activity is responsible for repolarization abnormalities in resting ECG of asymptomatic subjects two groups of cases were prospectively compared: Group A consisted of 35 asymptomatic subjects (10 men and 25 women, aged 51$\pm$8 years) with repolarization abnormalities without any clinical or instrumental evidence of organic heart disease and group B consisted of 35 healthy subjects, serving as controls, matched to group A for age and sex, with normal rest ECG. The comparative study comprised evaluation of cardiac adrenergic activity in basal condition using the indices: heart rate at rest, total electromechanical systole (QS_2), QT intervals, the QS_2/QT ratio, the ratio of preejection period to the left ventricular ejection time (PEP/QS_2). No differences were found, conserning the above indices, between the two groups. It is concluded that subjects with repolarization abnormalities in the resting ECG without evidence of organic heart disease do not exhibit any increase of adrenergic activity under basal condition.

Introduction

ST segment and T wave abnormalities in routine ECG of asymptomatic subjects without evidence of cardiopathies is not so so rare[1]. The precise physiologic mechanism responsible for these is obsure.

The aim of the study was to test the hypothesis that hyperadrenergic activity is responsible for these ECGphic changes.

Subjects and Methods

In a prospective study two groups of right-handed asymptomatic subjects were compared: Group A consisted of 35 subjects (10 men and 25 women), aged 51$\pm$8 years with ECGphic repolarization abnormalities in the rest ECG free of organic heart or nervous system disease. Group B consisted of 35 healthy subjects, serving as controls, matched to A for age and sex, with normal ECG. The exclusion of probability of organic condition in both groups was based on negative finding from the history, physical examination, X-rays, echo-investigation and exercise ECGphy (temporary reversion to normal of ST-T wave changes during or after the negative testing in group A). ST and T wave changes were defined as flat or inverted T waves in leads II, III, aVF and V_4 to 6 (n=19), deep T wave inversion particularly in leads V_2 to 6 (n=9) and minor ST segment depression in leads II, II, aVF and V_4 to 6 (n=7). Subjects with ST elevation due to early repolarization were not included. Maximal treadmill exercise testing was conducted using symptoms limited Bruce's protocol. The comparative study comprise evaluation of cardiac adrenergic activity in basal condition using the indices: 1) Heart rate (HR) at rest, 2) Total electromechanical systole (QS_2). 3) QT interval. 4) The QS_2/QT ratio[2]. 5) The ratio of preejection period to the left ventricular ejection time (PE/LVET). Systolic time intervals were measured conventionally[3]. From the systolic time intervals the duration of QT and QS_2 were calculated. The subjects were of medication. At least 5 cardiac cycles were averaged. The QS_2 and QT were corrected for heart rate (QSI and QT_c) employing the conventional Weissler[3] and Bazzett[4] equitations. Statistical evaluation was performed using the t-test.

Results

Exercise stress testing

The diverse parameters of the negative exercise stress testing did not show any difference between the two groups of subjects (Table 1).

Table 1. Exercise stress testing

	Group A (with ST-T changes)	Group B (with normal ECG)	P value
Duration (min)	9.7±2	9.2±3	NS
Max HR (beats/min)	160±15	153±19	NS
Max systolic blood pressure (mmHg)	170±21.7	168±17.8	NS

Evaluation of adrenergic activity

The evaluation of adrenergic activity in basal condition using non invasive indices showed no difference between the two groups (Table 2).

Table 2. Non invasive indices of adrenergic activity

	Group A (with ST-T changes)	Group B (with normal ECG)	P value
HR (bears/min)	78±14	74±12	NS
QS_2I (msec)	533.2±22.9	544.0±21.4	NS
QT_c (msec)	401.5±22.6	388.0±22.1	NS
QS_2/QT	1.09±0.06	1.04±0.05	NS
PEP/LVET	0.32±0.05	0.34±0.06	NS

Discussion

ST segment and T wave abnormalities in resting ECG of asymptomatic persons is not so rare. Atterhög et al[1] reported notced T waves in 4.4% and invested T waves in 0.9% of asymptomatic young men. Their prevalence is higher in some groups of top level athlets[5]. On the other hand many authors observed spontaneous or provoked idiopathic T wave abnormalities in normal untrained persons with a higher percent incidence in Negroes than in Caucasians[6]. Atterhög et al[7] provided evidence of increased sympathetic activity in these subjects. Taggart et al[8] on the other hand showed that an altered β-adrenoreceptor responsiveness in heart is more relevant than any catecholamine hypersecretion. This concept confirmed by other[9]. In the patients studied here the probability of ischaemic heart disease in the two groups, although coronary arteriogram was not performed is similar and very low (practically absent) because of absence of angina and the negative exercise stress testing[10] where all parameters were not different between the two groups (Table 1). The present study evaluate cardiac adrenergic activity in basal condition using the indices: HR, QS_2, QT, QS_2/QT and PEP/LVET that correlate with adrenergic activity[2,3]. Especially QS_2/QT ratio is a simple non invasive index of hyperadrenergic activity (normally $QS_2 > QT$) independent of heart rate. Only one subject with ST-T changes had $QT > QS_2$. Using these non invasive indices no significant difference was found between subjects with ST-T wave changes and subjects with normal ECG conserning adrenergic activity (Table 2). Probably there is, genetically, a functional asymmetry (some time latent) of cardiac sympathetic nerves that induce inequality of ventricular repolarization resulting in T wave abnormalities. The normalization of ventricular repolarization obtained by both isopreterenol infusion[5] and maximal exercise could be explained as due to a uniform enhancement of symapthetic tone at high levels wich overcomes functional asymmetry of resting sympathetic discharge. This regionally altered autonomic tone in the myocardium according to our work (see in this issue)[11] probably is centrally mediated.

In conclusion asymptomatic subjects with repolarization abnormalities in resting ECG without organic heart disease were found to have no evidence of hyperadrenergic activity.

References

1. J. H. Atterhög, L. C. Ekelound, G. Ericsson and B. Ahlborg, *Upsal. J. Med.* **85** (1980) 125.
2. H. Boudoulas, P. Geleris, R.P. Lewis and C. V. Leier, *Circulation* **64** (1981) 28.
3. A. M. Weissler, W. S. Harris and C. D. Shoefeld, *Am. J. Cardiol.* **23** (1969) 469.
4. H. L. Bazzet, *Heart* **7** (1919) 353.
5. P. Zeppili, M.M. Pirrami, M. Sassara and R. Fenici, *Am. Acart. J.* **100** (1980) 213.
6. R. G. His and L. E. Lamb, *Circulation* **25** (1962) 947.
7. J. H. Attherhög, K. Eliasson and P. Hjemdahl, *Br. Heart J.***46** (1981) 311.
8. P. Taggart, M. Carruthers, S. Joseph, et al, *Br. Heart J.* **41** (1979) 214.
9. J. Karjalainen, *Chest* **83** (1983) 869.
10. G. A. Diamond and J. S. Forrester, *New Engl. J. Med.* **300** (1979) 1350.
11. A. G. Economou, A. N. Fortos and L. I. Constantinou, *Proceedings of the 19th International Congress in Electrocardiology* (in this issue).

SPECIFIC POTENTIAL DOES NOT CORRELATE WITH LEFT VENTRICULAR PERFORMANCE IN HYPERTENSIVE PATIENTS

LJUBA BACHÁROVÁ

Research Institute of Medical Informatics, Jedľová 6
833 08 Bratislava, Czecho-Slovakia

and

JARMILA MELOTOVÁ
KATARÍNA SEDLÁKOVÁ
KATARÍNA JUREČKOVÁ

Research Institute of Medical Informatics, Jedľová 6
833 08 Bratislava, Czecho-Slovakia

EVA KELLEROVÁ

Institute of Normal and Pathological Physiology, Sienkiewiczova 1
813 71 Bratislava, Czecho-Slovakia

ABSTRACT

The specific potential, calculated as a ratio of maximum spatial QRS vector magnitude and left ventricular cross-sectional area was introduced as a parameter of myocardial status. The aim of this study was to evaluate the eventual relationship between the specific potential (SP) and echocardiographically ascertained hemodynamics in left ventricular hypertrophy (LVH) due to arterial hypertension. Frank lead electrocardiograms, as well as M-mode echocardiograms were recorded in a group of 67 hypertensive patients (aged from 16 to 68, average age 53.8). Group means of measured parameters were: systolic blood pressure 162.5 mmHg (S.D. 23.3), diastolic blood pressure 94.8 mmHg (9.7), maximum spatial QRS vector magnitude 1.543 mV (0.4), left ventricular mass 265.9 g (84.7), specific potential 0.76 uV/mm^2 (0.22), cardiac output 6.29 l/min (2.387), ejection fraction 69.92% (1.745), wall stress 59.75 dyn/cm^2 (2.54), diastolic function (A/E) 0.95 (0.965). 48 patients (71.6%) fulfilled the EchoCG criteria for LVH, but only 7 patients (10.4%) exceeded the VCG upper normal limit. No significant correlations were found between SP and hemodynamic parameters. Significant negative correlation was found between SP and LVM, ($r = -0.3835$, $p < 0.005$) and between SP and age ($r = -0.3888$, $p < 0.005$). Significant negative correlation was found between SP and age - SP could relfect the myocardial changes conditioned by age and the duration of presssure overload of left ventricle.

1. Introduction

In our previous studies[1,2] we introduced a new parameter - the specific potential - as a parameter of myocardial status, with the aim to describe the fact, that a small heart can be a strong generator of cardioelectric field, and vice versa, a large heart does not need to produce necessarily a strong electric field. SP was calculated as a ratio of maximum spatial QRS vector magnitude to the cross-sectional area of left ventricle. Theoretically, SP approximates the contribution of myocardial unit area to the total electric field represented by the maximum QRS vector. In other words, SP normalises the voltage to myocardial unit. The aim of this study was the evaluation of relationship between SP and echocardiographical hemodynamic parameters in left ventricular hypertrophy due to arterial hypertension.

2. Material and Methods

The study group was represented by 67 hypertensive patients (women 35, men 32) aged from 16 to 78 years, mean age 53.8. Values of systolic blood presuure ranged from 120 to 240 mmHg, mean 162.54, S.D. 23.46, values of diastolic blood pressure ranged from 80 to 120 mmHg, mean 94.81, S.D. 9.79. Orthogonal Frank lead electrocardiograms were recorded, the maximum spatial QRS vector magnitude was used as a vectorcardiographic parameter of left ventricular hypertrophy. Dimensions of interventricular septum, left ventricular end-diastolic diameter and left ventricular posterior wall thickness were measured from sector directed M-mode echocardiograms. The following parameters were calculated: left ventricular mass, left ventricular cross-sectional area, cardiac output, ejection fraction, wall stress and diastolic function. The correlations between vectorcardiographic and echocardiographic parameters were tested.

3. Results

The basic description of VCG and EchoCG parameters is listed in Table 1.

Table 1. Basic characteristics of vectorcardiographic and echocardiographic parameters and of the specific potential.

	min. - max.	mean	S.D.
$QRS_{max.}$ (mV)	0.312 - 2.897	1.543	0.421
LVM (g)	86.0 - 556.3	265.9	84.6
LVAA (mm^2)	11.0 - 34.0	20.8	0.45
CO (l/min.)	3.40 - 10.30	6.29	2.387
EF (%)	50 - 90	69.92	1.745
WS (dyn/cm^2)	25.2 - 194.1	59.75	2.541
DF	0.46 - 2.5	0.95	0.965
SP (uV/mm^2)	0.2 - 1.4	0.76	0.22

48 patients (71.6%) fulfilled the EchoCG criteria for LVH, but only 7 patients (10.4%) exceeded the VCG upper normal limit. There was slight significant correlation between QRSmax. and LVM ($r = 0.3027$, $p < 0.05$), anyway a considerable dispersion could be observed. No significant correlations were found between SP

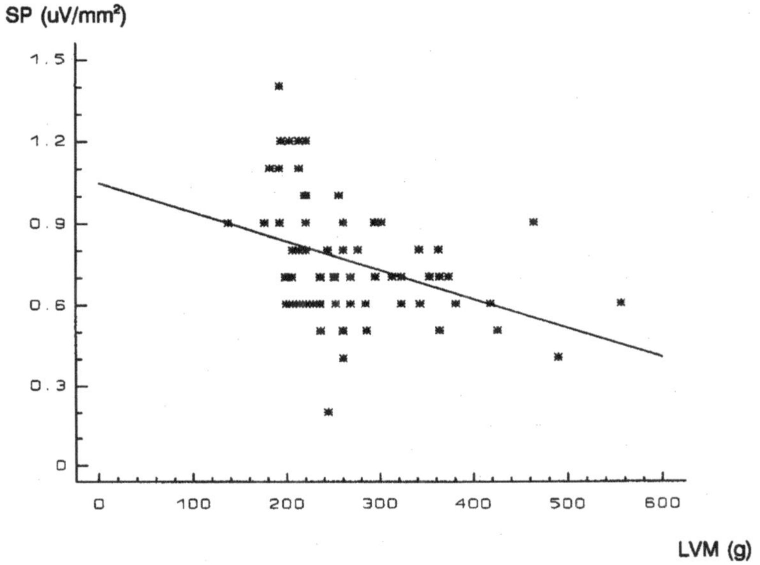

Figure 1. Relationship between specific potential and left ventricular mass. Significant negative correlation was found between these two variables ($r = -0.3835$, $p < 0.005$).

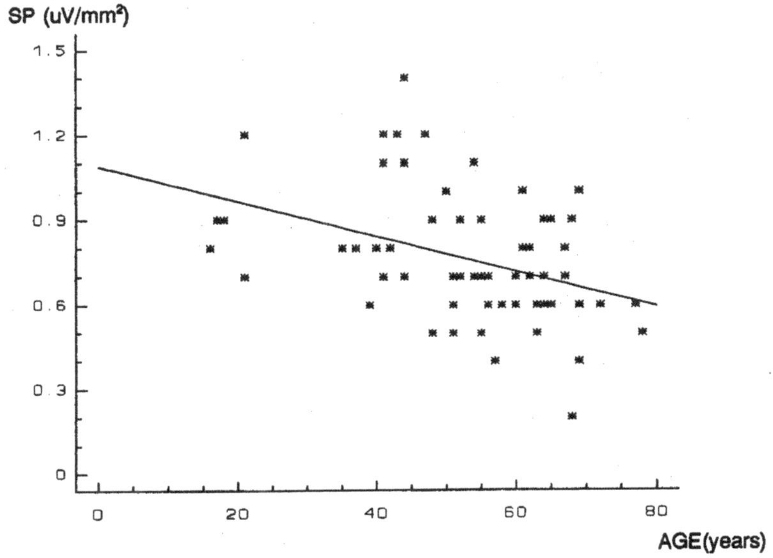

Figure 2. Relationship between specific potential and age. Significant negative correlation was found between these two variables ($r = -0.3888$, $p < 0.005$).

and hemodynamic parameters. Significant negative correlation was found between SP and LVM, ($r = -0.3835$, $p < 0.005$) (Figure 1) and between SP and age ($r = -0.3888$, $p < 0.005$) (Figure 2).

4. Discussion

With the aim to describe and quantify the discrepancies between ECG and EchoCG findings as well as to preserve both results, we introduced the index "specific potential". We used this method in two clinical studies for the evaluation of LVH in hypertensive patients[1,2] as well as in a retrospective evaluation of changes of cardioelectric field during the development of experimental left ventricular hypertrophy[3]. Main results of clinical studies were: SP values decreased with increasing values of LVM.

SP values were lower in hypertensive patients as compared to healthy persons, in contrast to higher values of $QRS_{max.}$ observed in hypertensive patients.

In experimental LVH due to volume overload in rabbits[4], values of the specific potential decreased during the whole follow-up period. They did not reach the initial values not even at the stage of developed hypertrophy, when the maximal increase of $QRS_{max.}$was observed.

It is obvious, that the myocardium as a generator of cardioelectric field is influenced by morphological, structural, biochemical and metabolic changes. Results of our study did not show significant correlation between SP and any hemodynamic parameters under study. Negative significant correlation was observed between SP and age. It supports the suggestion, that SP, which represents the potential contribution of myocardial unit to the total cardioelectric field, could reflect some changes of the myocardium due to developing left ventricular hypertrophy.

5. Conclusions

In agreement with our previous results, lower SP values were found in hypertensive patients. Negative correlation was found between SP and LVM, e.g. decreasing SP with increasing LVM. No significant correlations were found between SP and echocardiographically ascertained hemodynamic parameters. Significant negative correlation was found between SP and age.

6. References

1. Bachárová, L., Melotová, J., Sedláková, K., Hrušovská, K. in *Electrocardiology 1988*, ed. H. Abel (Elsevier, Excerpta Medica, Amsterdam 1989)
2. Bachárová, L. Gadžaeva, F.U., Melotová, J. in *Teorija i praktika avtomatizacii kardiologičeskich issledovanij*, ed. J. Blužas (K. Požely, Kaunas 199O)
3. Bachárová, L., Bernadič, M., Fízeľová, A. in *Electrocardiology 1991*, ed. J. Jagielski (World Scientific Publishing Co., London, in press)
4. Bernadič, M., Fízeľ, A., Fízeľová, A., Bakošová, M., Sapáková, E., *Bratisl. lek. Listy*, **84**(1985)638.

ELECTROCARDIOGRAPHIC CHANGES INDUCED BY TRANSIENT OCCLUSION OF THE LEFT CIRCUMFLEX CORONARY ARTERY

Pedro Abreu, José Baptista, Teresa Real,
R. Seabra-Gomes

Department of Cardiology - Santa Cruz Hospital
Carnaxide - Portugal

1. Introduction

Electrocardiographic (ECG) diagnosis of myocardial infarction (MI) due to occlusion of the circumflex (CX) coronary artery, is often a clinical challenge, because it is relativelly rare and because of the posterior location of circumflex artery.

Some studies have suggest ECG criteria for the circumflex related artery MI[1-5].

Coronary angioplasty (PTCA) with the transient occlusion of the coronary flow, could be the best way to evaluate ECG changes occured during acute MI[6,7].

2. Main purpose

Main purpose of this study were: 1) to evaluate ECG changes recorded during transient occlusion by PTCA of isolated CX artery; 2) to describe the relations between ECG changes in this study, and changes for CX related artery MI.

3. Study population, material and methods

We studied 45 patients, 40 males and 5 females, with a mean age of 53.3+/-9.6 years. All the patients had isolated CX coronary artery disease, and there were analysed in the 12 leads continuos ECG monitoring, the ECG changes (in the ST segment) during balloon inflation that produced the greatest of ST-segment deviation ("maximally ischemic periods"). The ST changes were defined when there was ST deviations equal or greater than 1 mm (80 mesec after J point).

Previous clinical and angiographyc data were as follows: Seventeen patients had previous myocardial infarction (antero-septal in 1, inferior in 9, and lateral in 7 patients). PTCA was performed in the proximal CX in 14 patients, distal CX in 15, obtuse marginals (OM) in 13, and a combination of CX and OMs in 3 patients. In 11 patients there was total occlusion (proximal CX in 4 patients, distal CX in 5, and OMs in 2 patients). Coronary circulation was considered as right dominance in 37 patients, left in 7, and ballanced in 1 patient.

4. Results

ECG changes occured only in 31 of the 45 patients (70%).

Concerning previous MI, 13 patients had ECG changes against 5 with no ECG changes (3 inferior and 2 lateral MI) - (NS). Relating vessels patency and PTCA site, ECG changes were less frequent (4 in 11 patients) when the segment was occluded ($p=0.02$), or when the dilated segment was the proximal CX (6 in 14 patients) , ($p=0.01$). Dominance was not related to any particular aspect concerning ECG changes - rigth dominance in 37 patients (24 with ECG changes and 13 with no ECG changes) - left dominance in 7 patients, with and without ECG changes in 6 and 1 patient respectivelly, and ballanced in 1 patient, with no ECG changes.

When we analysed the involved leads the results were: leads V5 and V6 were the more frequently involved, with 25 in 31 patients (80%), beeing in 60% ST elevation and in 40% ST depression, followed by leads V2-4 (in 71%), beeing ST elevation in 9% and ST depression in 91%, leads II-III-aVF (in 61.2%), with ST elevation in 63% and ST depression in 37% of the patients. ECG changes in lead aVL was present in 15 patients (50%), with ST depression in 10. When lead aVL had ECG changes, there was always ST elevation in inferior leads. The lead D-I, was the less frequently involved, only 2 patients, and one of them had left dominant coronary circulation ($p<0.001$).

The following criteria were tested: 1) ST segment elevation in inferior leads plus ST depression in lead aVL. We had 10 patients with this ECG changes during PTCA, in proximal CX in 1, distal CX in 5, OMs in 3 and lastly CX+OMs in 1 patient. 2) ST segment elevation in inferior leads plus ST depression in lead aVL, plus: a) ST elevation in leads V5-6 (6 patients, with proximal CX disease in 1, distal CX in 3, and OMs in 2 patients; b) ST depression in the same leads (3 patients, with proximal and distal CX disease in 1 and 2 patients respectivelly). 3) Only ischemia evidence: a) in precordial leads (6 patients, proximal CX, distal CX and OMs in 2 patients; b) in precordial leads plus inferior leads (3 patients, 1 with proximal CX and 2 patients with distal CX disease), and lastly c) in V5-6, only 1 patient in whom PTCA was performed in distal CX.

5. Discussion

The electrocardiographic diagnosis of the occlusion of CX coronary artery has a lower sensibility and specificity when compared with ECG diagnosis of the occlusion of the rigth or left descending coronary artery[1].

With thrombolysis for MI, some studies have been published concerning ECG paterns to identifie CX coronary artery related myocardial infarction[2-5].

Nevertheless, its rare frequency and posterior location of CX, increases the diagnostic ability[2].

In a study of Noel Bairey[3], with 41 patients with inferior MI, all the patients had ST elevation in inferior leads, and the diagnosis of CX occlusion versus right coronary occlusion was made by presence of ST elevation in leads aVL, V5-6 (Sensibility (S=83%); Specificity (SP=96%); Positive and Negative predictive value (PPV and NPV=91% and 93% respectivelly)).

Barry Huey[2], evaluating 241 patients with MI obtained a lower frequency in ECG changes during CX related artery MI, but whenever present, lateral leads were the most frequently involved.

Two studies in our hospital[4,5], were also in favour of the presence in inferior and lateral leads, and pratically no involvement of lead D-I (S=100%; SP=93% and 85%; PPV=25% and 78% and lastly NPV=100%).

Therefore, concerning the question of ECG patern relating occlusion of CX artery, these results show the great variability of ECG changes. Nevertheless, lateral and inferior leads seem to be the most frequently involved leads, and lead D-I, with almost no involvement, could make the diference between CX and right coronary artery occlusions during inferior myocardial infarction.

Our results concerning clinical and angiographyc profile reveal the diference between ECG changes when we analysed coronary patency or PTCA site. The presence of colaterals could explain the lower frequency of ECG changes when the dilated segment was occluded, but being the amount of ischemic myocardium greater when proximal CX is involved, it seems odd that there are less ECG changes during PTCA.

6. Conclusions

Although there is a great variability of ECG changes during occlusion of CX artery, there is a preferencial involvement of lateral and inferior leads with ST elevation, associated to ST depression in precordial leads and almost no involvement of lead D-I. On the other hand, PTCA could be an interesting moddel to evaluate ECG changes during myocardial infarction.

7. Bibliography

1. R.M.Fuchs, S.C.Achuff, B.A.Grunwald, F.P.Yin, L.C. Griffith. Circulation. **66** (1982) 1168.
2. B.L.Huey, G.A.Beller, D.L.Kaiser, R.S.Gibson. J Am Coll Cardiol **12** (1988) 456.
3. C.N.Bairey, P.K.Shah, A.S.Lew, S.Hulse. Am J Cardiol **60** (1987) 456.
4. M.J.Andrade, R.Ribeiras, J.Baptista, R.Seabra-Gomes. Rev Port Cardiol **7** Supl (1988) 19:26 (abstr.)
5. P.F.Abreu, V.Gil, J.A.Silva, R.Seabra-Gomes. Rev Port Cardiol **11** (1992) 127.
6. N.B.Wagner, D.C.Sevilla, M.W.Krucoff, K.S.Pieper, K.L.Lee,R.D.White, K.M.Kent, R.Renzi, R.W.Selvester, G. Wagner. Am J Cardiol **63** (1989) 1208.
7. M.Dellborg, H.Emanuelsson, M.Riha, K.Sweedberg. Coronary arterry disease **2** (1991) 43.

SOFTWARE BASED NEURAL NETWORKS IN COMPUTER BASED ECG INTERPRETATION

P.W. Macfarlane.
University Dept. of Medical Cardiology, Royal Infirmary, Glasgow, Scotland.

ABSTRACT

Software based neural networks have recently become more readily available. This paper provides a very brief introduction to the technique applied in computer assisted ECG interpretation. Some of the theoretical background is presented together with results from early studies using the technique.

A variety of techniques has been used to enhance methods for computer assisted reporting of electrocardiograms. Of most recent interest, is the application of neural networks which have now become more widely available in software based form following the solution of a problem that had held back their widespread use for over twenty years. In this review, some of the early attempts at using neural networks in ECG interpretation are considered briefly. The concept of a neural network is first introduced.

A neural network is so-called because its design is based on the neural structure of the brain; both have many highly interconnected neurons[1]. There are two types of neural network, namely:

a) Biological, e.g. a network inside the human brain.
b) Artificial, e.g. a model network that simulates a biological neural network.

In the biological situation, impulses are transmitted forwards to synapses which can have an excitatory (positive) or inhibitory (negative) effect. The net result is an output signal from the neuron which is then transmitted along the axon.

In a similar situation in a model neural network, measurements such as ECG amplitudes and durations can be input to a "neuron" where an individual measurement is multiplied by a weighting factor which may have a positive or negative influence and then summed together with other weighted inputs to enable the output of the neuron to be calculated. This output can then be fed forwards(Figure 1).

The output from a neuron is scaled to have a value between 0 and 1 and this is most often achieved using a sigmoidal type of function. Mathematically, if the sums of the measurements I input to a single neuron multiplied by the corresponding weights W is

$$S = I_1 W_1 + I_2 W_2 \ldots = \Sigma I_i W_i$$

then the neuron output is given by

$$\text{output} = \frac{1}{1 + e^{-s}}$$

The discussion above has related to input and output from only one neuron. In practice there may be any number of inputs to multiple neurons which gives rise to the concept of layers of a neural network(Figure 2). Measurements from the input layer are fed forward to the layer of neurons called the "hidden layer" where the processing described above is carried out. The hidden layer usually contains one or two rows of neurons as illustrated in Figure 2. The outputs from the hidden layer(s) are then fed forward to the output layer which may contain one or more neurons depending on the application under consideration. If, for example, it is desired to know whether an ST-T pattern is consistent with "LV Strain" or not, then there need only be one output neuron. If this achieves a value > 0.5, then LV strain may be said to be present. If on the other hand, it is desired to discriminate between normal and six abnormal ST-T segments, there could be seven output neurons and the one with the highest value (< 1) after processing, would indicate the desired classification. Alternatively, this particular network could have six abnormal output neurons and if none exceeded a critical value, then the decision would be made that a normal STT segment was present.

One major point in all of this discussion is the estimation of the weighting factors. This is achieved through a training process whereby the measurements from ECGs with a known classification are fed to a network together with the classification. A process known as "back propagation" allows calculation of the weighting factors[2]. The training procedure may take several hours or days of computer calculation depending on the complexity of the network and the size of the training set but thereafter, the analysis of a new test ECG requires only a fraction of a second.

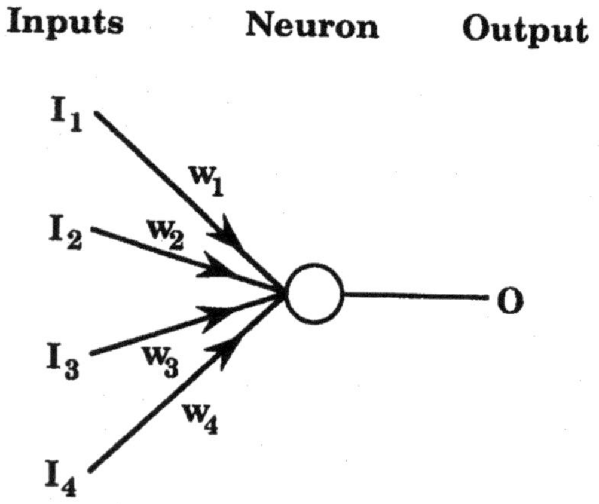

Fig. 1: Schematic illustration of inputs to a neuron with the output (o) calculated as described in the text.

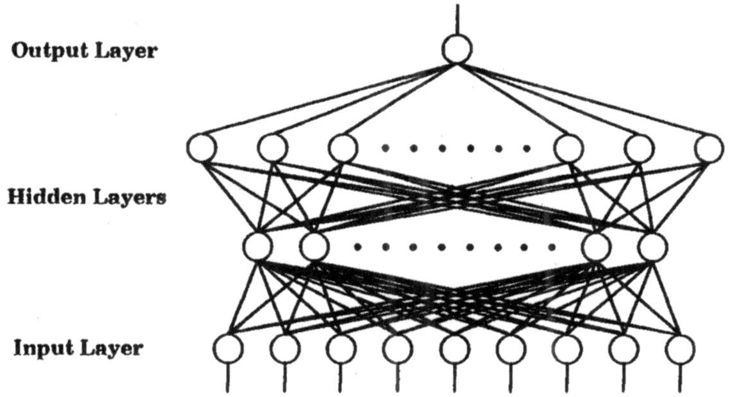

Fig. 2: Schematic illustration of a neural network with one input layer, two hidden layers and a single output.

Some basic factors should be mentioned. For a given application, the training set can be fed to a variety of networks to decide which one gives the best performance. In general terms, there is a levelling off of the number of hidden neurons beyond which any benefit can be obtained. Likewise, there is also a limit to the value of the number of input neurons that contribute to the classification[3].

APPLICATIONS IN ELECTROCARDIOGRAPHY

A number of different applications of neural networks have been described. These include pattern recognition[3], diagnostic interpretation[4,5], rhythm analysis[6] and data compression of the Holter ECG[7]. Only the first two are discussed here while the third can be found elsewhere in these Proceedings.

a) Pattern Recognition

Macfarlane, Edenbrandt and Devine recently assessed the use of neural networks for classification of electrocardiographic ST-T segments[8]. 1,000 ST-T segments from V4 to V6 were classified singly by each of two experienced electrocardiographers into one of eight groups and consensus obtained where necessary. The classified ECGs were divided into two equally structured sets of 500. The first was used for training neural networks and the second for testing. 500 ECGs in the test set were classified blindly for a second time by one of the electrocardiographers.

The training set was processed by an established program[9] which produced a variety of ST-T measurements. These included the time normalised ST-T amplitudes, the maximum positive and negative T wave amplitudes, the ST slope and the amplitude of the J point. The network with the best results in the training set had 12 neurons in the input layer, 10 in the hidden layer and 8 in the output layer. In the test set, the network classified 79.8% of the ECGs correctly while the electrocardiographer classified 85.6%, i.e. when viewing the 500 blindly for a second time.

In a separate study[3], Edenbrandt, Devine and Macfarlane showed that a neural network could classify eight STT patterns chosen from V2 to V4 with an accuracy of up to 95%. There were some surprising misclassifications, however, but one of the drawbacks of a neural network is that it is difficult to determine why a misclassification is made.

b) Diagnostic Interpretation

Bortolan and colleagues have studied classification of the complete ECG using neural networks[4]. They used a network with 39 neurons in the input layer, 7 in the hidden layer and 5 in the output layer. The latter consisted of outputs for normal, LVH, RVH, anterior and inferior myocardial infarction. If LVH and RVH both produced a positive result, then BVH was diagnosed. Likewise, if anterior and inferior infarction were positive, mixed infarction was recorded. There were 2,446 ECGs in the training set and 820 in the test set. The overall accuracy of classification was 66.3% which compared with accuracies of 67.2 and 66.3% using linear discriminant analysis and logistic discriminant analysis respectively.

In a second paper[5], these authors also studied the effect of combining different networks but showed that little could be gained using this approach.

CONCLUSIONS

Neural networks are unlikely to prove a panacea for computer assisted ECG analysis. However, if used carefully they may prove helpful in selected areas of computer based ECG interpretation.

References

1. J. Stanley. In: *Introduction to Neural Networks*(California) Scientific Software, Sierra Madre, 1990) p9.
2. D.E. Rumelhart, G.E. Hinton, R.J. Williams, In: *Parallel Distributed Processing*, Vol. 1. eds. D.E. Rumelhart and J.L. McLelland. (MIT Press, Cambridge MA, 1988) p318.
3. L. Edenbrandt, B. Devine, P.W. Macfarlane, *J. Electrocardiology*, 25. (1992) 167.
4. G. Bortolan, R. Degani and J.L. Willems, Computers in Cardiology,1990, (IEEE Computer Society, Washington DC, 1991), p269.
5. G. Bortolan, R. Degani, J. Willems, Computers in Cardiology, 1991, (IEEE Computer Society Press, Washington DC, 1992), p177.
6. T.F. Yang, B. Devine and P.W. Macfarlane, In: Electrocardiology '92, eds. P.W. Macfarlane, F. de Padua, (World Scientific Publishing, London, 1993).
7. A. Iwata, Y. Nagasaka and N. Suzumura, *I.E.E.E. Eng. Med. Biol.* (1990) 53.
8. P.W. Macfarlane, L. Edenbrandt, B. Devine, *J.A.C.C.*19 (1992) 5A.
9. P.W. Macfarlane, B. Devine, S. Latif, S. McLaughlin, D.B. Shoat, M .P. Watts, *Methods of Information in Medicine*, 29 (1990) 354.

AUTHORS INDEX

www.ingramcontent.com/pod-product-compliance
Lightning Source LLC
La Vergne TN
LVHW082254241026
850861LV00008B/46